MR Imaging of the Adnexa

Editors

ERICA B. STEIN
KIMBERLY L. SHAMPAIN

MAGNETIC RESONANCE IMAGING CLINICS OF NORTH AMERICA

www.mri.theclinics.com

Consulting Editors
SURESH K. MUKHERJI
LYNNE S. STEINBACH

February 2023 • Volume 31 • Number 1

ELSEVIER

1600 John F. Kennedy Boulevard • Suite 1800 • Philadelphia, Pennsylvania, 19103-2899

http://www.mri.theclinics.com

MAGNETIC RESONANCE IMAGING CLINICS OF NORTH AMERICA Volume 31, Number 1
February 2023 ISSN 1064-9689, ISBN 13: 978-0-323-98767-7

Editor: John Vassallo (j.vassallo@elsevier.com)
Developmental Editor: Arlene Campos

Magnetic Resonance Imaging Clinics of North America (ISSN 1064-9689) is published quarterly by Elsevier Inc., 360 Park Avenue South, New York, NY 10010-1710. Months of issue are February, May, August, and November. Business and Editorial Offices: 1600 John F. Kennedy Blvd., Ste. 1800, Philadelphia, PA 19103-2899. Customer Service Office: 3251 Riverport Lane, Maryland Heights, MO 63043. Periodicals postage paid at New York, NY and additional mailing offices. Subscription prices are $408.00 per year (domestic individuals), $783.00 per year (domestic institutions), $100.00 per year (domestic students/residents), $455.00 per year (Canadian individuals), $1021.00 per year (Canadian institutions), $573.00 per year (international individuals), $1021.00 per year (international institutions), $100.00 per year (Canadian students/residents), and $275.00 per year (international students/residents). International air speed delivery is included in all *Clinics* subscription prices. All prices are subject to change without notice. **POSTMASTER:** Send address changes to *Magnetic Resonance Imaging Clinics*, Elsevier Health Sciences Division, Subscription Customer Service, 3251 Riverport Lane, Maryland Heights, MO 63043. Customer Service (orders, claims, online, change of address): Elsevier Health Sciences Division, Subscription **Customer Service, 3251 Riverport Lane, Maryland Heights, MO 63043. Tel:1-800-654-2452 (U.S. and Canada); 314-447-8871 (outside U.S. and Canada). Fax: 314-447-8029. E-mail: journalscustomerservice-usa@elsevier.com (for print support); journalsonlinesupport-usa@elsevier.com (for online support).**

Reprints. For copies of 100 or more of articles in this publication, please contact the Commercial Reprints Department, Elsevier Inc., 360 Park Avenue South, New York, NY 10010-1710. Tel.: 212-633-3874; Fax: 212-633-3820; E-mail: reprints@elsevier.com.

Magnetic Resonance Imaging Clinics of North America is covered in the *RSNA Index of Imaging Literature, MEDLINE/PubMed (Index Medicus),* and *EMBASE/Excerpta Medica.*

Contributors

CONSULTING EDITORS

SURESH K. MUKHERJI, MD, MBA, FACR
Clinical Professor of Radiology and Radiation
Oncology, University of Illinois, Robert Wood
Johnson Medical School, Rutgers University,
Faculty, Otolaryngology Head Neck Surgery,
Michigan State University, National Director of
Head and Neck Radiology, ProScan Imaging,
Carmel, Indiana, USA

LYNNE S. STEINBACH, MD, FACR
Emeritus Professor of Radiology on Full Recall,
Department of Radiology and Biomedical
Imaging, University of California, San
Francisco, California, USA

EDITORS

ERICA B. STEIN, MD
Clinical Assistant Professor of Radiology,
Director of Body CT, Department of Radiology,
Michigan Medicine, Ann Arbor, Michigan, USA

KIMBERLY L. SHAMPAIN, MD
Clinical Assistant Professor of Radiology,
Director of GI/Fluoro, Department of
Radiology, Michigan Medicine, Ann Arbor,
Michigan, USA

AUTHORS

SUSAN M. ASCHER, MD
Professor, Department of Radiology, Vice
Chair, Research MedStar Georgetown
University Hospital, Washington, DC, USA

MYRA K. FELDMAN, MD
Assistant Professor, Imaging Institute, Section
of Abdominal Imaging, Cleveland Clinic,
Cleveland, Ohio, USA

JOANIE GARRATT, MD
Assistant Professor, Department of Radiology,
University of Pennsylvania, Philadelphia,
Pennsylvania, USA

NICOLE HINDMAN, MD
Department of Radiology and Surgery, New
York University Grossman School of Medicine,
New York, New York, USA

JEANNE M. HOROWITZ, MD
Department of Radiology, Northwestern
University Feinberg School of Medicine,
Chicago, Illinois, USA

AURÉLIE JALAGUIER-COUDRAY, MD
Service de Radiologie, Institut Paoli Calmettes,
Marseille, France

PRIYANKA JHA, MBBS
Associate Professor, Department of Radiology
and Biomedical Imaging, University of
California, San Francisco, California, USA

PWINT P. KHINE, MD
Clinical Fellow, Abdominal Imaging and
Ultrasound, Department of Radiology and
Biomedical Imaging, University of California,
San Francisco, California, USA

AOIFE KILCOYNE, MB BCh, BAO
Department of Radiology, Massachusetts
General Hospital, Harvard Medical School,
Boston, Massachusetts, USA

NANCY KIM, MD
Assistant Professor, Department of Radiology,
MedStar Georgetown University Hospital,
Washington, DC, USA

SUSANNA I. LEE, MD, PhD
Department of Radiology, Massachusetts
General Hospital, Harvard Medical School,
Boston, Massachusetts, USA

KIRA MELAMUD, MD
Department of Radiology, New York University
Grossman School of Medicine, New York, New
York, USA

JOHN D. MILLET, MD, MHS
Department of Radiology, Division of
Abdominal Imaging, Clinical Assistant
Professor of Radiology, Michigan Medicine,
University of Michigan, Ann Arbor, Michigan,
USA

JACOB R. MITCHELL, MD
Abdominal Imaging Fellow, Department of
Radiology, University of Pennsylvania Health
System, Philadelphia, Pennsylvania, USA

MALLIKA MODAK, PhD
Department of Radiology, Northwestern
University Feinberg School of Medicine,
Chicago, Illinois, USA

TARA MORGAN, MD
Associate Professor, Department of Radiology
and Biomedical Imaging, University of
California, San Francisco, California, USA

PREETHI RAGHU, MD
Assistant Professor, Department of Radiology
and Biomedical Imaging, University of
California, San Francisco, California, USA

ANDREA G. ROCKALL, MRCP, FRCR
Clinical Chair in Radiology, Division of Cancer
and Surgery, Faculty of Medicine, Imperial
College London, London, United Kingdom;
Hon Consultant Radiology, Department of
Radiology, Imperial College Healthcare NHS
Trust, London, United Kingdom

MOLLY E. ROSELAND, MD
Department of Radiology, Division of
Abdominal Imaging, Clinical Assistant
Professor of Radiology, Michigan Medicine,
University of Michigan, Ann Arbor, Michigan,
USA

ELIZABETH SADOWSKI, MD
Department of Radiology and Obstetrics and
Gynecology, University of Wisconsin School of
Medicine, Madison, Wisconsin, USA

MICHELLE D. SAKALA, MD
Assistant Professor, Department of Radiology,
Division of Abdominal Imaging, University of
Michigan-Michigan Medicine, Ann Arbor,
Michigan, USA

KIMBERLY L. SHAMPAIN, MD
Clinical Assistant Professor of Radiology,
Director of GI/Fluoro, University of Michigan
Department of Radiology, Ann Arbor,
Michigan, USA

EVAN S. SIEGELMAN, MD
Professor of Radiology, Department of
Radiology, University of Pennsylvania Health
System, Philadelphia, Pennsylvania, USA

ERICA B. STEIN, MD
Clinical Assistant Professor of Radiology,
Director of Body CT, Department of Radiology,
University of Michigan, Ann Arbor, Michigan,
USA

KARTHIK M. SUNDARAM, MD, PhD
Assistant Professor of Radiology, Department
of Radiology, University of Pennsylvania Health
System, Philadelphia, Pennsylvania, USA

MYLES T. TAFFEL, MD
Assistant Professor, Department of Radiology,
New York University Langone Health, New
York, New York, USA

**ISABELLE THOMASSIN-NAGGARA, MD,
PhD**
Professor, Service de Radiologie, Hôpital
Tenon, Assistance Publique-Hôpitaux de Paris,
Institute for Computing and Data Sciences,
Sorbonne Université, Paris, France

JULIANA J. TOBLER, MD
Department of Radiology, University of
Cincinnati, Cincinnati, Ohio, USA

ANGELA TONG, MD
Assistant Professor, Department of Radiology,
New York University Langone Health, New
York, New York, USA

TUGCE AGIRLAR TRABZONLU, MD
Department of Radiology, Northwestern
University Feinberg School of Medicine,
Chicago, Illinois, USA

SHAUN A. WAHAB, MD
Department of Radiology, University of
Cincinnati, Cincinnati, Ohio, USA

ASHISH P. WASNIK, MD
Professor of Radiology, Director, Division of
Abdominal Radiology, Chair, Medical Student

Research in Radiology, Michigan Medicine,
University of Michigan, University Hospital, Ann
Arbor, Michigan, USA

LIMIN XU, MD
Department of Radiology, Boston Children's
Hospital, Harvard Medical School, Boston,
Massachusetts, USA

Contents

> The ovary resides in the pelvic cavity and is a dynamic organ with physiologic changes from birth to menopause. The imaging features of the normal ovary depend on the physiologic changes through puberty, reproductive age, and menopause. It is important for radiologists to understand the imaging features of normal physiologic changes in the ovaries and differentiate them from disease states.

> Constituting a broad spectrum of developmental abnormalities of the female genital tract, Müllerian duct anomalies (MDAs) are present in up to 7% of the general population and in up to 25% of women who present with infertility and a history of miscarriage. Imaging plays an important role in narrowing the diagnostic considerations in these patients. In this article, we review the normal embryologic development of the female genital tract followed by the MR imaging techniques and protocol recommendations to evaluate such patients. The differential diagnoses and the MR imaging features of MDAs are also reviewed.

> MR imaging has an important role in imaging evaluation of fallopian tube (FT) pathology, ranging from benign to malignant conditions. Congenital Mullerian anomalies of FTs such as accessory tubal ostia and unicornuate uterus and associated pathology are well assessed by MR imaging. Benign diseases include hydrosalpinx, pelvic inflammatory disease, and its manifestations including salpingitis, pyosalpinx, tubo-ovarian abscess, and tubal endometriosis manifesting as hematosalpinx. Acute benign conditions include isolated FT torsion and ectopic pregnancy. Neoplastic conditions include benign paratubal cysts to malignant primary FT carcinomas.

> Benign and borderline epithelial ovarian tumors represent a substantial proportion of incidental adnexal lesions and familiarity with the typical imaging features on MR imaging can aid in their diagnosis and management. Clinical information such as menstrual status, age, and associated conditions is also important considerations when

evaluating an adnexal lesion. Radiologists play an integral role in the preoperative evaluation process and can help guide treatment, particularly in those with lesions demonstrating benign or borderline features and those who may be candidates for fertility-sparing surgery.

MR imaging shows high sensitivity and specificity for discriminating benign from malignant lesions, thereby aiding in cancer management from assessing the initial extent of disease to subsequent treatment response. Understanding the utility and application of advanced imaging techniques allows better lesion characterization. Subtypes of epithelial ovarian tumors are presented, along with characteristic imaging findings, and illustrated with examples. Select mimics of malignancy are also presented.

MR imaging is useful in the detection and characterization of adnexal lesions. This review discusses the clinical findings and MR imaging appearances of two types of ovarian neoplasms: germ cell and sex cord stromal tumors. The most common of these lesions, mature cystic teratomas, is characterized by the presence of bulk fat on MR imaging. Some of the other germ cell neoplasms and sex cord stromal tumors may have suggestive clinical, laboratory, or MR imaging features (eg, lipid and fibrosis) to establish a diagnosis. The ability to differentiate benign tumors from possible malignancy can aid in patient management.

MR imaging plays a key role in the characterization of adnexal lesions of indeterminate malignant potential found at ultrasound. Recently, the Ovarian-Adnexal Reporting and Data Systems (O-RADS) MRI lexicon and scoring system was developed to aid in standardization of reporting and interpretation of adnexal lesions, allowing for risk stratification based on MR imaging findings. This in turn can help improve communication between radiologists and referring providers, and potentially aid the selection of optimal treatment options. This article provides a detailed review of the lexicon and the scoring rubric of the O-RADS MRI risk stratification system.

Ovarian metastases tend to arise in young women, either in patients with known cancer or as the first presentation of a previously occult extraovarian malignancy. Although imaging cannot always differentiate between secondary and primary ovarian neoplasms, and pathologic confirmation is generally required, it is important to recognize suggestive imaging features on pelvic MR imaging. Ovarian metastases are commonly described as bilateral, solid, heterogenous, and hypervascular. Features vary based on the tumor origin and histology. Knowledge of these features, plus the appropriate clinical context, can help guide radiologists to include metastases in their differential diagnosis for atypical adnexal masses.

Acute pelvic pain is a common presenting symptom in women, but the etiology is often not readily apparent. The differential diagnosis varies greatly for pre versus postmenopausal and pregnant versus nonpregnant women. In addition to physical examination and laboratory evaluation, imaging plays an important role in narrowing the differential diagnosis. Pelvic ultrasound (US) is the first-line imaging modality, but occasionally pelvic magnetic resonance imaging (MRI) is used for problem-solving in the acute setting. The aim of this article is to educate radiologists on the appearance of acute adnexal pathologies that can be definitively diagnosed at MRI.

Endometriosis is the presence of ectopic endometrial glands outside of the uterus. MR imaging is particularly useful for characterizing deep infiltrating endometriosis but can also be useful in characterizing endometriomas and hematosalpinges, characterizing broad ligament deposits, assessing for endometriosis-associated malignancy, and differentiating malignancy from decidualized endometriomas. Masses and cysts with hemorrhagic or proteinaceous contents can sometimes be difficult to distinguish from endometriomas. Imaging protocols should include pre-contrast T1-weighted imaging with fat saturation, T2-weighted imaging without fat saturation, opposed- and in-phase or Dixon imaging, administration of contrast media, and subtraction imaging.

Mimics of adnexal masses can include uterine leiomyomas, intraperitoneal cystic and solid masses of mesenteric or gastrointestinal origin, and extraperitoneal cystic and solid masses. When a pelvic mass is discovered on imaging, a radiologist should recognize these mimics to avoid mischaracterization of a mass as ovarian for optimal patient management. Knowledge of pelvic anatomy, determining whether a mass is intraperitoneal or extraperitoneal, and troubleshooting with MR imaging can help determine the etiology and origin of a pelvic mass. Imaging characteristics and keys to diagnosis of these adnexal mass mimics are reviewed in this article.

MR imaging has a high diagnostic accuracy and reproducibility to classify adnexal masses as benign or malignant, using a risk stratification scoring system, the Ovarian-Adnexal Reporting and Data System (O-RADS) MR imaging score. The first step in achieving high accuracy is to ensure high technical quality of the MR scan. The sequences needed are clearly described in this article, with tips for handling difficult cases. This information will assist in obtaining the best possible images, to allow for accurate use of the O-RADS MR imaging risk score.

MAGNETIC RESONANCE IMAGING CLINICS OF NORTH AMERICA

FORTHCOMING ISSUES

May 2023
Musculoskeletal MRI-Ultrasound Correlation
Jan Fritz

August 2023
MR Angiography: From Head to Toe
Prashant Nagpal and Thomas M. Grist, *Editors*

November 2023
Clinical Value of Hybrid PET/MRI
Minerva Becker and Valentino Garibotto,
Editors

RECENT ISSUES

November 2022
Postoperative Joint MR Imaging
Luis Beltran, *Editor*

August 2022
MR in the Emergency Room
John Conklin and Michael H. Lev, *Editors*

May 2022
MR Imaging of the Knee
Mary K. Jesse

SERIES OF RELATED INTEREST

Advances in Clinical Radiology
Neurologic Clinics
PET Clinics
Radiologic Clinics

VISIT THE CLINICS ONLINE!
Access your subscription at:
www.theclinics.com

PROGRAM OBJECTIVE

The goal of *Magnetic Resonance Imaging Clinics of North America* is to keep practicing physicians up to date with current clinical practice by providing timely articles reviewing the state of the art in patient care.

TARGET AUDIENCE

All practicing physicians and healthcare professionals who provide patient care utilizing findings from Magnetic Resonance Imaging.

LEARNING OBJECTIVES

Upon completion of this activity, participants will be able to:
1. Review how normal physiologic changes in the uterus and associated reproductive organs differ from disease-related changes.
2. Discuss the benefits of using MRI in conjunction with standardized protocols and scoring systems when diagnosing and managing diseases of the uterus and related reproductive organs.
3. Recognize MRI as a first-line tool for identifying abnormalities and disease states in the uterus and reproductive organs.

ACCREDITATION

The Elsevier Office of Continuing Medical Education (EOCME) is accredited by the Accreditation Council for Continuing Medical Education (ACCME) to provide continuing medical education for physicians.

The EOCME designates this journal-based CME activity enduring material for a maximum of 12 *AMA PRA Category 1 Credit*(s)™. Physicians should claim only the credit commensurate with the extent of their participation in the activity.

All other healthcare professionals requesting continuing education credit for this enduring material will be issued a certificate of participation.

DISCLOSURE OF CONFLICTS OF INTEREST

The EOCME assesses conflict of interest with its instructors, faculty, planners, and other individuals who are in a position to control the content of CME activities. All relevant conflicts of interest that are identified are thoroughly vetted by EOCME for fair balance, scientific objectivity, and patient care recommendations. EOCME is committed to providing its learners with CME activities that promote improvements or quality in healthcare and not a specific proprietary business or a commercial interest.

The planning committee, staff, authors and editors listed below have identified no financial relationships or relationships to products or devices they or their spouse/life partner have with commercial interest related to the content of this CME activity:

Tugce Agirlar Trabzonlu, MD; Susan M. Ascher, MD; Myra K. Feldman, MD; Joanie Garratt, MD; Nicole Hindman, MD; Jeanne M. Horowitz, MD; Aurélie Jalaguier-Coudray, MD; Priyanka Jha, MD; Pwint Phyu Khine, DO; Aoife Kilcoyne, MB BCh, BAO; Nancy Kim, MD; Pradeep Kuttysankaran; Susanna I. Lee, MD, PhD; Kira Melamud, MD; John D. Millet, MD, MHS; Jacob R. Mitchell, MD; Mallika Modak, PhD; Tara Morgan, MD; Preethi Raghu, MD; Andrea G. Rockall, MRCP, FRCR; Molly E. Roseland, MD; Elizabeth Sadowski, MD; Michelle Sakala, MD; Kimberly L. Shampain, MD; Evan S. Siegelman, MD; Erica B. Stein, MD; Karthik M. Sundaram, MD, PhD; Myles Taffel, MD; Doreen Thomas-Payne, MSN, BSN, RN, PMHNP-BC; Isabelle Thomassin-Naggara, MD, PhD; Juliana J. Tobler, MD; Angela Tong, MD; Shaun A. Wahab, MD; Ashish P. Wasnik, MD; Limin Xu, MD

UNAPPROVED / OFF-LABEL USE DISCLOSURE

The EOCME requires CME faculty to disclose to the participants:
1. When products or procedures being discussed are off-label, unlabelled, experimental, and/or investigational (not US Food and Drug Administration [FDA] approved); and
2. Any limitations on the information presented, such as data that are preliminary or that represent ongoing research, interim analyses, and/or unsupported opinions. Faculty may discuss information about pharmaceutical agents that is outside of FDA-approved labelling. This information is intended solely for CME and is not intended to promote off-label use of these medications. If you have any questions, contact the medical affairs department of the manufacturer for the most recent prescribing information.

TO ENROLL

To enroll in the *Magnetic Resonance Imaging Clinics of North America* Continuing Medical Education program, call customer service at 1-800-654-2452 or sign up online at http://www.theclinics.com/home/cme. The CME program is available to subscribers for an additional annual fee of USD 281.00.

METHOD OF PARTICIPATION

In order to claim credit, participants must complete the following:
1. Complete enrolment as indicated above.
2. Read the activity.
3. Complete the CME Test and Evaluation. Participants must achieve a score of 70% on the test. All CME Tests and Evaluations must be completed online.

CME INQUIRIES/SPECIAL NEEDS

For all CME inquiries or special needs, please contact elsevierCME@elsevier.com.

Foreword

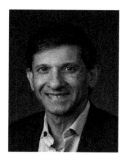 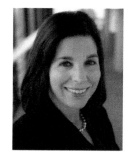

Suresh K. Mukherji, MD, MBA, FACR   Lynne S. Steinbach, MD, FACR

Consulting Editors

When we first started our radiology residency (in the last century!), the only modality that could reliably visualize the ovaries was ultrasound. Advances in CT have allowed this modality to better visualize these structures. However, MR has taken ovarian imaging to a new level. Initial imaging with pelvic ultrasound remains the mainstay, and the role of MR imaging of the adnexa has expanded and is very important in the diagnosis and treatment of both benign and malignant pathologies.

It was with this in mind that we invited Drs Erica Stein and Kimberly Shampain to guest edit this issue of *Magnetic Resonance Imaging Clinics of North America*. This issue of *Magnetic Resonance Imaging Clinics of North America* is authored by gynecologic radiology experts and covers a wide range of pathology and topics that include normal anatomy, neoplasms, congenital anomalies, inflammatory, and "mimics." There are also specific articles devoted to optimization of imaging techniques and O-RADS.

We would like to thank all the contributing authors for their wonderful articles and exquisite images. The article authors are world-renowned in their domain expertise, and we are grateful for their time and commitment to create such

wonderful content. Finally, we would like to thank Drs Stein and Shampain for guest editing this wonderful issue. I know everyone is "overcommitted," and we thank everyone for their dedication to develop such a terrific issue. On a personal note, Erica was a resident when I (S.K.M.) was Neuroradiology Division Director at University of Michigan. Erica was a "Superstar," and I am *delighted* to be able to collaborate with her on this important issue. Congratulations again to both Erica and Kim, and best wishes for continued success!

Suresh K. Mukherji, MD, MBA, FACR
University of Illinois & ProScan Imaging Carmel
IN 46074, USA

Lynne S. Steinbach, MD, FACR
Department of Radiology and Biomedical Imaging
University of California
San Francisco 505 Parnassus, San Francisco, CA
9413-0628, USA

E-mail addresses:
sureshmukherji@hotmail.com (S.K. Mukherji)
lynne.steinbach@ucsf.edu (L.S. Steinbach)

Magn Reson Imaging Clin N Am 31 (2023) xiii
https://doi.org/10.1016/j.mric.2022.09.004
1064-9689/23/© 2022 Published by Elsevier Inc.

Preface
Value Added: MR of the Adnexa

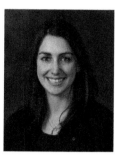 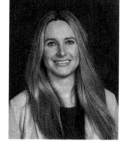

Erica B. Stein, MD   Kimberly L. Shampain, MD

Editors

MR imaging of the adnexa has become increasingly important in the diagnosis and treatment of both benign and malignant pathologies. Initial imaging with pelvic ultrasound remains the mainstay, but multimodality analysis utilizing MR imaging is a critical component to the disease-focused approach. As this type of imaging is utilized on a more widespread scale, the expectations of the radiologist have intensified as well. Our goal with this issue is to provide a primer to aid with the acquisition and interpretation of these examinations.

This issue of *Magnetic Resonance Imaging Clinics of North America* is authored by gynecologic radiology experts and covers a wide range of pathologic conditions and topics. The first article focuses on the anatomical MR appearance of the ovaries in patients of all ages. A range of adnexal developmental anomalies and variants are then presented, followed by a dedicated article on fallopian tubes. A detailed discussion of ovarian neoplasms, including benign, borderline, malignant, and germ cell, and sex-cord stromal lesions then follows.

An article dedicated to O-RADS MRI reviews the lexicon and classification system of these aforementioned neoplasms. The imaging appearance of metastatic disease to the adnexa is then discussed as are imaging findings of acute adnexal pathology condition, adnexal endometriosis, and mimics of adnexal pathology condition. Characterization and risk stratification of many of these entities requires excellent MR technique and image acquisition, which are summarized last (as we are referring to an article here).

We would like to thank all our contributing authors for their well-written articles and beautiful imaging examples. We are incredibly grateful for their time, commitment, and expertise on this topic. We would also like to thank our gynecologic oncology colleagues and all the members of the UM Gynecologic Oncology tumor board, who we have learned so much from over the years. In addition, we thank our dedicated MR imaging technologists, who are always willing to troubleshoot with us to optimize our exams. We are incredibly appreciative of the editorial staff at Elsevier for their guidance, support, and patience throughout this process as well as Dr. Suresh Mukherji and Dr. Lynne Steinbach for inviting us to edit this important issue. Last, yet most importantly, we thank our family for their continued support and encouragement. We hope that you will find this issue to be enjoyable and informative and that it allows

Magn Reson Imaging Clin N Am 31 (2023) xv–xvi
https://doi.org/10.1016/j.mric.2022.09.003
1064-9689/23/© 2022 Published by Elsevier Inc.

you to more easily and accurately interpret
adnexal MR images.

Erica B. Stein, MD
Department of Radiology
Division of Abdominal Imaging
Michigan Medicine, University of Michigan
University Hospital B1 D502
1500 East Medical Center Drive
Ann Arbor, MI 48109, USA

Kimberly L. Shampain, MD
Department of Radiology
Division of Abdominal Imaging
Michigan Medicine, University of Michigan
University Hospital B1 D502
1500 East Medical Center Drive
Ann Arbor, MI 48109, USA

E-mail addresses:
erst@med.umich.edu (E.B. Stein)
kshampai@med.umich.edu (K.L. Shampain)

MR Imaging of the Ovaries
From Puberty to Menopause

Nancy Kim, MD*, Susan M. Ascher, MD

KEYWORDS

• MR imaging • Normal ovary • Puberty • Reproductive age • Menopause

KEY POINTS

- The ovary is a dynamic organ with various physiologic changes from birth to menopause.
- It is important for the radiologist to understand the imaging features of normal physiologic findings in the ovary through puberty, reproductive age, and menopause.
- The imaging appearance of the normal ovary in women of reproductive age varies depending on the menstrual cycle phase.
- Post-menopausal ovaries can be difficult to visualize on MR imaging due to atrophy and lack of follicles, but occasionally contain simple cysts.

INTRODUCTION

The ovary, along with the fallopian tubes and ligaments, makes up the adnexa. It is a dynamic organ with physiologic changes from birth to menopause. The imaging manifestations of normal ovarian physiology should not be mistaken for pathology on imaging. The goal of this review is to highlight the imaging features of the normal ovary throughout the lifespan.

Normal Anatomy

The ovaries reside in the pelvic cavity completely surrounded by peritoneum and are bound to the uterus by the ovarian ligaments. Laterally, the ovaries are bound to the pelvic wall by the suspensory ligaments of the ovary also known as the infundibulopelvic ligaments, which are sometimes visible on MR imaging.[1] The ovaries are close in proximity to the fimbriae and infundibulum of the fallopian tubes.

On histology, the outer most layer of the ovary is the surface epithelium. The ovarian parenchyma is composed of a cortex and medulla. The peripheral aspect, the cortex, is composed of the stroma and ovarian follicles and is encased by the tunica albuginea. The inner aspect of the ovarian parenchyma, the medulla, is composed of vessels.[2] The ovaries have a dual blood supply from the ovarian and uterine arteries. The ovarian artery arises laterally from the aorta just distal to the renal arteries and courses inferiorly toward the pelvis through the suspensory ligament of the ovary. The uterine artery, a branch of the internal iliac artery, gives rise to an ovarian branch which courses through the ovarian ligament. The right ovarian vein drains directly into the inferior vena cava and the left ovarian vein drains into the left renal vein.[3,4]

Embryology (for a comprehensive discussion of embryology, refer to Refs.[5,6]).

The development of the ovary during fetal life can be divided into 4 stages: indifferent gonad, stage of differentiation, stage of oogonal multiplication, and oocyte formation, the stage of primordial follicle formation.[5]

The *indifferent stage* occurs during the first 6 weeks following fertilization. Primordial germ cells migrate from the yolk sac to the urogenital ridge. In the absence of testis determining factor, the primordial germ cells become the cortex.

The *differentiation stage* begins after the sixth week when, in women, the paired mesonephric (Wolffian) ducts regress due to the absence of

Department of Radiology, MedStar Georgetown University Hospital, CCC Building Ground Floor, CG 201 3800 Reservoir Road, NW, Washington, DC 20007, USA
* Corresponding author.
E-mail address: Nancy.Kim@gunet.georgetown.edu

Magn Reson Imaging Clin N Am 31 (2023) 1–10
https://doi.org/10.1016/j.mric.2022.07.001
1064-9689/23/© 2022 Elsevier Inc. All rights reserved.

anti-Mullerian hormone (AMH) and sex determining region Y gene. The absence of AMH allows for development of the paramesonephric (Mullerian) ducts, which will give rise to the upper third of the vagina, cervix, fallopian tubes, and the uterus.[5,6]

The *stages of oogonal multiplication and oocyte formation* occurs during the second to the early third trimesters of pregnancy. The primordial germ cells divide into small clusters with intervening stromal tissue extending from the medulla to the cortex. These small groups of primitive germ cells proliferate and develop into oogonia. The oogonia enter meiosis and form oocytes.

Follicle formation, the final phase, occurs when the oocytes are surrounded by a layer of epithelial cells to become primordial follicles. Women are born with approximately 400,000 primordial follicles, which decrease progressively through life as they undergo folliculogenesis and atresia. Only approximately 400 primordial follicles will mature to the point of ovulation during a woman's lifespan.[5–7]

Puberty

Physiology
Puberty begins when the hypothalamic–pituitary–gonadal axis is activated and the hypothalamus releases small amounts of gonadotropin-releasing hormone (GnRH). The pulsatile release of GnRH causes the pituitary gland to secrete luteinizing hormone (LH) and follicle-stimulating hormone (FSH). In early puberty, FSH levels are higher than LH, which increases estrogen production and promotes granulosa cell growth and proliferation. This results in an increase in antral follicle size and number. As puberty progresses, LH levels become elevated, which increases circulation of androgens and promotes further follicular maturation. Eventually, the circulation of both estradiol and progesterone leads to an LH surge, which causes ovulation leading to menarche.[2] The age of menarche has been decreasing over the years with the median age at 11.9 years.[8]

MR Imaging
Most pediatric and adolescent imaging is performed with ultrasound; however, at times MR imaging can be helpful especially in visualizing the full morphology of the ovaries when transvaginal ultrasound is contraindicated.[9] In early puberty, the ovarian volume increases reflecting FSH predominance and concomitant increase in size and number of antral follicles. Normal ovarian volume in pre-menarchal girls ages 11 to 12 years ranges from 2 to 4 cm^3 and 2.5 to 20 cm^3 in post-menarchal girls.[10] On imaging, the ovaries can have a multi-follicular appearance, which sometimes can be mistaken for polycystic ovaries (**Fig. 1**).

The normal zonal anatomy of the ovary is best seen on the T2-weighted images. The cortex has a lower signal intensity than the centrally located medulla. The cortex will contain small follicles that are hyperintense on T2-weighted images and hypointense on T1-weighted images (**Fig. 2**). On T1-weighted post-contrast images, the ovarian parenchyma will be hypoenhancing compared with pre-menopausal uterine myometrium (**Fig. 3**).[11]

Reproductive age

Physiology
Women have an average reproductive window of approximately 36 years from menarche to menopause. The average menstrual cycle is approximately 28 days with a range of 26 to 35 days and is broken down into 3 phases: follicular, ovulation, and luteal phases.[12] The follicular phase of the menstrual cycle, also known as the proliferative phase, takes place from days 1 to 14, based on a 28-day cycle. Estradiol is the dominant hormone during this phase and stimulates follicle maturation and endometrial proliferation. A primordial follicle matures into a Graafian follicle, a precursor to ovulation. The ovulation phase occurs 14 days before menstruation with an LH surge causing a mature follicle to rupture and release an oocyte. The collapsed follicle becomes the corpus luteum. The last phase of the menstrual cycle is the luteal or secretory phase, which occurs from days 14 to 28. Progesterone, secreted by the corpus luteum, is the dominant hormone during this phase and prepares the endometrium for possible implantation of the blastocyst. If fertilization occurs, the corpus luteum persists and maintains hormone levels during the first trimester of pregnancy. If fertilization does not occur, the corpus luteum involutes into a corpus albicans and hormone levels decrease rapidly causing the endometrium to break down and menstruation begins. The cycle then repeats and enters the follicular phase.[13,14]

MR Imaging
The imaging appearance of the ovary changes throughout the menstrual cycle. The number and size of cysts, as well as signal intensity of the ovary on diffusion weighted imaging (DWI) varies.

Physiologic Follicles
In the follicular phase, dominant pre-ovulatory follicles can enlarge up to 1.7 to 2.5 cm in size.[15] Physiologic follicles in various stages of development are usually 3 cm or smaller. On MR imaging,

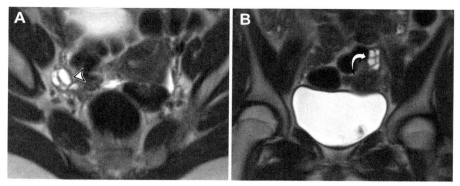

Fig. 1. Normal pre-menarchal ovaries in a 13-year-old girl. (*A*) Axial and (*B*) coronal T2-weighted half-Fourier acquisition single-shot turbo spin-echo images show multiple small thin-walled hyperintense follicles in the right (*arrowhead*) and left (*curved arrow*) ovaries, respectively.

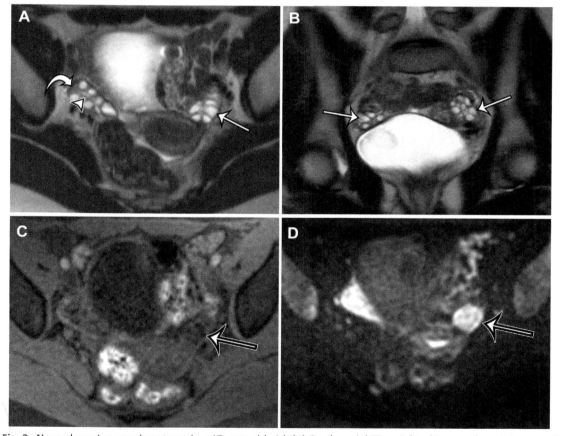

Fig. 2. Normal ovarian zonal anatomy in a 17-year-old girl. (*A*) On the axial T2-weighted image, there is increased T2 signal in the medulla (*arrowhead*) and intermediate T2 signal in the cortex (*curved arrow*). The cortex contains small follicles that are hyperintense on T2-weighted images (*arrow*). (*B*) Coronal T2-weighted images of normal ovaries with multiple small T2 hyperintense follicles (*arrows*). (*C*) Normal follicles are hypointense on T1-weighted fat saturated pre-contrast images (*arrow*), and (*D*) demonstrate increased signal on diffusion weighted images (*arrow*).

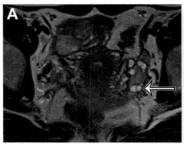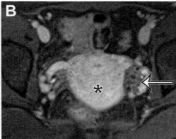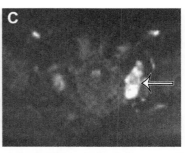

Fig. 3. Normal ovary in a 41-year-old woman. (*A*) Normal left ovary with physiologic follicles in the left ovary with thin imperceptible wall (*arrow*). (*B*) On T1-weighted fat saturated post-contrast images, the ovarian parenchyma (*arrow*) is hypoenhancing compared with the uterine myometrium (*asterisk*). (*C*) The ovarian parenchyma in women of reproductive age is hyperintense on DWI, especially during the luteal phase of the menstrual cycle (*arrow*).

they are hypointense on T1-weighted images, hyperintense on T2-weighted images, and have an imperceptible thin wall.[11,16] Normal reproductive age ovaries have relatively high signal intensity on DWI especially during the luteal phase of the menstrual cycle (see **Fig. 3**).[17,18]

Follicular cysts
When follicles fail to regress or ovulate during the follicular phase, they can develop into follicular cysts (**Fig. 4**). Follicular cysts can contain simple fluid or blood products and can range in size from 3 to 8 cm; however, rarely exceeds 5 cm.[15] They are usually hypointense on T1-weighted pre-contrast images, hyperintense on T2-weighted images, and have thin enhancing walls on T1-weighted post-contrast images.[19]

Corpus luteal cysts
During the luteal phase after ovulation and oocyte release, a corpus luteal cyst remains in the ovarian cortex. These are usually singular and typically 1 to 3 cm in size; however, they can range up to 6 cm in diameter.[15] The appearance of corpus luteal cysts varies on MR imaging due to possible hemorrhage and collapse. Typically, they are hypointense on T1-weighted pre-contrast images and hyperintense on T2-weighted sequences. Following contrast, their thick, irregular, crenulated wall is hyperemic (**Fig. 5**). If there is hemorrhage, there may be increased signal on T1-weighted pre-contrast images and variable signal on T2-weighted images.[20]

Hemorrhagic cysts
Hemorrhagic ovarian cysts occur following bleeding into a follicular or a corpus luteal cyst. Corpus luteal cysts are more likely to bleed due to increased wall vascularity than follicular cysts. Hemorrhagic cysts have increased signal intensity on T1-weighted pre-contrast images, intermediate-to-high signal

on T2-weighted images, and do not demonstrate enhancement on post-contrast T1-weighted images (**Fig. 6**).[21] When small, hemorrhagic cysts can be difficult to distinguish from endometriomas on MR imaging. A unilateral, single, hyperintense lesion in the ovary on T1-weighted fat suppressed pre-contrast images favors a hemorrhagic cyst, whereas multiple hyperintense lesions favor endometriomas (**Fig. 7**).[22] In addition, hemorrhagic cysts will usually resolve in 6 to 8 weeks, whereas endometriomas will persist.[20]

Menopause

Physiology
Menopause is the permanent cessation of menstruation secondary to loss of ovarian follicular activity. Clinically, menopause is considered to have occurred after 12 consecutive months of amenorrhea. The age range for onset of menopause is 40 to 60 years with the average age between 51 and 53 years.[23,24] Before full menopause, there are various stages of the perimenopausal state based on The Stages of Reproductive Aging Workshop staging system. The early perimenopausal stage is characterized by persistent irregularity of the menstrual cycle. The late perimenopausal stage is characterized by amenorrhea of greater than or equal to 60 days in the prior 12-month period.[25,26] During perimenopause, there is marked hormonal instability with various patterns of hormone levels. Ultimately, there is progressive increase in FSH and decrease in estradiol at the time of last menstrual cycle. In the postmenopausal state, there are increased levels of FSH and LH with low levels of estradiol and progesterone which result in absence of folliculogenesis.[25]

MR Imaging
Ovarian volume decreases in the postmenopausal woman ranging from 1.2 to 5.8 cm^3 depending on

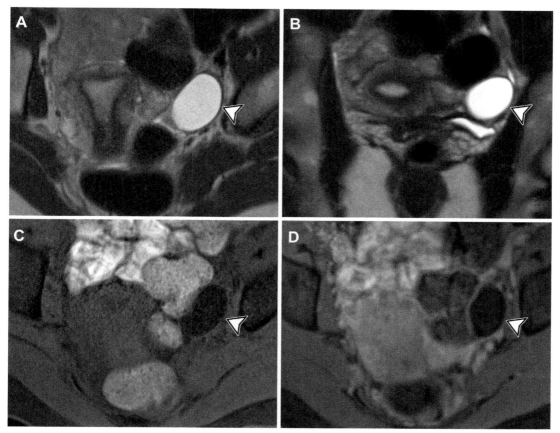

Fig. 4. A 35-year-old woman with a follicular cyst in the left ovary. On axial (*A*) and coronal (*B*) T2-weighted images, there is a well-circumscribed T2 hyperintense cyst in the left ovary (*arrowhead*). (*C*) On pre-contrast T1-weighted fat saturated images, the cyst is hypointense (*arrowhead*). (*D*) On post-contrast T1-weighted fat saturated images, there is mild enhancement of the thin wall without internal enhancement (*arrowhead*).

the hormonal status and stage of menopause. An ovarian volume greater than 8 cm^3 is considered abnormal.[27,28]

Ovaries may be difficult to identify in postmenopausal women on MR imaging due to atrophy and lack of follicles. However, if identified, they demonstrate homogeneous intermediate-to-hypointense signal on T1-weighted images and homogenously hypointense signal on T2-weighted images. On T1-weighted post-contrast images, the enhancement

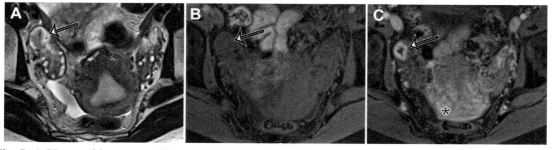

Fig. 5. A 35-year-old woman with a non-hemorrhagic corpus luteal cyst in the right ovary. (*A*) On axial T2-weighted images, there is a collapsed lesion in the right ovary with an intermediate signal thick crenulated wall (*arrow*). (*B*) On axial T1-weighted fat saturated pre-contrast images, the lesion is hypointense (*arrow*). On post-contrast images (*C*), there is avid enhancement of the thick crenulated wall (*arrow*) that is similar in enhancement to the uterine myometrium (*asterisk*) with central nonenhancement most compatible with a corpus luteal cyst. Small amount of physiologic free fluid is present.

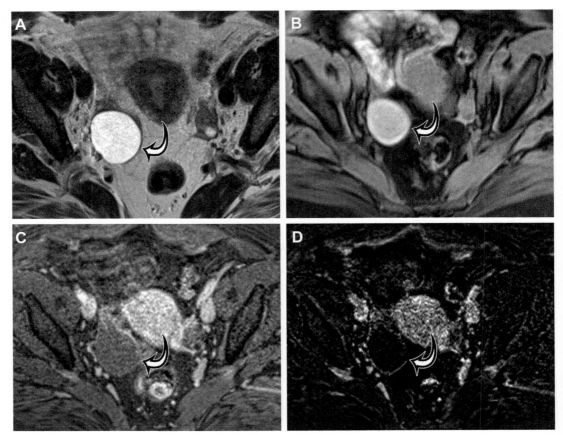

Fig. 6. A 48-year-old woman with hemorrhagic cyst in the right ovary. (*A*) The axial T2-weighted MR image shows a well-circumscribed T2 hyperintense cyst in the right ovary (*curved arrow*). (*B*) On the axial T1-weighed fat saturated pre-contrast image, there is increased signal within the cyst compatible with hemorrhage (*curved arrow*). The hemorrhagic cyst (*curved arrow*) does not enhance on the T1-weighted fat saturated post-contrast (*C*) and subtraction (*D*) images.

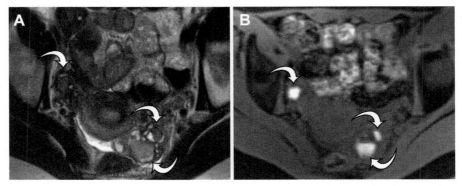

Fig. 7. A 29-year-old woman with bilateral endometriomas. (*A*) On the axial T2-weighted image, there are bilateral T2 intermediate signal lesions in bilateral ovaries with "T2-shading" (*curved arrows*) due to recurrent hemorrhage. (*B*) On the axial T1-weighted fat saturated pre-contrast image, these lesions contain hyperintense signal compatible with blood products (*curved arrows*). Unlike hemorrhagic cysts that are usually singular, multiple hemorrhagic lesions in bilateral ovaries are most consistent with endometriomas. Trace free fluid is present in the pelvis.

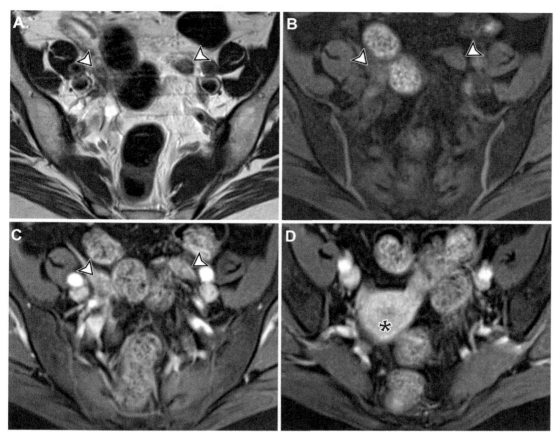

Fig. 8. Normal post-menopausal ovaries in a 63-year-old woman. (*A*) On the axial T2-weighted image, the ovaries demonstrate homogeneous hypointense signal (*arrowheads*). (*B*) On the axial T1-weighted fat saturated pre-contrast image, the ovaries are homogeneous with intermediate signal intensity (*arrowheads*). (*C, D*) On axial T1-weighted post-contrast images, the ovaries demonstrate homogeneous enhancement (*arrowheads*), which is similar to the uterine myometrial enhancement (*asterisk*).

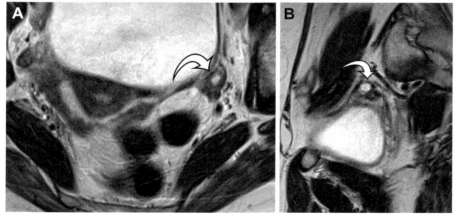

Fig. 9. A 53-year-old postmenopausal woman with small simple cyst in the left ovary. On axial (*A*) and coronal (*B*) T2-weighted images, there is a small T2 hyperintense simple cyst in the T2-intermediate signal postmenopausal left ovary (*curved arrow*). Given the small size of the cyst, no further follow up is necessary.

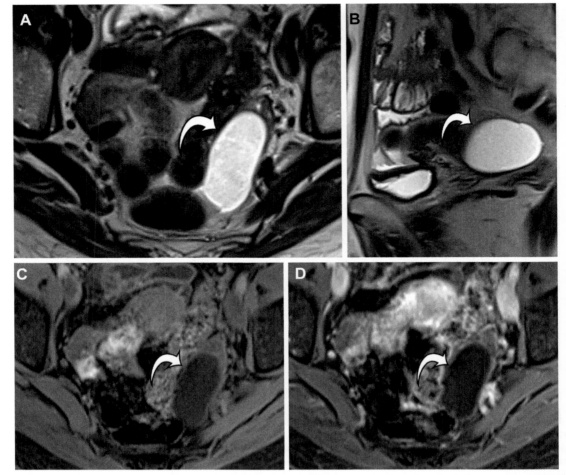

Fig. 10. A 54-year-old postmenopausal woman with a greater than 5 cm simple cyst in the left ovary. On axial (*A*) and coronal (*B*) T2-weighted images, there is a well circumscribed, thin-walled cyst in the left ovary (*curved arrow*). (*C*) On the T1-weighted fat saturated pre-contrast axial image, the cyst demonstrates hypointense signal (*curved arrow*). (*D*) On T1-weighted post-contrast images, the cyst does not enhance and is most consistent with a simple cyst (*curved arrow*). Given large size of the simple cyst, this cyst is being followed and has remained stable for 1 year.

of the ovaries is similar to, or less than, the uterine myometrium (**Fig. 8**).[23,29]

Although folliculogenesis no longer occurs in the postmenopausal ovaries, simple ovarian cysts can still occur, likely secondary to an occasional ovulatory event during the perimenopausal and early menopausal periods. On MR imaging, this manifests as simple cysts that are usually smaller than 3 cm. A large study of women above 55 years of age showed that 14% of women had cysts on initial ultrasound. In total, 32% of the cysts resolved on subsequent imaging and the incidence of developing a new simple cyst at 1 year follow up was 8%.[30,31] These cysts are hyperintense on T2-weighted images and hypointense on T1-weighted images without enhancement on post-contrast T1-weighted images (**Fig. 9**).[19,23] If simple cysts in the post-menopausal ovary are greater than 3 cm and equal to, or less than, 5 cm, no further imaging follow up is necessary. However, if the simple cyst is larger than 5 cm, then ultrasound follow up is advised (**Fig. 10**).[31,32]

SUMMARY

The ovary is a hormonally sensitive, dynamic organ that changes throughout a woman's life. It is important for radiologists to understand the imaging features of these physiologic changes and differentiate them from disease states.

CLINICS CARE POINTS

- When unable to find the ovaries on the T2-weighted sequences, consider looking for them on diffusion weighted images.
- When evaluating ovaries in a woman of reproductive age, consider the various physiologic changes of the ovary during the menstrual cycle.
- When assessing a simple ovarian cyst in a postmenopausal woman, consider size and consult the Ovarian-Adnexal Reporting & Data System.

DISCLOSURES

The authors have nothing to disclose.

REFERENCES

1. Kaniewska M, Gołofit P, Heubner M, et al. Suspensory ligaments of the female genital organs: MRI evaluation with intraoperative correlation. Radiographics 2018;38(7):2195–211.
2. Colvin CW, Abdullatif H. Anatomy of female puberty: The clinical relevance of developmental changes in the reproductive system. Clin Anat 2013;26(1):115–29.
3. Hricak H, Akin O, Sala E, et al. Diagnostic imaging: Gynecology. Amirsys 2007;7-1-7-15.
4. Ssi-Yan-Kai G, Rivain AL, Trichot C, et al. What every radiologist should know about adnexal torsion. Emerg Radiol 2018;25(1):51–9.
5. Fritz MA, Speroff L. The Ovary - Embryology and Development. In: Clinical Gynecologic Endocrinology and Infertility. 9th edition. United States: Wolters Kluwer; 2020. p. 59–70.
6. Kurman R, Fu Y. Embryology of the Female Genital TRact and Disorders of Abnromal Sexual Development, . Blaustein's pathology of the Female Genital Tract. 4th edition. New York. NY: Springer-Verlag; 1994. p. 3–11.
7. Cunha GR, Robboy SJ, Kurita T, et al. Development of the human female reproductive tract. Differentiation 2018;103:46–65.
8. Martinez GM. National Health Statistics Reports. 1995. Number 146, September 10, 2020 Available at: https://www.cdc.gov/nchs/products/index.htm.
9. Brown M, Park AS, Shayya RF, et al. Ovarian imaging by magnetic resonance in adolescent girls with polycystic ovary syndrome and age-matched controls. J Magn Reson Imaging 2013;38(3):689–93.
10. Garel L, Dubais J, Grignon A, et al. US of the pediatric female pelvis: A clinical perspective. Radiographics 2001;21(6).
11. Woodfield CA, Siegelman ES. MR Imaging of Benign Ovarian Lesions. Contemp Diagn Radiol 2006;29(2):1–5.
12. Mihm M, Gangooly S, Muttukrishna S. The normal menstrual cycle in women. Anim Reprod Sci 2011;124(3–4):229–36.
13. Broekmans FJ, Soules MR, Fauser BC. Ovarian aging: Mechanisms and clinical consequences. Endocr Rev 2009;30(5):465–93.
14. Silberstein SD, Merriam GR. Physiology of the menstrual cycle. Cephalalgia 2000;20(3):148–54.
15. Tamai K, Koyama T, Saga T, et al. MR features of physiologic and benign conditions of the ovary. Eur Radiol 2006;16(12):2700–11.
16. Vargas HA, Barrett T, Sala E. MRI of ovarian masses. J Magn Reson Imaging 2013;37(2):265–81.
17. Morisawa N, Kido A, Koyama T, et al. Changes of the normal ovary during menstrual cycle in reproductive age on the diffusion-weighted image. J Comput Assist Tomogr 2012;36(3):319–22.
18. Duarte AL, Dias JL, Cunha TM. Armadilhas em imagem ponderada em difusão da pelve feminina. Radiol Bras 2018;51(1):37–44.
19. Outwater EK, Mitchell DG. Normal ovaries and functional cysts: MR appearance. Radiology 1996;198(2):397–402.
20. Bonde AA, Korngold EK, Foster BR, et al. Radiological appearances of corpus luteum cysts and their imaging mimics. Abdom Radiol 2016;41(11).
21. Jeong Y-Y, Outwater EK, Kang HK. Imaging Evaluation of Ovarian Masses. RadioGraphics 2000;20(5):1445–70.
22. Siegelman ES, Oliver ER. MR imaging of endometriosis: Ten imaging pearls. Radiographics 2012;32(6):1675–91.
23. Langer JE, Oliver ER, Lev-Toaff AS, et al. Imaging of the female pelvis through the life cycle. Radiographics 2012;32(6):1575–97.
24. Te Velde ER, Pearson PL. The variability of female reproductive ageing. Hum Reprod Update 2002;8(2):141–54.
25. Burger HG. Physiology and endocrinology of the menopause. Medicine (Baltimore) 2006;34(1):27–30.
26. Monteleone P, Mascagni G, Giannini A, et al. Symptoms of menopause - Global prevalence, physiology and implications. Nat Rev Endocrinol 2018;14(4):199–215.
27. Cohen HL, Tice HM, Mandel FS. Ovarian volumes measured by US: Bigger than we think. Radiology 1990;177(1):189–92.

28. Aviram R, Gassner G, Markovitch O, et al. Volumes of normal ovaries, ovaries with benign lesions, and ovaries with cancer in menopausal women: Is there an optimal cut-off value to predict malignancy? J Clin Ultrasound 2008;36(1):1–5.

29. Outwater EK, Schiebler ML. Magnetic resonance imaging of the ovary. Magn Reson Imaging Clin N Am 1994;2(2):245–74.

30. Greenlee RT, Kessel B, Williams CR, et al. Prevalence, incidence, and natural history of simple ovarian cysts among women >55 years old in a large cancer screening trial. Am J Obstet Gynecol 2010;202(4):373.e1–9.

31. Patel MD, Ascher SM, Horrow MM, et al. Management of Incidental Adnexal Findings on CT and MRI: A White Paper of the ACR Incidental Findings Committee. J Am Coll Radiol 2020;17(2): 248–54.

32. Levine D, Gosink BB, Wolf SI, et al. Simple adnexal cysts: The natural history in postmenopausal women. Radiology 1992;184(3):653–9.

MR Imaging of Müllerian Anomalies

Joanie Garratt, MD*, Evan S. Siegelman, MD

KEYWORDS

- Duct anomalies • Uterine anomalies • Primary amenorrhea • Endometriosis
- Reproductive outcomes • Infertility

KEY POINTS

- MR imaging is a comprehensive imaging technique for evaluating individuals with amenorrhea and anomalies. MR imaging can determine the absence or presence of the uterus, cervix, and proximal vagina as well as depict complications of functional obstruction of menstrual blood in those with functioning endometrium.
- As the management and therapeutic interventions are different for septate and bicornuate anomalies of the uterus, it is imperative to accurately distinguish between these diagnoses on imaging.
- Renal and Mullerian anomalies can be associated with one another. One should consider including a larger field of view set of MR images when evaluating those with uterine anomalies to confirm the presence of orthotopic kidneys.

INTRODUCTION

Constituting a broad spectrum of developmental abnormalities of the female genital tract, Mullerian duct anomalies (MDAs) are more common than previously thought[1]. Earlier literature estimated that 1% of all females and 3% of females with poor reproductive outcomes had MDAs.[2] Recent literature estimates that the prevalence of developmental anomalies involving the uterus and upper vagina is 7% in the general population and that this number rises to nearly 25% in women who present with infertility and miscarriage.[1,3–7] More accurate and widely available imaging methods may be in part responsible for the recent increase in diagnosis.[4,8] However, because many patients are asymptomatic and will go undiagnosed, the precise prevalence remains unknown.

As there is a broad spectrum of MDAs, the clinical features and presentations of these patients are also diverse. Many patients may not present until after puberty, despite an anomaly existing since birth.[5,9] Other patients will present later in life with infertility or pregnancy loss.[10]

MDAs are just one potential etiology of infertility and pregnancy loss. It has been suggested that women with MDAs do not have problems with conceiving but do have higher rates of pregnancy complications and loss, including spontaneous abortion and preterm delivery. Reproductive outcomes, however, vary depending on the specific MDA. Septate uterus, for instance, reportedly has the highest rate of spontaneous abortion, estimated to be 65%.[5,6,11]

MDAs are also associated with renal and urinary tract anomalies, occurring in nearly 30–40% of patients with genital tract anomalies.[12] In a patient diagnosed with a renal anomaly, such as renal agenesis, ectopic ureter, or multicystic dysplastic kidney, one should evaluate for a concomitant genital tract anomaly.[4] Conversely, when evaluating someone for an MDA, one should ensure that the patient has normal kidneys.

EMBRYOLOGY

During normal embryologic development, paired Mullerian ducts (MDs) are the primordial components of the female reproductive tract and give rise to the fallopian tubes, uterus, cervix, and upper two-thirds of the vagina. If there is a disruption in the formation (organogenesis), failure of fusion,

Department of Radiology, University of Pennsylvania, 3400 Spruce Street/1 Silverstein, Philadelphia, PA 19103, USA
* Corresponding author.
E-mail address: Joanie.Garratt@pennmedicine.upenn.edu

Magn Reson Imaging Clin N Am 31 (2023) 11–28
https://doi.org/10.1016/j.mric.2022.06.002
1064-9689/23/© 2022 Elsevier Inc. All rights reserved.

mri.theclinics.com

or incomplete septal resorption of these paired ducts, MDAs result.[6,11,13,14]

In embryos of both genders before 6 weeks, both Wolffian (mesonephric) and Mullerian (paramesonephric) ducts are present. After 6 weeks, the MDs will grow with concomitant regression of the Wolffian ducts if there is no Mullerian-inhibiting factor (MIF), which is associated with the Y chromosome.[6,13–15] Aplasia or hypoplasia of the Mullerian structures, such as uterine agenesis and unicornuate uterus, results if organogenesis is interrupted.[14]

The MDs will subsequently grow, migrate toward the midline, and fuse to form the uterovaginal primordium. Fusion anomalies, such as uterine didelphys and bicornuate uterus, result if development is interrupted at this time. The uterovaginal septum intervening between the fused MDs is then resorbed between 9 and 12 weeks. Partial and complete resorption anomalies, including the septate and arcuate uterus, are the result of interruption during this period of development.[6,14,15]

The lower one-third of the vagina and vaginal introitus develops from the urogenital sinus, which invaginates and fuses vertically with the developing Mullerian ductal system.[14,16,17] Interruption of vertical fusion can result in vaginal atresia, transverse vaginal septum, or cervical atresia.[18]

Both the MDs and the primordial structures of the urinary tract originate from the same mesodermal ridge.[15] The ureteral bud arises from the Wolffian (mesonephric) ducts, is responsible for prompting organogenesis of the kidneys and is the embryological precursor of the renal collecting tubules, renal calices, and ureters.[13] This association of the MDs and the urinary tract underlies combined genitourinary malformations.

IMAGING OF MULLERIAN DUCT ANOMALIES

Initial imaging evaluation of the female reproductive system is most often performed with ultrasonography (US) and/or hysterosalpingography (HSG). In the evaluation of infertility, the gold standard to evaluate fallopian tube patency is HSG; however, HSG is not typically indicated in adolescents and it does not assess the external fundal contour.[13,19] It may be possible to diagnose genital tract anomalies with HSG or US in some patients; transvaginal three-dimensional (3D) ultrasound, in particular, is accurate.[4,14,20] Nonetheless, MR imaging is often used as a problem-solving tool for further classification of MDAs.

With diagnostic accuracy of nearly 100%, MR imaging is typically considered the gold standard in imaging suspected uterine anomalies.[3,15,20,21] In comparison to other modalities, MR imaging

has superior soft-tissue contrast, allowing detailed imaging of the zonal anatomy of the uterus as well as the external fundal contour. It also allows specific characterization of tissue and fluid as well as imaging of the entire female pelvis.[3] As there can be considerable overlap in features of MDAs and accurate diagnosis is crucial, MR imaging is often needed for classification.[4] Furthermore, MR imaging allows evaluation of the entire female pelvis, such as for endometriosis and presurgical planning, and the upper abdomen for renal anomalies.[10,13]

The drawbacks of MR imaging include relative higher cost, sensitivity to patient motion, long acquisition time, poor tolerance in claustrophobic patients, and contraindication in patients with certain metallic foreign bodies or implanted medical devices. MR imaging is particularly useful in adolescent patients who are not sexually active, as transabdominal US alone may be inconclusive, especially in the evaluation of Mullerian remnants.[3,4,20]

MR IMAGING TECHNIQUE

MR imaging for suspected uterine anomaly can be performed at 1.5 T or 3 T, although 3 T does provide a better signal-to-noise ratio.[4,19] Intravenous contrast is not required. In adult patients, a vaginal gel can assist in delineating the vaginal canal and identifying potential septa or other anomalies.[14] Glucagon or buscopan may also be given to reduce motion artifacts from the adjacent bowel.[21] In addition, patients should void before the exam to reduce motion and ghosting artifacts from a full bladder.[21] A sample protocol is provided in **Table 1**.

When evaluating the female pelvis with MR imaging, it is essential to include T2-weighted sequences which show the zonal anatomy of the uterus.[4,14,19,22] Studies should include thin section oblique T2-weighted images that are oriented along the long axis of the uterus; the initial T2-weighted images in the sagittal plane may be used to identify the orientation and position of the uterus for these oblique sequences (**Fig. 1**).[4,14,23] The fundal contour is best depicted on the long axis T2 images through the uterus, which is used to differentiate septate from the bicornuate uterus (discussed in more detail later). Alternatively, obtaining a 3D T2-weighted sequence permits one to obtain any desired long axis through post-processing.[3,4,19,24]

On T2-weighted MR imaging, the zonal anatomy of the normal uterus shows the following signal intensities: hyperintense endometrium, hypointense junctional zone/inner myometrium, and intermediate

Table 1
Recommendations for MR imaging protocol in the evaluation of uterine anomalies

Sequence Descriptions	FOV (cm)	TE	Slice Thickness (mm)	Comments
Three-plane localizer				
Coronal T2-weighted single-shot fast spin echo larger field-of-view (FOV)	38–40	90	4–5	Large FOV to evaluate kidneys
Sagittal T2-weighted fast spin echo	22–24	90–110	4–5	
Coronal oblique long axis T2-weighted	22–24	90–110	4–5	Long axis to uterus
Axial oblique short axis T2-weighted	22–24	90–110	4–5	Short axis to uterus
Axial T1-weighted two-dimensional dual echo SPGR	22–24		4–5	Phase encoding left to right
Axial T2-weighted two-dimensional SPGR fat-suppressed	22–24		4–5	
Axial balanced GRE	22–24		4–5	Best Sequence for outlining bowel

outer myometrium (see **Fig. 1**).[2,4,15,19,22] The junctional zone normally measures 8 to 12 mm, with varying thickness depending on the phase of menses and age.[15] The layers of the cervix are contiguous with those of the uterus and have a similar appearance on MR imaging. The vaginal mucosa is hyperintense and the submucosa and surrounding vaginal musculature are hypointense on T2-weighted imaging.[19]

Unless dilated or outlined by fluid, the fallopian tubes are not normally visualized on MR imaging. Attached to the posterior aspect of the broad ligament and located along the lateral pelvic wall, the paired ovaries are identified by hyperintense follicles on T2-weighted imaging.[13]

T1-weighted imaging with fat suppression is useful in the evaluation of endometriomas and hematometrocolpos, which can occur in women who have functional obstruction of the antegrade flow of menstrual blood. Blood products, hematosalpinx, and endometriomas will typically be hyperintense on T1-weighted imaging. The uterus is homogenous on T1-weighted imaging, precluding evaluation of the zonal anatomy.[2,4,10,14,15,19,22]

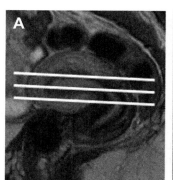 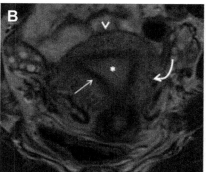 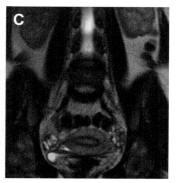

Fig. 1. MR imaging of a normal uterus. (A) Sagittal T2-weighted image of the pelvis shows the orientation plane (white lines) of long axis imaging through the uterus. (B) T2-weighted image through the long axis of the uterus. Normal zonal anatomy includes hyperintense endometrium (asterisk), hypointense junctional zone/inner myometrium (thin arrow), and intermediate outer myometrium (curved arrow). Note the normal external fundal contour (arrowhead). (C) Large field of view coronal T2-weighted image allow evaluation of the kidneys. The ovaries and uterus (short axis view) are present.

The kidneys and collecting systems should be evaluated in patients with MDAs, given the associations with genitourinary malformations.[4,14,20,25–27] A large field of view sequence that covers the upper abdomen allows evaluation of the kidneys (see **Fig. 1**), performed at our institution as a coronal fast T2-weighted sequence.[4,23] If there is a renal anomaly, it is ipsilateral to the side of functional obstruction of menstrual blood or absent uterine moiety. Representative anomalies include hydronephrosis, renal ectopia, hypoplastic kidney, multicystic dysplastic kidney, and unilateral agenesis.[4,12]

AMENORRHEA

Worldwide, the prevalence of amenorrhea is approximately 3%–4%, excluding amenorrhea from pregnancy, lactation, or menopause.[18] Amenorrhea is defined as the absent or abnormal cessation of menstrual bleeding. For the diagnosis of primary amenorrhea, one of the following must be true:

- Absence of menarche at age 16 with normal secondary sexual characteristics
- Absence of menarche at age 14 without normal secondary sexual characteristics[16,18]

Secondary amenorrhea, by comparison, refers to the absence of menses for 3 mo or more in a female who has had menses in the past. The physiology of the female reproductive axis is complex and disruption of any link in the chain may cause amenorrhea, resulting in a broad differential diagnosis. In this study, we focus on primary amenorrhea. Although the imaging findings of congenital MDAs and their mimics are complex, a systematic approach (**Fig. 2**) assists in narrowing the broad differential diagnosis.[14] Treatment is dependent upon the underlying etiology.

The most common causes of primary amenorrhea include anomalies of the hypothalamic–pituitary axis, gonadal dysgenesis, and anomalies of the outflow tract. Of these diagnoses, gonadal dysgenesis is most frequent, accounting for half of the cases of primary amenorrhea. Congenital structural anomalies that result in outflow obstruction are responsible for nearly 20%, whereas another 25% are explained by anomalies of the hypothalamic–pituitary axis. Other less common etiologies include polycystic ovarian syndrome and congenital adrenal hyperplasia.[16,18]

GONADAL DYSGENESIS

Gonadal dysgenesis, defined by partial or complete deformation of the gonads, is the most frequent cause of primary amenorrhea. It is associated with both normal and abnormal karyotypes. Although there are several types, pure gonadal dysgenesis in the setting of Turner syndrome accounts for two-third of the cases.[16,18] The remaining patients with gonadal dysgenesis have either 46XX or 46XY karyotype.[16]

Turner Syndrome

Affecting 1:2000 to 1:4000 live-born girls and 1:15 spontaneous abortions, Turner syndrome is a chromosomal abnormality in which there is a partial or complete loss of an X chromosome (most often 45XO).[16,28,29] Clinically, patients with Turner syndrome present short stature, a webbed neck, short fourth metacarpals, low-set ears, and widely spaced nipples. Secondary sex characteristics are absent. Patients will usually present with primary amenorrhea if not diagnosed prenatally or in childhood. In patients who have 45X/46XY mosaicism, the gonads are removed as there is an increased risk of malignant transformation, nearly 30% by age 30.[16] Patients with Turner syndrome may have associated cardiovascular and renal anomalies, as well as autoimmune disorders, such as thyroiditis and diabetes.[29]

Normal pubertal development is possible if the patient is diagnosed early and treated with hormone replacement. Although possible with assisted reproductive technologies, pregnancies in patients with Turner syndrome are considered high risk. Potential fetal and maternal complications include fetal chromosomal abnormalities, miscarriage, prematurity, and maternal morbidity and mortality from cardiovascular conditions.[16,28]

On imaging, the uterus is small and hypoplastic because of gonadal failure. The ovaries are most often small or streak in size (**Fig. 3**).[16,18] MR imaging is useful to evaluate if there are functional follicles when the patients are 46XY. Treatment involves oophorectomy given the risk for gonadoblastoma, particularly in patients with a Y chromosome.[29]

ANOMALIES OF THE OUTFLOW TRACT

A patent outflow tract is required for normal menses. Primary amenorrhea may result from congenital structural anomalies of the outflow tract.[16] Once again, a systematic approach assists in narrowing the broad differential diagnosis (see **Fig. 1**).

First, evaluate whether the MD derivatives are present, hypoplastic, or absent. If the uterus and other MD derivatives are absent, then diagnostic considerations include androgen insensitivity syndrome (AIS) and Mayer–Rokitansky–Kuster–

Diagnosis of Primary Amenorrhea

Primary Amenorrhea

- Gonadal Dysgenesis
- Central Anomalies
  Hypothalamic-Pituitary Axis
- Anomalies of the Outflow Tract
- Other
  PCOS, Adrenal Hypoplasia

- Pure
  - 45 XO Turner Syndrome
  - 46 XX
  - 46 XY Swyer Syndrome
- Partial
- Mixed

Uterus Present?

No   Yes

Ovaries Present?   Where is Obstruction?

Yes   No

Meyer-Rokitansky-Kuster-Hauser
Müllerian Agenesis

Androgen Insensitivity Syndrome
46 XY, Retained Testes

Cervix

Vagina
Transverse Septum

Hymen
Imperforate Hymen

Fig. 2. Systematic approach in the evaluation of primary amenorrhea.

Hauser (MRKH) syndrome. To differentiate between these diagnoses, determine if the ovaries are present or absent. If the ovaries are also absent, then AIS is the most likely diagnosis. If the ovaries are present, MRKH syndrome is the suspected diagnosis.[14,18,30] MRKH syndrome is discussed in detail later.

Androgen Insensitivity Syndrome

A mimic of MDAs, AIS is an X-linked inherited disorder of sex development affecting 1:20,000 to 1:64,000 individuals.[14,18,31] A mutation in the androgen receptor gene (Xq11-q12 region) results in complete unresponsiveness of target tissues to androgens.[15,31] The diagnosis of AIS is dependent upon a male karyotype (46XY), female phenotype, normal but undescended testes, and complete absence of receptor activity.[15,31,32] Although most often secondary to AIS, there is a differential diagnosis for female phenotype with a male karyotype (46XY).[31]

Embryologically, the fetal testes develop normally in patients with AIS. The fetal testes secrete testosterone, triggering the MDs to regress. However, the male genitalia do not develop because of insensitivity to circulating androgens. Normal female external genitalia result from aromatization of testosterone into estrogen in peripheral tissues, although puberty is typically delayed. The ovaries and uterus are both absent and the vagina is foreshortened because the testes also produce MIF.

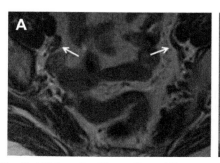
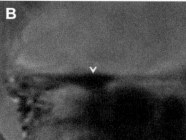
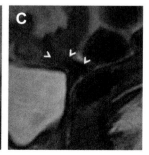

Fig. 3. MR imaging illustration of Turner syndrome in a 20-year-old woman with primary amenorrhea. (A) Axial T2-weighted image of the pelvis shows "streak ovaries" (arrows). (B) Axial and (C) sagittal T2-weighted imaging of the pelvis shows an atrophic uterus (arrowheads) and cervix. Genetic testing showed Turner syndrome.

Axillary and pubic hair is usually decreased or absent.[18,32]

Early identification of patients with AIS is essential to inform patients and their parents.[31] If a prenatal ultrasound shows female external genitalia in a fetus with 46XY karyotype on prenatal genetic screening tests, parents should be referred to a genetic counselor. Further testing at birth is required to confirm the diagnosis, including hormonal tests, karyotype analysis, and ultrasound.[31]

AIS may be diagnosed in infancy in females who present with bilateral inguinal masses from retained testes, accounting for 0.8%–2.4% of young girls with bilateral inguinal hernias.[31] Most often, the diagnosis of AIS is made at puberty in the setting of primary amenorrhea. The patients are phenotypically female, meaning that they have female external genitalia and normal breast development.[14,15,18,31]

Imaging confirms the absence of Mullerian structures while allowing the identification of retained testes and a blind-ending vagina.[15,32] On MR imaging, testes are normally hyperintense on T2-weighted imaging and hypointense on T1-weighted imaging. Retained testes may be small in size and have a hypointense rim from the tunica albuginea.[14,31] Paratesticular cysts are also common.[14] The location of these retained testes is variable, although 50% are found in the inguinal canals; if located in the pelvic cavity, they can be mistaken for uterine buds from MRKH syndrome.[14,18] The absence of normal ovaries in AIS is the distinguishing feature that separates it from MRKH.[31]

Management of AIS is multidisciplinary. The retained testes increase the risk for testicular germ cell tumor, requiring imaging surveillance or prophylactic gonadectomy with hormonal replacement.[14,15,32,33] Psychological concerns and decisions regarding the type of hormonal therapy also present challenges in treatment.[16]

Outflow Tract Obstruction

If the MD derivatives are present or hypoplastic, then determine the level of outflow obstruction. Isolated dilation of the uterine cavity (hematometra) suggests obstruction at the upper vagina or cervix, usually from an MDA. Dilation of the uterine and cervical cavities and vagina (hematometrocolpos) suggests outflow obstruction at the distal vagina or hymen, from a transverse vaginal septum or imperforate hymen. Because of its thin walls, the vagina is more distensible than the endometrial cavity.[18]

No matter the level of obstruction, postpubertal patients can present with cyclic pain secondary to cryptomenorrhagia from the accumulation of blood products. Patients otherwise have pubertal development.[16]

Transverse Vaginal Septum

The transverse vaginal septum is a developmental defect that occurs at the junction of the urogenital sinus and the MD component of the vagina. This anomaly likely results from incomplete or failed vertical fusion and resorption of the vaginal plate as it joins the MD derivatives.[9,14,16]

The prevalence of transverse vaginal septum is between 1:2100 and 1:72,000 in females.[16] It can occur anywhere along the vaginal canal, although nearly half occur in the upper vagina. The lower vagina is the least common site, accounting for only 15 to 20% of cases. A transverse vaginal septum can be associated with either vaginal duplication—a longitudinal vaginal septum—and/or other uterine anomalies. Thus, one needs to carefully evaluate the remainder of the vagina as well as the cervix and uterine configuration in these patients.[9,16,18]

On physical examination, the vagina is short and blind-ending. Unlike imperforate hymen, there is no bulging at the vaginal introitus with Valsalva maneuvers. The membrane will be entirely pink.[9,14] On MR imaging, the vagina is markedly distended with blood products (hematocolpos) (**Figs. 4** and **5**). The septum is best appreciated on T2-weighted imaging as a hypointense structure that can measure up to 5 mm. Sagittal imaging can differentiate an imperforate hymen from a transverse vaginal septum; however, the former will show distended blood to the level of the introitus and the latter will have a more proximal transition.

Treatment is surgical resection with vaginal end-to-end anastomosis. Postsurgical stenosis may occur in some patients. After resection, reproductive outcomes are most successful in patients with a lower vaginal septum. In those with an upper vaginal septum, successful pregnancy occurred in only 20% of patients, likely related to endometriosis.[9,16,21]

CLASSIFICATION

In 2021, the American Society of Reproductive Medicine (ASRM) published an updated classification for Mullerian anomalies.[30] One goal of the updated classification system was to provide more anatomic information and include anomalies that would otherwise be difficult to classify, including female genital tract anomalies that are not Mullerian in origin.[5,17,18]

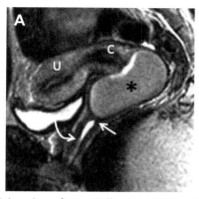
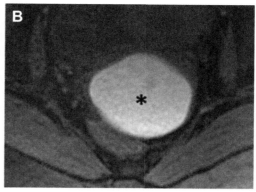

Fig. 4. MR imaging of a partially obstructing mid-transverse vaginal septum (*arrow*). (*A*) Sagittal T2-weighted image shows normal uterus (U) and cervix (C). There is a distended proximal vagina (*) containing low to intermediate signal intensity material. Note the distal vagina is normal (*curved arrow*). (*B*) Axial fat-suppressed T1-weighted image at the level of the proximal vaginal canal shows T1 hyperintense subacute blood (*). Two weeks after the MR imaging, the patient had resection of the transverse septum with evacuation of blood products within the proximal vagina.

As diagnosis guides treatment, it is important to accurately classify female genital tract anomalies.[4,8] Many classification systems have been proposed, none of which is flawless or universally accepted.[8,34,35] The classification scheme developed in 1988 by the American Fertility Society, now known as the ASRM, has been the most widely utilized.[5,14,15,36]

Müllerian Agenesis

Accounting for approximately 5 to 10% of all MDAs, MRKH syndrome is the most common cause of hypoplasia or agenesis of the MD derivatives, including the fallopian tubes, uterus, cervix, and upper two-thirds of the vagina.[5,12,14,15,18,37] These patients have normal secondary sex characteristics, female karyotype (46XX), and normal functional ovaries.[12,14,15,37] The prevalence of MRKH is 1:4000 in females and it is the second most common cause of primary amenorrhea after gonadal dysgenesis.[12,14] Differential considerations include gonadal dysgenesis (Turner syndrome), AIS, and male pseudohermaphroditism.[21]

Clinically, MRKH is a diagnosis of exclusion.[14] Primary amenorrhea is the most common clinical

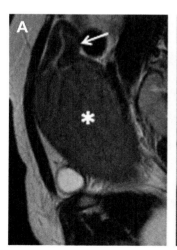
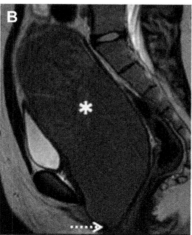
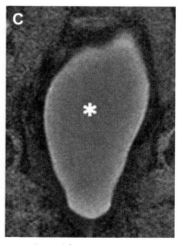

Fig. 5. MR imaging of a low transverse vaginal septum in a 14-year-old girl presenting with primary amenorrhea. (*A, B*) Two adjacent sagittal T2-weighted images show a normal uterus and cervix (*arrow*) and a markedly distended vaginal canal containing low to intermediate signal intensity blood products (*). The level of the obstruction is just above the introitus (*dashed arrow*). On both MR imaging and at physical exam, it was difficult to differentiate a low transverse septum from an imperforate hymen; the former was found at surgery. (*C*) Coronal fat-suppressed T1-weighted image shows the vaginal canal distended with hyperintense subacute blood (*).

presentation; MRKH is one of the few MDAs that cause primary amenorrhea.[14,18,37] The most severe form of MRKH is a complete absence of MD derivatives; many patients, however, will have Mullerian remnants in the setting of partial agenesis.[37] If there is a rudimentary uterus with functioning endometrium, then patients may present with cyclic pain; surgical removal of functioning uterine tissue will prevent cyclic hematometra and the development of endometriosis.[5,16,38]

MR imaging findings of Mullerian remnants include laterally located uterine buds connected by fibrous bands to a midline triangular soft tissue focus that overlies the bladder and may abut an atrophic vagina. A rudimentary uterus or uterine bud will appear as a soft tissue mass with no zonal anatomy and similar signal intensity to myometrium (**Fig. 6**). Although the uterus is normally located in the midline, the uterine remnants in MRKH patients are localized laterally underneath the ovaries. The fibrous tissue will be hypointense on T2-weighted imaging.[14] If there is functioning endometrium, it will be T2 hyperintense; one should look for associated complications of retrograde menstruation, including hematosalpinx and endometriomas.

Treatment of patients with MRKH is multidisciplinary, including psychosocial counseling. Except in the rare case of uterine transplantation (see **Fig. 6**), patients with MRKH are infertile. Pregnancy can be achieved with egg donation to a surrogate. Surgical procedures allow normal sexual function, such as lengthening of a distal vagina or creation of a neovagina.[5,9,12,29]

Cervical Agenesis

Cervical agenesis has been reported in less than 100 cases. Patients typically present with primary amenorrhea, cyclic pain, and normal secondary sexual characteristics. Because of retrograde menstruation, it is commonly associated with endometriosis and hematosalpinx.[9,38]

Imaging shows hematometra and the absence of the cervix (**Fig. 7**). Treatment is usually hysterectomy given the complexity of reconstruction,

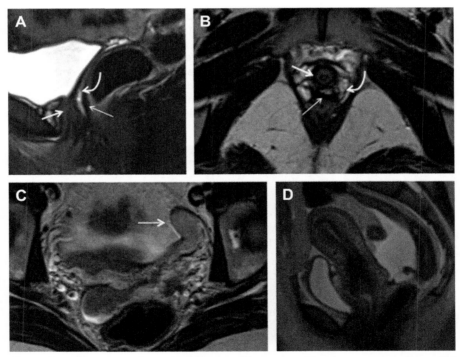

Fig. 6. MR illustration of MRKH syndrome in a 32-year-old woman with primary amenorrhea. (*A*) Sagittal fat-suppressed T2-weighted image through the midline pelvis shows a normal urethra (*arrow*), high signal intensity paravaginal veins (*curved arrow*) and low signal intensity fibrous tissue (*thin arrow*) in the expected location of the vagina. No cervix or uterine tissue is present in the midline. (*B, C*) Axial T2-weighted imaging through the low and midline pelvis shows a rudimentary left uterine horn (*double arrow*) without identifiable endometrial tissue in the lateral pelvis. Inferiorly, the normal urethra (*arrow*), paravaginal venous plexus (*curved arrow*), and fibrous hypoplastic vagina (*thin arrow*) are present. (*D*) Three years later, the patient underwent uterine transplantation. Sagittal T2-weighted image shows normal uterus, cervix and proximal vagina.

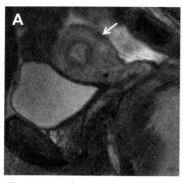
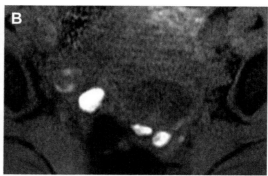

Fig. 7. MR illustration of MRKH with cervical agenesis in a 22-year-old-woman with primary amenorrhea, and endometriosis. (A) Sagittal T2-weighted image shows normal zone anatomy of a hypoplastic uterus (arrow). The endometrial complex is surrounded by T2 hypointense junctional zone without any visualized endocervix or fibrous cervical stroma. No cervix was identified on speculum exam. (B) Axial fat-suppressed T1-weighted image shows bilateral multiple T1 hyperintense adnexal lesions, representing endometriomas. Women with obstruction of functioning endometrial tissue are at increased risk of developing endometriosis.[38] This patient chose to be treated with hormonal suppression as opposed to laparoscopic resection of the uterus.

potential infectious complications, and poor reproductive outcomes in patients with a neocervix.[9]

Unicornuate Uterus

Comprising 20% of all MDAs, unicornuate uterus occurs when there is a normal development of one of the paired MDs and partial or complete failed development of the contralateral duct. Four subtypes of the unicornuate uterus have been described:

- No rudimentary horn
- Noncavitary rudimentary horn (no functioning endometrium)
- Noncommunicating cavitary rudimentary horn
- Communicating cavitary rudimentary horn[5,14,15]

A cavitary rudimentary horn with functional endometrium is present in nearly half of patients, most of which do not communicate with the larger uterine moiety. This subtype is associated with dysmenorrhea.[4,5,15,38] Patients with the other subtypes are typically diagnosed incidentally, sometimes during an infertility evaluation.[14]

The unicornuate uterus also has the greatest association with renal and urinary tract anomalies, usually ipsilateral to the absent or rudimentary horn. Concomitant unilateral renal agenesis, for instance, has been reported in up to 70% of these patients.[5,14]

On MR imaging, the fully developed horn of the unicornuate uterus is located lateral to the midline, contains normal zonal anatomy, and is curved or banana-shaped.[14,15] If present, the imaging appearance of the rudimentary horn is dependent

upon the subtype. MR imaging is the most sensitive modality to evaluate for functioning endometrium.

A noncavitary rudimentary horn seems as a homogenous hypointense mass on T2-weighted imaging (Fig. 8). Rudimentary horns that contain endometrium have normal zonal anatomy (Fig. 9). Imaging often demonstrates hematometra, unilateral hematosalpinx, and endometriosis because of retrograde menstrual flow from the endometrium of a noncommunicating rudimentary horn. These blood products will be hyperintense on T1-weighted imaging.[9,15,38]

Given the association between increased risk of obstetric complications and endometrium within a communicating rudimentary horn, surgical resection of the rudimentary horn is performed. Surgical resection also prevents potential complications from endometriosis-related to active endometrium within a noncommunicating rudimentary horn.[14,15,38] If the rudimentary horn is communicating, then the uterine cavity must be reconstructed to permit future pregnancy.[9]

Uterine Didelphys

Representing approximately 5% of MDAs, uterine didelphys is the complete failure of fusion of the MDs. Each duct fully develops, resulting in two separate uterine horns and two cervices; in many cases, there is duplication of the proximal vagina, separated by a longitudinal septum.[5,15] In the absence of functional obstruction of menstrual flow, uterine didelphys is rarely of clinical importance and the diagnosis is often made incidentally in asymptomatic patients.[5,14,15]

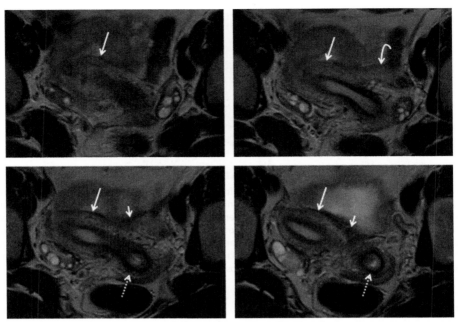

Fig. 8. MR illustration of unicornuate uterus with noncommunicating horn with no functioning endometrium. Four consecutive axial T2-weighted images show right-sided uterine horn (*arrow*) that is continuous with a midline cervix (*dashed arrow*). Small volume tissue consisting of smooth muscle (*curved arrows*) contains no high signal intensity endometrial tissue. The hypoplastic left uterus horn is continuous with the normal right uterine horn via a thin muscular band (*small arrows*).

When classifying an MDA on MR imaging, evaluate the outer fundal contour. A cleft is measured by drawing an orthogonal line from the outer myometrium to the outer myometrium at the level of the left and right fundus (**Fig. 10**). Fusion anomalies, including didelphys and bicornuate uterus, have a cleft deeper than 10 mm, distinguishing them from resorption anomalies, including the septate uterus. It is an important distinction to make because surgical treatments are not needed for fusion anomalies.[5,15]

On MR imaging, uterine didelphys appear as two widely divergent uterine horns and two cervices with no communication of the uterine canals (**Fig. 11**). Duplication of the upper vagina is seen in most patients. However, zonal anatomy is normal.

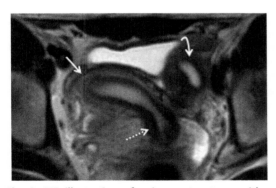

Fig. 9. MR illustration of unicornuate uterus with a noncommunicating horn with functioning endometrium in a 31-year-old woman. Axial T2-weighted image shows normal right uterine moiety (*arrow*) and cervix (dashed *arrow*). There is a left uterine horn (*curved arrow*) that has similar zonal anatomy as the right uterus. No communication to the cervix was present on other images. The left kidney was developmentally absent. The left uterine horn was surgically removed in part to prevent endometriosis (which was found at surgery).

Bicornuate Uterus

Bicornuate uterus constitutes approximately 10% of MDAs. It is the result of a partial fusion of the MDs, characterized by two divergent uterine horns that fuse near the uterine isthmus. A single or duplicated cervix may be present, described as unicollis and bicollis, respectively. An associated longitudinal vaginal septum occurs in a small portion of patients (see the section titled, "Longitudinal vaginal septum").[15] Patients are often asymptomatic. Further, although less common than other MDAs, coexisting renal anomalies can occur, most often ipsilateral renal agenesis.[15]

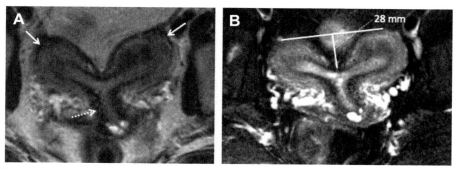

Fig. 10. MR imaging of a bicornuate uterus in a 36-year-old woman. (*A*) Axial T2-weighted image shows the presence of two separate uterine horns (*arrows*). There is a shared lower uterine segment and cervix (*dashed arrow*). (*B*) Measurement confirms a cleft of >2.5 cm between the two uterine horns. When measuring the cleft on MR imaging, draw an orthogonal line from outer myometrium to outer myometrium at the level of the left and right fundus.

Imaging of the bicornuate uterus shows two divergent uterine horns that fuse near the lower uterine segment and have normal zonal anatomy (see **Fig. 10**). Distinguishing uterine didelphys from the bicornuate bicollis uterus can be challenging, particularly if there is a longitudinal vaginal septum; however, there is little clinical significance in differentiating between these two entities as neither is treated with surgery unless there is a vaginal septum. However, because the septate uterus is managed differently, it is imperative to accurately distinguish the bicornuate from the septate uterus.[4] A cleft deeper than 10 mm differentiates bicornuate and didelphys anomalies from the septate uterus.[5]

Septate Uterus

The most common of the MDAs, the septate uterus is a resorption anomaly, occurring when there is a partial or complete failure of resorption of the urovaginal septum.[5] The septum can be of

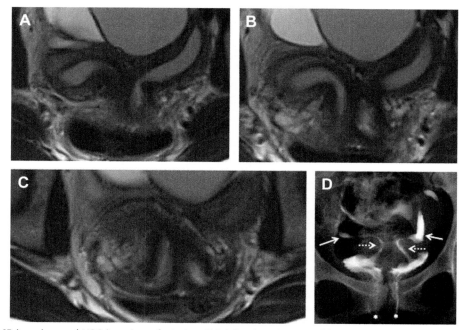

Fig. 11. MR imaging and HSG imaging of uterine didelphys in a 34-year-old woman. (*A–C*) Consecutive axial T2-weighted images show distinct separate right and left uteri and cervices. (*D*) Corresponding HSG shows opacification of separate uterine cavities (*arrow*), endocervical canals (*dashed arrow*), and vaginal fornixes (*). Separate cannulations of the left and right vaginal canals were required.

variable length; a complete septum extends to the cervix or upper vagina (**Fig. 12**). The septum is composed of fibrous tissue, myometrium, or both; it is important to determine the composition of the septum because the surgical approach differs depending on the composition.[15] A fibrous septum can be removed via a hysteroscope while surgeons often perform laparoscopic excision of a muscular septum to minimize bleeding complications.

The septate uterus has the strongest correlation with obstetric complications. The estimated spontaneous abortion rate is 65% and the fetal survival rate is 30%.[5,14] Other complications include intrauterine growth restriction, premature birth, and fetal malpresentation. Studies have suggested that reproductive outcomes improve after hysteroscopic resection. Concomitant urinary tract anomalies do occur, but less so compared with other MDAs.[5,15]

On imaging, the external fundal contour of a septate uterus may be convex, flat, or have a cleft less than 10 mm; the external fundal contour is a key distinguishing feature between resorption (septate) and fusion (bicornuate) anomalies (**Fig. 13**).[14,15] The ASRM criteria for the septate uterus include an indentation depth of more than 10 mm, as measured from an orthogonal line down from a line extending from endometrial complex to endometrial complex (not the outer uterine contour to outer fundal uterine contour), and indentation angle of less than 90° (**Fig. 14**).[5] The zonal anatomy and uterine size are normal. Fibrous tissue composition of a septum is hypointense on both T1-and T2-weighted imaging, whereas myometrial tissue composition is isointense to the remaining myometrium.[15]

Arcuate Uterus

If one considers resorption anomalies a spectrum, the arcuate uterus is on one end of the spectrum as it represents near-complete resorption of the uterovaginal septum.[14] By comparison, a complete septate uterus is a complete failure of resorption and would be at the other end of the spectrum.

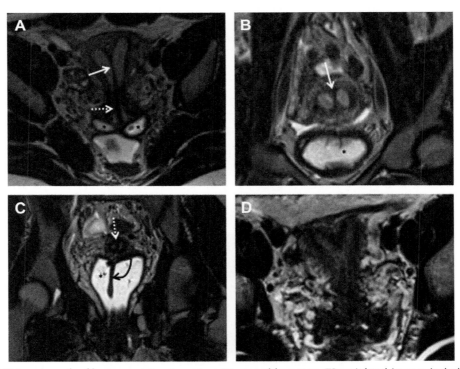

Fig. 12. MR imaging of a fibrous septate uterus in a 21-year-old woman. T2-weighted images include an axial oblique along the long axis of the uterus and cervix (*A*), coronal oblique along the short axis of the uterus (*B*), and coronal oblique along the short axis of the cervix (*C*). The upper vagina is also seen (*), distended with a vaginal gel. A septum involves the uterus (*arrows*), cervix (*dashed arrows*), and vagina (*curved arrow*). It is predominantly hypointense, suggesting a fibrous tissue. (*D*) Axial oblique T2-weighted image shows the uterus following resection of a 4 cm uterine septum.

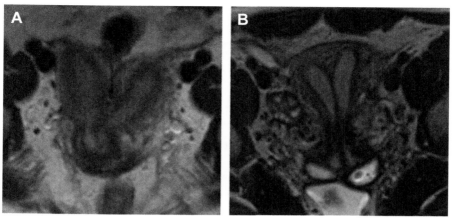

Fig. 13. MR illustration of (*A*) bicornuate uterus versus (*B*) septate uterus. It is necessary to distinguish between these two entities because septate uterus is treated surgically, whereas bicornuate uterus is not.

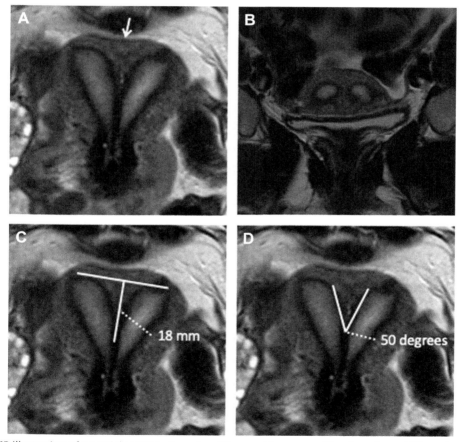

Fig. 14. MR illustration of a partial septate uterus in a 32-year-old woman with miscarriage at 20 weeks gestation. (*A*) T2-weighted axial oblique image along the long axis of the uterus shows a normal external contour (*arrow*) and a septum that does not extend to the cervix (partial septum). (*B*) T2-weighted image along the short axis of the uterus. (*C*) Smooth indentation of the fundal endometrial canal more than 10 mm (measured from the *line* drawn between the tubal ostia) and (*D*) an acute angle of 50° between the uterine cavities, in keeping with a septate uterus.

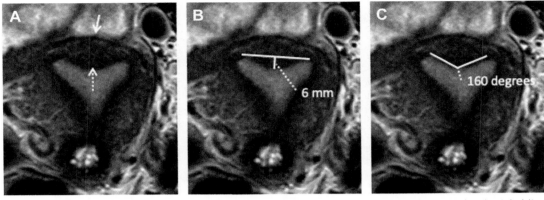

Fig. 15. MR illustration of an arcuate uterus in a 33-year-old woman with infertility. (A) T2-weighted axial oblique image through the uterus shows a normal external fundal contour (arrow), (B) a smooth indentation of the fundal endometrial canal less than 10 mm (dashed arrow), and (C) an obtuse angle of 160° between the uterine cavities, in keeping with the arcuate uterus.

Patients with an arcuate uterus are asymptomatic. This anomaly has no known clinical significance and is often thought of as a normal variant. Imaging demonstrates a normal external fundal contour and mild, smooth prominence of the myometrium at the internal fundal contour (Fig. 15).[5]

COMPLEX ANOMALIES

The ASRM classification for Mullerian anomalies 2021 improved upon prior arrangements by allowing the inclusion of anomalies that would have traditionally been difficult to categorize. For instance, a patient with a combined bicornuate and septate uterus (Fig. 16) can be classified as a complex anomaly using the new classification scheme.

Herlyn–Werner–Wunderlick syndrome or obstructed hemivagina and ipsilateral renal anomaly

Obstructed hemivagina and ipsilateral renal anomaly (OHVIRA) is a rare presentation of a uterine didelphys, transverse hemivagina septum, and ipsilateral renal anomaly. A transversely oriented septum involving one side of a duplicated proximal vagina (Fig. 17) results in outflow obstruction of one uterine horn and retrograde menstrual flow.

Clinically, patients most often present after puberty with symptoms of dysmenorrhea and pelvic pain from the obstructing hemivagina septum and associated retrograde menstruation and/or endometriosis.[15,38] As one uterine horn is not obstructed, patients will not present with primary amenorrhea. A pelvic exam may show a vaginal bulge from hematocolpos extrinsically compressing the nonobstructed hemivagina.[39] When

obstructed, uterine didelphys is often associated with ipsilateral congenital renal and urinary tract anomalies, most commonly renal agenesis or multicystic dysplastic kidney.[14]

On MR imaging, one uterine horn and the obstructed proximal vagina (hemihematometrocolpos) distend the menstrual blood that is hyperintense on T1-weighted imaging. Describing the distance from the hematocolpos to the perineum

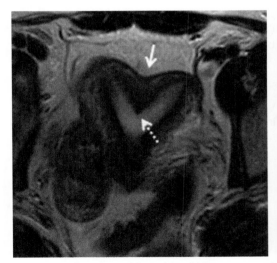

Fig. 16. MR illustration of combined bicornuate and septate uterus in a 30-year-old patient. T2-weighted axial oblique image through the uterus shows that an external fundal contour with deep cleft measuring more than 10 mm (arrow), in keeping with a bicornuate uterus, as well as smooth indentation of the fundal endometrial canal more than 10 mm (dashed arrow), in keeping with a septate uterus.

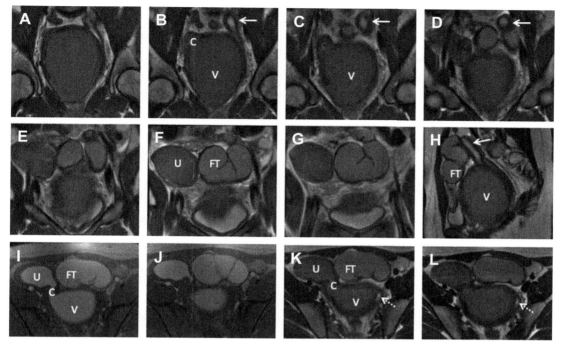

Fig. 17. MR illustration of Herlyn–Werner–Wunderlich syndrome, known as OHVIRA, in a 15-year-old girl with painful menses and solitary left kidney on prenatal ultrasound. T2-weighted (A–G) consecutive coronal images through the pelvis from posterior to anterior, (H) sagittal image, and (K, L) axial images show uterine didelphys. The right uterine horn (U), cervix (C), and hemivagina (V) are dilated with blood products (hematometrocolpos). There is an associated right hematosalpinx (FT). (I, J) Axial T1-weighted images confirm the presence of blood products from transverse vaginal septum obstructing the vaginal vault. The left uterine horn (arrow) has normal zonal anatomy. The normal, unobstructed vagina is displaced to the left (dashed arrow). FT, fallopian tube.

assists in surgical planning.[39] Treatment of OHVIRA is vaginoplasty; hemihysterectomy may be necessary in complicated cases.[39]

VAGINA

Vaginal anomalies may occur with or without uterine anomalies. Embryologically, the vagina has

two origins: the upper two-third is a MD derivative, whereas the lower one-third is derived from the urogenital sinus.[4,9] Transverse vaginal septum is discussed elsewhere in this article.

Longitudinal Vaginal Septum

Congenital longitudinal vaginal septum likely results from the incomplete or failed lateral fusion of the

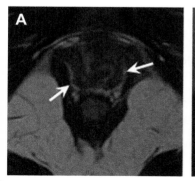
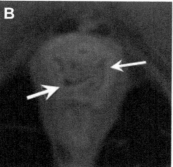
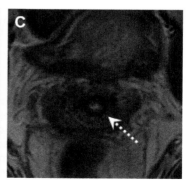

Fig. 18. MR illustration of congenital duplication of the vagina in a 26-year-old patient with abnormal pelvic exam. Axial (A) T2-weighted image and (B) T1-weighted post-gadolinium image through the low pelvis show two distinct separate vaginal canals (arrows). A single normal uterus and cervix (C) were present.

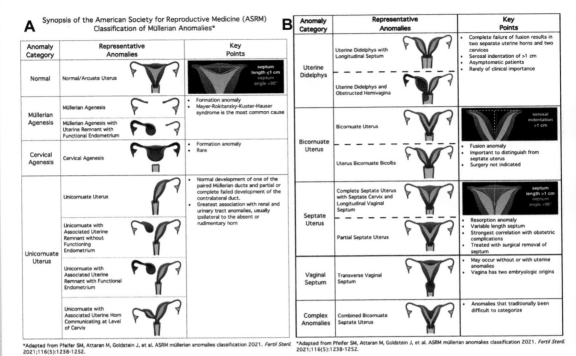

Fig. 19. Synopsis of the ASRM classification of Mullerian anomalies. (*Data from* Ref. [30].)

MDs or from incomplete resorption of the vaginal septum.[9,14,16] This septum may be partial or complete. Approximately, 75% of patients with uterine didelphys will have a longitudinal vaginal septum.[21]

Patients most often present with difficulty inserting tampons or controlling menstrual flow with one tampon. Other patients describe dyspareunia. Occasionally, it may be found incidentally on a physical examination.[9] Excision of the septum is usually recommended.

On imaging, a longitudinal vaginal septum is best delineated when a vaginal gel is used to distend the vagina. It appears as a thin structure that is hypointense on T2-weighted imaging.[21] Vaginal duplication, by comparison, shows two distinct vaginal canals separated by paravaginal connective tissue (**Fig. 18**).

SUMMARY

MDAs constitute a broad spectrum of developmental abnormalities of the female genital tract (**Fig. 19**). MR imaging is typically considered the gold standard in imaging of suspected uterine anomalies as it can determine the absence or presence of the uterus, cervix, and proximal vagina as well as depict complications of functional obstruction of menstrual blood in those with functioning endometrium.

CLINICS CARE POINTS

- Differentiating a septate uterus from a bicornuate uterus is clinically important. Women with a septate uterus have a significantly increased risk of early pregnancy loss. Excision of septal tissue improves outcomes for future pregnancies.

- Long axis T2-weighted images through the uterus are ideal for differentiating between septate and bicornuate uterus.

- Independent of which classification you employ, evaluate and describe the presence, absence, or duplication of the vagina, cervix, and uterus in patients with potential Mullerian duct anomalies as well as any complications of blockage of antegrade menstrual flow. A survey depiction of the retroperitoneum will assist in excluding an associated renal anomaly.

- MR imaging is an ideal single imaging modality that can provide a comprehensive evaluation of individuals with primary amenorrhea.

DISCLOSURE

The authors have nothing to disclose.

REFERENCES

1. Rivas AG, Epelman M, Ellsworth PI, et al. Magnetic resonance imaging of Müllerian anomalies in girls: concepts and controversies. Pediatr Radiol 2022; 52(2):200–16.

2. Marcal L, Nothaft MA, Coelho F, et al. Mullerian duct anomalies: MR imaging. Abdom Imaging 2011; 36(6):756–64.

3. Gould SW, Epelman M. Magnetic resonance imaging of developmental anomalies of the uterus and the vagina in pediatric patients. Semin Ultrasound CT MRI 2015;36(4):332–47.

4. Epelman M, Dinan D, Gee MS, et al. Müllerian duct and related anomalies in children and adolescents. Magn Reson Imaging Clin N Am 2013;21(4):773–89.

5. Merritt BA, Behr SC, Khati NJ. Imaging of infertility, Part 2. Radiol Clin North Am 2020;58(2):227–38.

6. Robbins JB, Broadwell C, Chow LC, et al. Müllerian duct anomalies: embryological development, classification, and MRI assessment. J Magn Reson Imaging 2015;41(1):1–12.

7. Dietrich JE, Millar DM, Quint EH. Non-Obstructive müllerian anomalies. J Pediatr Adolesc Gynecol 2014;27(6):386–95.

8. Acién P, Acién MI. The history of female genital tract malformation classifications and proposal of an updated system. Hum Reprod Update 2011;17(5): 693–705.

9. Edmonds DK. Congenital malformations of the genital tract and their management. Best Pract Res Clin Obstet Gynaecol 2003;17(1):19–40.

10. Wu V, Mar W, Milad MP, et al. magnetic resonance imaging in the evaluation of female infertility. Curr Probl Diagn Radiol 2022;51(2):181–8.

11. Robbins JB, Parry JP, Guite KM, et al. MRI of pregnancy-related issues: M??llerian duct anomalies. Am J Roentgenol 2012;198(2):302–10.

12. Morcel K, Camborieux L. Programme de Recherches sur les Aplasies Müllériennes (PRAM), Guerrier D. Mayer-Rokitansky-Küster-Hauser (MRKH) syndrome. Orphanet J Rare Dis 2007;2(1): 13.

13. Merritt BA, Behr SC, Khati NJ. Imaging of Infertility, Part 1. Radiol Clin North Am 2020;58(2):215–25.

14. Yoo RE, Cho JY, Kim SY, et al. A systematic approach to the magnetic resonance imaging-based differential diagnosis of congenital Müllerian duct anomalies and their mimics. Abdom Imaging 2015;40(1):192–206.

15. Coleman AD, Arbuckle JL. Advanced imaging for the diagnosis and treatment of coexistent renal and müllerian abnormalities. Curr Urol Rep 2018; 19(11):89.

16. Marsh CA, Grimstad FW. Primary amenorrhea: diagnosis and management. Obstet Gynecol Surv 2014; 69(10):603–12.

17. Servaes S, Victoria T, Lovrenski J, et al. Contemporary pediatric gynecologic imaging. Semin Ultrasound CT MRI 2010;31(2):116–40.

18. Teo SY, Ong CL. A systematic approach to imaging the pelvis in amenorrhea. Abdom Radiol 2021;46(7): 3326–41.

19. Church DG, Vancil JM, Vasanawala SS. Magnetic resonance imaging for uterine and vaginal anomalies. Curr Opin Obstet Gynecol 2009;21(5):379–89.

20. Santos XM, Krishnamurthy R, Bercaw-Pratt JL, et al. The utility of ultrasound and magnetic resonance imaging versus surgery for the characterization of müllerian anomalies in the pediatric and adolescent population. J Pediatr Adolesc Gynecol 2012;25(3): 181–4.

21. Grant LA, Sala E, Griffin N. Congenital and acquired conditions of the vulva and vagina on magnetic resonance imaging: a pictorial review. Semin Ultrasound CT MRI 2010;31(5):347–62.

22. Olpin JD, Moeni A, Willmore RJ, et al. MR imaging of müllerian fusion anomalies. Magn Reson Imaging Clin N Am 2017;25(3):563–75.

23. Dykes TM, Siegel C, Dodson W. Imaging of congenital uterine anomalies: review and self-assessment module. Am J Roentgenol 2007;189(3_supplement):S1–10.

24. Behr SC, Courtier JL, Qayyum A. Imaging of müllerian duct anomalies. RadioGraphics 2012;32(6): E233–50.

25. Junqueira BLP, Allen LM, Spitzer RF, et al. müllerian duct anomalies and mimics in children and adolescents: correlative intraoperative assessment with clinical imaging. RadioGraphics 2009;29(4): 1085–103.

26. Jaramillo D, Lebowitz RL, Hendren WH. The cloacal malformation: radiologic findings and imaging recommendations. Radiology 1990;177(2):441–8.

27. Blask AR, Sanders RC, Gearhart JP. Obstructed uterovaginal anomalies: demonstration with sonography. Part I. Neonates and infants. Radiology 1991; 179(1):79–83.

28. Bouet PE, Godbout A, El Hachem H, et al. Fertility and pregnancy in turner syndrome. J Obstet Gynaecol Can 2016;38(8):712–8.

29. Sybert VP. Turner's syndrome. N Engl J Med 2004; 351(12):1227–38.

30. Pfeifer SM, Attaran M, Goldstein J, et al. ASRM müllerian anomalies classification 2021. Fertil Steril 2021;116(5):1238–52.

31. Russo G, di Lascio A, Ferrario M, et al. 46,XY karyotype in a female phenotype fetus: a challenging diagnosis. J Pediatr Adolesc Gynecol 2012;25(3): e77–9.

32. Lanciotti L, Cofini M, Leonardi A, et al. different clinical presentations and management in complete androgen insensitivity syndrome (CAIS). Int J Environ Res Public Health 2019;16(7):1268.

33. Khan S, Mannel L, Koopman CL, et al. The use of MRI in the pre-surgical evaluation of patients with androgen insensitivity syndrome. J Pediatr Adolesc Gynecol 2014;27(1):e17–20.

34. Grimbizis GF, Gordts S, Di Spiezio Sardo A, et al. The ESHRE/ESGE consensus on the classification of female genital tract congenital anomalies. Hum Reprod Oxf Engl 2013;28(8):2032–44.

35. Grimbizis GF, Di Spiezio Sardo A, Saravelos SH, et al. The Thessaloniki ESHRE/ESGE consensus on diagnosis of female genital anomalies. Gynecol Surg 2016;13:1–16.

36. Bhagavath B, Greiner E, Griffiths KM, et al. uterine malformations: an update of diagnosis, management, and outcomes. Obstet Gynecol Surv 2017;72(6):377–92.

37. Hall-Craggs MA. Mayer-rokitansky-kuster-hauser syndrome: diagnosis with MR Imaging. Genitourin IMAGING 2013;269(3):6.

38. Pitot MA, Bookwalter CA, Dudiak KM. Müllerian duct anomalies coincident with endometriosis: a review. Abdom Radiol 2020;45(6):1723–40.

39. Gungor Ugurlucan F, Dural O, Yasa C, et al. Diagnosis, management, and outcome of obstructed hemivagina and ipsilateral renal agenesis (OHVIRA syndrome): Is there a correlation between MRI findings and outcome? Clin Imaging 2020;59(2):172–8.

MR of Fallopian Tubes
MR Imaging Clinics

Pwint P. Khine, MD, Preethi Raghu, MD, Tara Morgan, MD, Priyanka Jha, MBBS*

KEYWORDS

- MR imaging • Fallopian tube • Ultrasound • Pelvic inflammatory disease • fallopian tube cancer
- fallopian tube torsion

KEY POINTS

- Pelvic inflammatory disease is the most common pathologic condition of the FT encountered on imaging. Pyosalpinx is manifested by enhancing tubal wall with surrounding inflammatory changes.
- FTs can be involved with endometriosis and sometimes hematosalpinx may be the only MR imaging finding in some women.
- Isolated FT torsion should be considered in the setting of normal ovaries with hydrosalpinx in a patient with acute lower abdominal pain.
- The presence of an extraovarian mass in a patient with positive pregnancy test is highly suspicious for an ectopic pregnancy. Hematosalpinx and hemoperitoneum in a patient with positive pregnancy test and no intrauterine pregnancy is highly suspicious for a ruptured ectopic pregnancy, especially when an extrauterine gestational sac is not identified.
- Primary FT cancer is usually associated with hydrosalpinx, and intratubal fluid secreted by the tumor can decompress into the uterine cavity or into the peritoneal cavity. In contrast, ovarian cancers are usually not associated with hydrosalpinx or intrauterine fluid accumulation.

INTRODUCTION

Fallopian tube (FT) evaluation is an important component of the imaging of the female reproductive tract. Although normal FTs are challenging to visualize on MR imaging, pathologic conditions of FT, ranging from benign to malignant conditions, can render them identifiable on imaging. Familiarity with relevant anatomy and imaging features of these conditions are crucial for making an accurate diagnosis and guide appropriate management. The knowledge of embryology and normal anatomy of FTs is also fundamental for understanding FT diseases. The authors review these principles and discuss the imaging modalities for FT evaluation and MR imaging findings of various benign and malignant conditions related to FT and their mimics.

IMAGING MODALITIES FOR EVALUATING FALLOPIAN TUBE DISEASES

Ultrasound (US) is the initial modality for evaluation of suspected FT pathology. MR imaging is usually performed as a complementary problem-solving tool.[1] Sometimes, FT pathology can be identified incidentally on imaging performed for other indications. Other imaging techniques include hysterosalpingo-contrast-sonography (HyCoSy), which involves injection of microbubbles into the endometrium and FTs under US-guidance; hysterosalpingography (HSG) that involves injection of contrast into the endometrium and FTs under fluoroscopic guidance; and computed tomography (CT) of the abdomen and pelvis. Applications and benefits of each imaging modality are described in **Table 1**.

Department of Radiology & Biomedical Imaging, University of California, San Francisco (UCSF), 513 Parnassus Avenue, Room S-261, Box 0628, San Francisco, CA 94143-0628, USA
* Corresponding author.
E-mail address: priyanka.jha@ucsf.edu

Magn Reson Imaging Clin N Am 31 (2023) 29–41
https://doi.org/10.1016/j.mric.2022.06.008
1064-9689/23/© 2022 Elsevier Inc. All rights reserved.

ANATOMY, EMBRYOLOGY, AND PHYSIOLOGY OF THE FALLOPIAN TUBES
Normal Anatomy and Physiology of Fallopian Tubes

FTs are paired organs that extend laterally within the mesosalpinx of the broad ligament from the anterosuperior aspect of the uterine fundus and terminate near the ipsilateral ovary.[2] The primary function of the FTs is to transport the mature ovum from the ovary to the uterus for implantation.

The FTs comprise four main anatomic segments: the interstitial segment is the most proximal and located within the myometrium at the level of the uterine cornua. The next adjacent segment is the isthmus, which is the narrowest segment of the FT followed by the ampulla. The ampulla is the widest portion of the tube, and ectopic pregnancy (EP) usually occurs within this segment. The infundibulum is the most lateral segment located close to the ovary, which opens into the peritoneal cavity and has multiple fimbriae to catch the released oocyte during ovulation with each menstrual cycle. FTs have dual arterial supply with the proximal two-thirds perfused by uterine arteries and the lateral one-third perfused by ovarian arteries. The uterine veins drain blood from the FTs to the internal iliac vein and the pampiniform plexus in the broad ligaments drains blood to the ovarian veins. The para-aortic and internal lymph nodes include the lymphatic drainage.[3]

Embryology

During the first 5 to 6 weeks of development, both male and female embryos demonstrate paired mesonephric (Wolffian or male genital) ducts and paramesonephric (Mullerian or female genital) ducts. After 6 weeks, the mesonephric ducts regress in female embryos. The paramesonephric ducts continue to develop and the cranial portions of the ducts become the precursors for formation of the FT and the caudal portions grow and fuse to form the uterus. Fusion of the paramesonephric ducts also creates the broad ligaments that attach the lateral aspect of the uterus to the pelvic side walls. The cranial end of the FT is open to the peritoneal cavity via fimbriae, which are fingerlike projections at the free edge of the FTs. The caudal end is continuous with the uterine cornua.[3]

CONGENITAL ANOMALY

Congenital anomalies of FTs include accessory tubal ostia, which are rare normal variants. They occur when ectopic fimbriae are formed more proximally within the FT than its normal fimbriated end,[4] resulting in more than one communication with the uterine endometrium. Other congenital Mullerian anomalies of FTs include agenesis, hypoplasia, or aplasia of one of the paired FTs resulting in unicornuate uterus. A rudimentary uterine horn is most commonly associated with unicornuate uterus, which can be noncavitary, cavitary noncommunicating (often associated with pelvic pain caused by increased prevalence of endometriosis, Fig. 1), and cavitary communicating (which has an increased risk of EP, miscarriage, and preterm labor). MR imaging is the imaging modality of choice for accurate diagnosis and classification of Mullerian anomalies and rudimentary uterine horn. Imaging findings include deviation of unicornuate uterus to one side of the pelvis with an elongated

---

Table 1
Various imaging modalities available for evaluation of fallopian tube pathology

Imaging Modality	Applications	Benefits
	Applications of Various Imaging Modalities for Evaluation of Fallopian Tubes	
US	Primary imaging modality	Grayscale US: evaluation of dilated, thickened tubes, mass, cysts, or fluid collection Color and spectral Doppler US: evaluation of hyperemia, torsion, or neovascularity HyCoSy: morphologic evaluation of uterus and FT patency
MR imaging	Problem-solving	Origin of adnexal pathology Tissue characterization
HSG	Tubal patency	Evaluation for infertility, tubal ligation, or after reversal of tubal ligation
CT	Emergent pelvic evaluation Malignancy staging	Pelvic symptoms or staging

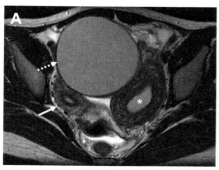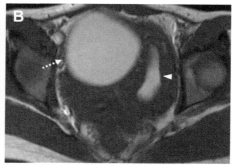

Fig. 1. Unicornuate uterus with a cavitary noncommunicating rudimentary horn. A 19-year-old woman with chronic pelvic pain. (*A*) Axial T2-weighted and (*B*) axial T1-weighted MR images demonstrate a right unicornuate uterus (*arrow*) and left rudimentary horn with distinct cavity (*asterisk*) without communication with the right endometrium. The left noncommunicating rudimentary horn is distended with hemorrhage (T1-hyperintense fluid) (*arrowhead*). Note a large endometrioma with T1 hyperintensity and T2 shading (*dotted arrow*).

shape often described as a "banana shape." A unicornuate uterus can be associated with renal agenesis ipsilateral to the side of the rudimentary horn (**Fig. 2**).[5]

BENIGN FALLOPIAN TUBE PATHOLOGY
Pelvic Inflammatory Disease

Pelvic inflammatory disease (PID) is the infection of the upper female genital tract and is the most common disease of the FT.[6] PID results from superior extension of vaginal and cervical infection to the uterus, FTs, and eventually the peritoneal cavity. The spectrum includes salpingitis, pyosalpinx, and tubo-ovarian abscess (TOA). The most common organisms are *Chlamydia trachomatis, Neisseria gonorrhoeae, and Mycoplasma genitalium.* Other less common organisms include gram-negative bacteria/polymicrobial infections,

tuberculosis, and actinomycosis.[7] Young age, multiple sexual partners, intrauterine device (IUD) use, and history of gynecologic surgeries are the most common risk factors.[8] Patients typically present with mucopurulent vaginal discharge, pelvic pain, fever, dyspareunia, leukocytosis, and elevated erythrocyte sedimentation rate or C-reactive protein. Although diagnosis of the PID is mainly based on clinical symptoms, imaging may be required in cases with nonspecific symptoms, no clinical improvement with treatment, or abscess evaluation. US is the initial imaging modality for evaluation of PID. Although MR imaging is not traditionally used in acute settings, its superior spatial and contrast resolution helps differentiate FTs from ovaries, pyosalpinx from hematosalpinx, and peritoneal inclusion cyst from adnexal masses.[1]

Salpingitis
Salpingitis is inflammation of the FT without pus or obstruction. It can be associated with PID-related infertility and EP.[6] Salpingitis itself may not be apparent on US as the tubes are not distended. When thickened tubes are identified, color Doppler imaging can show hypervascularity. However, the inflamed FTs can be more conspicuous on contrast-enhanced MR imaging due to wall thickening, mucosal hyperenhancement, and surrounding inflammatory fat stranding (**Fig. 3**).

Pyosalpinx
Pyosalpinx is the next stage of salpingitis in the setting of PID and results from obstruction of infected FTs caused by peritubal adhesions secondary to inflammation. As the obstructed fimbrial end is unable to drain fluid, the FT gets distended with pus. On US, the distended ampullary segments and fimbriae can mimic a complex multiloculated adnexal mass and

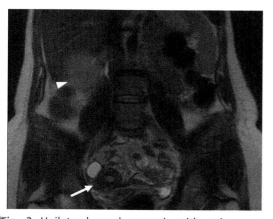

Fig. 2. Unilateral renal agenesis with unicornuate uterus. A 34-year-old women with infertility. Coronal T2-weighted MR image shows a right unicornuate uterus (*arrow*) with a solitary right kidney (*arrowhead*). A normal left kidney is not identified in the renal fossa.

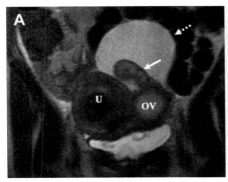 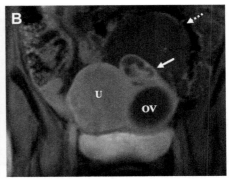

Fig. 3. Salpingitis and peritoneal inclusion cyst. A 49-year-old woman with recent IUD placement followed by acute left-sided pain and leukocytosis. (*A*) Coronal T2-weighted and (*B*) T1-weighted contrast-enhanced MR images show left FT with thickened hyperenhancing wall, consistent with salpingitis (*arrow*). Also seen is a T2-hyperintense cyst which conforms to peritoneal contours, suggestive of a peritoneal inclusion cyst (*dotted arrow*). OV, ovary; U, uterus.

history and temporal course of symptoms can help with the diagnosis. On MR imaging, pyosalpinx appears as a dilated tubular structure arising from the uterine cornua extending to the ipsilateral ovary. The fluid within the tube demonstrates variable T1 signal and T2 hyperintensity with absence of shading, which differentiates from hematosalpinx. The fluid may also demonstrate reduced diffusion (**Fig. 4**). Thick enhancing tubal wall with surrounding inflammatory changes also helps differentiate pyosalpinx from hematosalpinx and hydrosalpinx.[1,3]

Tubo-ovarian abscess

Worsening PID can lead to further progression of pyosalpinx and infection can spread from the FT to the adjacent ovary and peritoneal cavity leading to formation of the TOA. The FT and ovary can no

longer be separately identified and ovarian parenchymal necrosis can occur, which can mimic an ovarian mass, with solid, hypervascular components. TOA rupture can lead to life-threatening peritonitis and Fitz–Hugh–Curtis syndrome.[9] The early diagnosis and imaging is important for timely diagnosis and management.

TOA appears as a nonspecific, hypervascular adnexal mass with debris on US, and interpretation in conjunction with the clinical presentation is essential. MR imaging findings of TOA similarly include an adnexal mass with T2 hyperintensity and variable T1 signal intensity based on the abscess contents. The fluid within the cystic component and the walls of the mass may demonstrate reduced diffusion. Contrast-enhanced imaging shows thickened enhancing rim around the mass with septal hyperenhancement and non-

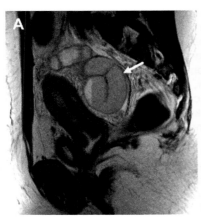 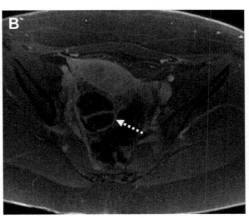

Fig. 4. Pyosalpinx. A 25-year-old woman with history of pelvic inflammatory disease. (*A*) Sagittal T2-weighted and (*B*) axial T1-weighted contrast-enhanced MR images show a dilated right fallopian tube with fluid-fluid level (*arrow*) and thick hyperenhancing wall (*dotted arrow*), consistent with pyosalpinx in a patient with pelvic inflammatory disease.

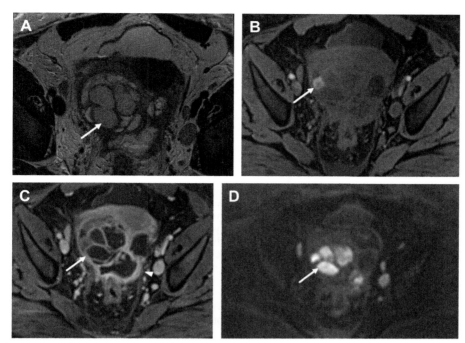

Fig. 5. Tubo-ovarian abscess. A 22-year-old woman with history of pelvic inflammatory disease. (*A*) Axial T2-weighted, (*B*) axial T1-weighted precontrast, (*C*) axial T1-weighted contrast-enhanced, and (*D*) axial diffusion-weighted MR images show a multiloculated collection consistent with the tubo-ovarian abscess (*arrows*). Collection shows T2-hyperintensity, T1 hypointensity with some areas of T1 hyperintensity, rim enhancement, and restricted diffusion. Note the adjacent soft tissue enhancement in the pelvis (*arrowhead*), indicating inflammation. Separate right ovary is not identified.

enhancement of internal contents (**Fig. 5**).[3] A lack of internal enhancement helps differentiate from a solid adnexal mass.

Salpingitis Isthmica Nodosa

Salpingitis isthmica nodosa (SIN), also known as FT diverticulosis, is commonly seen in patients with infertility and ectopic pregnancies. Although the cause is unknown, it is widely believed that SIN is related to chronic PID. The disease is bilateral in 85% of cases and diverticula can completely obstruct the tubal lumen in severe cases.[2] On HSG, contrast medium can be seen outlining small tubal diverticula affecting one or both tubes (**Fig. 6**).[2] MR imaging findings of SIN include small intramural cystic changes, from fluid within the obstructed diverticula (**Fig. 7**). FT tuberculosis and endometriosis should also be considered in the differential diagnosis of SIN.

Hydrosalpinx

Hydrosalpinx is a dilated, fluid-filled FT resulting from intraluminal fluid accumulation from obstruction, most commonly, caused by adhesions from

chronic PID.[10] Other less common causes include endometriosis, adhesion from prior procedures, tubal neoplasm, and tubal EP. Some patients may be asymptomatic, whereas others experience recurrent pelvic pain. Owing to impeded tubal function, infertility is a common symptom.[11]

Imaging findings of hydrosalpinx include a dilated tubular structure that arises from the upper lateral margin of the uterine fundus, with incomplete septations. A cog wheel appearance can be seen with *en face* imaging. Tubal fluid demonstrates T2 hyperintensity and variable T1 signal intensity depending on the fluid contents. A large hydrosalpinx can stimulate a multilocular ovarian tumor such as cystadenoma and presence of incomplete septations points to the correct diagnosis.[3] MR imaging can also help differentiate hydrosalpinx from ovarian tumor by identifying a separate ipsilateral ovary (**Fig. 8**).[3] The incomplete longitudinal folds within the tubular cystic structure represent mucosal or submucosal plicae, which can aid with the diagnosis of a hydrosalpinx (see **Fig. 8**).[12]

Tubal Endometriosis

Endometriosis is defined as the presence of ectopic endometrial tissue outside the uterine

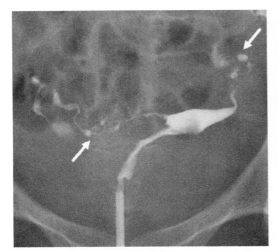

Fig. 6. Salpingitis isthmica nodosa. A 28-year-old woman for infertility workup. Anteroposterior fluoroscopic hysterosalpingogram image after intrauterine iodinated contrast administration shows diverticula arising from the isthmic portions of the fallopian tubes (*arrow*).

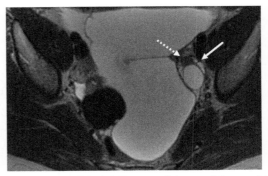

Fig. 7. Salpingitis isthmica nodosa. A 26-year-old woman with history of pelvic inflammatory disease. Axial T2-weighted MR image demonstrates small cystic structures along the intramural component of the left fallopian tube (*arrow*). A separate normal left ovary was present (*dotted arrow*).

cavity and patients present with pelvic pain and infertility.[13] The disease affects approximately 10% of women of reproductive age and is diagnosed in about 20% to 50% of infertile women.[14] Extraluminal and intraluminal endometriosis are two recognized forms of tubal deep endometriosis. In extraluminal tubal endometriosis, the serosal implants cause repeated episodes of hemorrhage and fibrosis, leading to peritubal adhesions and resultant hydrosalpinx.[15] Intraluminal tubal endometriosis, which is less common, is the implantation of endometrial tissue in the fimbriated lining and muscular wall of the FT. Bleeding into the lumen from these tubal implants can lead to hematosalpinx, which may be the only MR imaging finding of deep endometriosis in some women.[16]

Hematosalpinx is diagnosed by the presence of intrinsic T1 hyperintensity in a dilated FT. T2 shading as seen with endometriomas may not be typically present in hematosalpinx (**Fig. 9**).[11] Malignant transformation of endometriosis is a rare complication and should be considered when thickened septa or enhancing nodules are seen in the hematosalpinx (**Fig. 10**).

Isolated Fallopian Tube Torsion

Isolated FT torsion is defined as torsion of the FT without ovarian torsion. It is exceedingly rare, has a prevalence of one in 1.5 million women, and occurs in adolescent girls and women of reproductive age.[3,17] Similar to ovarian torsion, the presence of masses such as paratubal cysts predisposes to torsion. Right FT torsion is more common than the left due to the fixation of the left tube by the sigmoid mesentery. Other risk factors include PID, hydrosalpinx, hypermotility of the FT, prior tubal ligation, tubal neoplasm, adhesions, trauma, and adjacent ovarian masses.[1] Patients typically present with acute onset pelvic pain and may be accompanied by peritoneal signs, nausea, and vomiting. A diagnosis of isolated FT torsion can be challenging as the clinical symptoms can mimic other conditions. If isolated FT torsion is not treated in a timely manner, necrosis of the tube with gangrenous transformation can lead to superinfection and peritonitis.[3,17]

Initial imaging is usually performed with US in these cases, where a hydrosalpinx with "whirlpool" sign and non-enlarged ipsilateral ovary can be seen.[1,3] Although rare, it is important to recognize the possibility of isolated FT torsion in the setting of normal ovaries with hydrosalpinx in a patient with acute lower abdominal pain. MR imaging is helpful in challenging cases with FT torsion which will show a dilated, thick-walled tube with minimal or absent mural enhancement and a separate normal ovary (**Fig. 11**). Thickened wall of the torsed FT may also show restricted diffusion. Swirling appearance of the tube without ipsilateral ovarian enlargement can help clinch the diagnosis. The absence of wall enhancement on intravenous contrast administration can suggest necrosis and loss of viability of the FT, although findings at laparoscopy provide the final assessment for viability.[3,18] Management includes laparoscopic detorsion in viable FT or salpingectomy in cases with FT necrosis.[3]

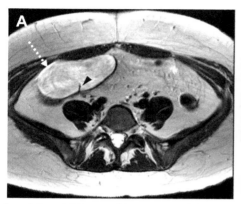
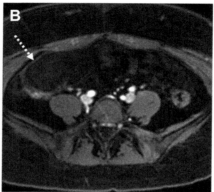

Fig. 8. Hydrosalpinx. A 30-year-old woman with history of pelvic inflammatory disease and right ovarian mass seen on ultrasound. (A) Axial T2-weighted and (B) axial T1-weighted contrast-enhanced MR images show a cystic mass with incomplete septation, consistent with a right hydrosalpinx. A normal right ovary was present (not shown). Incomplete septation represents a submucosal plica (arrowhead) within the hydrosalpinx. The wall of the hydrosalpinx is thin without hyperenhancement (dotted arrow).

Ectopic Pregnancy

EP is defined as the implantation of a blastocyst outside the endometrium and it is the leading cause of death during the first trimester of pregnancy.[19,20] Ninety-five percent of EPs are tubal with the ampulla being the most common location (75%) followed by isthmus (13%) and fimbriae (12%).[21,22] Major risk factors for EP are prior EP, PID, and tubal surgery.[20] EP should be considered in women with 5 to 9 week history of amenorrhea, sudden onset of pelvic pain, and vaginal spotting in the setting of a positive pregnancy test or elevated β-human chorionic gonadotropin (hCG) level.

The initial evaluation of suspected EP entails serum β-hCG and transvaginal US. The presence of an extraovarian mass in a patient with positive pregnancy test is highly suspicious for an EP. Usually, MR imaging is not necessary and can be complementary in workup of pregnancy of unknown location and noncontributory US. MR imaging findings include hematosalpinx with T1 hyperintensity and T2 hypointensity from blood products (Fig. 12). Frequently, a heterogeneously enhancing, saclike cystic structure with thick, enhancing walls can be seen. Hemorrhage can be seen adjacent to the FT with tubal rupture, and a large volume hemoperitoneum can ensue.[23] Identifying the ectopic gestational sac can become challenging after rupture. In fact, the presence of hematosalpinx and hemoperitoneum with a positive pregnancy test, and no intrauterine pregnancy is highly suspicious for EP, even when an extrauterine gestational sac is not identified.

Management of tubal EP includes methotrexate treatment or laparoscopic resection, based on size, laboratory values, and presence of

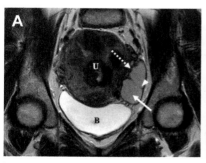
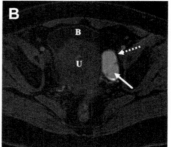
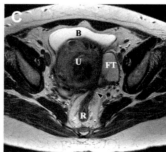

Fig. 9. Hematosalpinx. A 33-year-old woman with infertility and deep infiltrating endometriosis. (A) Coronal T2-weighted and (B) axial T1-weighted fat-suppressed MR images show hematosalpinx with T2 hypointensity and T1 hyperintensity (arrow), suggestive of hemorrhagic contents. The tube contains an incomplete septation (white arrowhead) and thin wall (dotted arrow). (C) Axial T2-weighted image shows tethering of the left hematosalpinx to the anterior rectal wall (black arrowhead), which can be seen with deep endometriosis. B, bladder; FT, fallopian tube; R, rectum; U, uterus.

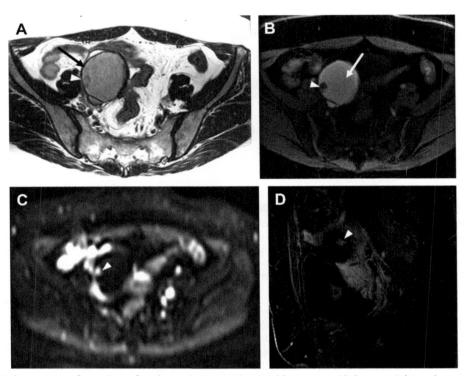

Fig. 10. Malignant transformation of endometrioma. A 46-year-old woman with known right endometrioma and severe right pelvic pain. Ultrasound (not shown) detected increased size of the right ovarian endometrioma with new mural nodule and MR imaging was recommended for further evaluation. Clear cell cancer was diagnosed at surgery. (*A*) Axial T2-weighted, (*B*) axial T1-weighted fat suppressed, (*C*) axial diffusion-weighted, and (*D*) sagittal T1-weighted contrast-enhanced subtraction MR images demonstrate a right ovarian endometrioma with T1 hyperintensity and T2 hypointensity, consistent with T2-shading within an endometrioma (*arrow*). Solid mural nodule with restricted diffusion and contrast enhancement (*arrowhead*) is suspicious for malignant transformation.

embryonic cardiac activity. Methotrexate is the preferred treatment option for patients with hemodynamic stability, serum β-hCG level ≤5000 mIU/mL, ectopic mass less than 3 to 4 cm, and no cardiac activity detected on transvaginal US.[24] Surgery is performed in situations when methotrexate is contraindicated, such as patients with hemodynamic instability, heterotopic pregnancy, or signs of impending or ongoing rupture of EP.

FALLOPIAN TUBE NEOPLASMS

FT neoplasms are rare and consist of benign and malignant neoplasms. Benign neoplasms include paratubal cysts (most common), and

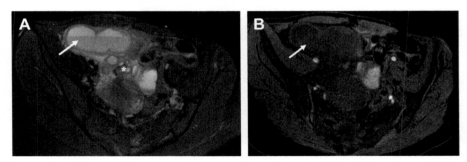

Fig. 11. Tubal torsion. A 25-year-old woman with severe right pelvic pain. (*A*) Axial T2-weighted MR image shows a dilated right fallopian tube with fluid-fluid level and dependent layering fluid demonstrating T2 hypointensity (*arrow*). Note the normal right ovary (*asterisk*). (*B*) Axial T1-weighted contrast-enhanced MR image shows minimal tubal wall enhancement (*arrowhead*), suggestive of tubal torsion and poor perfusion to the tube. Intraoperatively, patient was found to have tubal torsion and salpingectomy was performed due to ischemic changes.

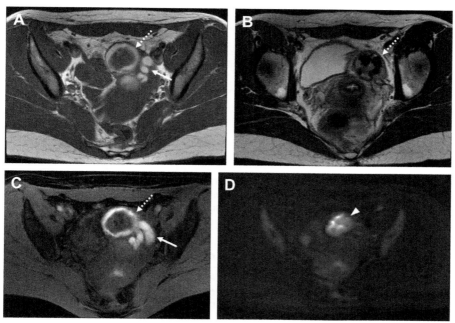

Fig. 12. Tubal ectopic pregnancy. A 36-year-old woman with positive pregnancy test and a large mass seen on US. (*A*) Axial T1-weighted nonfat saturated, (*B*) axial T2-weighted, (*C*) axial fat-suppressed contrast-enhanced, and (*D*) axial diffusion-weighted MR images show a cystic mass with thick rim within the distal tube (*dotted arrow*). The mass has peripheral rim T1 hyperintensity and T2 hypointnesity, suggestive of hemorrhage with proximal hematosalpinx (*arrow*). Nodular hypointense components represent the chorion within the gestational sac, which demonstrates restricted diffusion (*arrowhead*).

other rare masses such as leiomyoma, teratoma, mucosal polyp, and fibroma. Malignant neoplasms are most commonly adenocarcinoma, including serous tubal intraepithelial carcinoma (STIC), which can progress to primary FT carcinoma.[1,3]

Benign Neoplasm

Paratubal cyst

Paratubal cysts, also referred to as paraovarian cysts, constitute approximately 10% of all adnexal masses. They commonly originate from the mesothelium of the broad ligament and less commonly from the paramesonephric or mesonephric remnants.[3] Paratubal cysts are predominantly seen in women in third to fourth decades of life and are rarely symptomatic.[25] Symptoms develop in large cysts greater than 5 cm and those with hemorrhage, rupture, infection, torsion, or neoplastic transformation.[26]

Paratubal cysts are incidentally detected on MR imaging and are typically simple cysts with high T2 hyperintensity, T1 hypointensity,

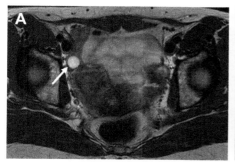
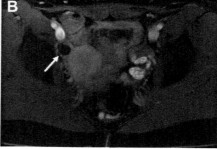

Fig. 13. Paratubal cyst. A 33-year-old woman with myomatous uterus. (*A*) Axial T2-weighted and (*B*) axial T1-weighted contrast-enhanced MR images show a right paratubal cyst with T2 hyperintenity and no enhancement (*arrow*), adjacent to but separate from the right ovary.

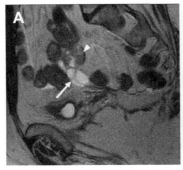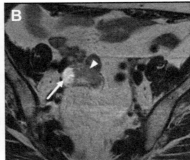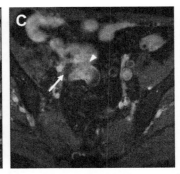

Fig. 14. Primary fallopian tube cancer. A 66-year-old women with right pelvic pain, watery vaginal discharge, and vaginal bleeding. (*A*) Sagittal T2-weighted, (*B*) axial T2-weighted, and (*C*) axial contrast-enhanced MR images demonstrate hydrosalpinx (*arrow*) with intratubal soft tissue (*arrowhead*) that demonstrates contrast enhancement, consistent with primary fallopian tube cancer.

and no internal contrast enhancement (**Fig. 13**). Hemorrhage or proteinaceous cystic contents can result in T1 hyperintensity and variable T2 intensity. Soft tissue nodularity or mass within the cyst may indicate a benign or malignant neoplasm (cystadenoma or cystadenocarcinoma). Differential diagnosis for paratubal cyst includes ovarian cyst, peritoneal inclusion cyst, and hydrosalpinx. On MR imaging, identification of the cyst adjacent to but separate from the ovary is a key diagnostic feature.[27] Management is similar to ovarian cysts.

Malignant Neoplasms

Primary fallopian tube carcinoma and serous tubal intraepithelial carcinoma

Primary FT carcinoma (PFTC) is a rare malignancy accounting for 1.8% of all gynecologic malignancies. Recent data have shown that serous epithelial ovarian carcinoma arises from the fimbrial end of the FTs.[28] As papillary serous carcinoma of PFTC is histologically similar to serous ovarian carcinoma, it has been challenging to identify the primary site of malignancy with advanced stage. These STIC lesions are believed

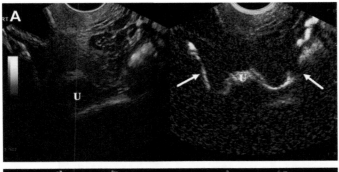
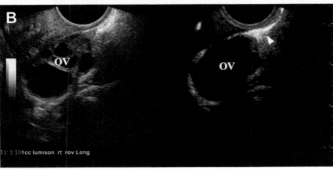

Fig. 15. Fallopian tube patency. A 31-year-old woman with infertility presents for evaluation of tubal patency. (*A*) HyCoSy dual images with grayscale image on left and contrast-mode image on right after intraluminal US contrast instillation shows contrast-opacified fallopian tube (*arrows*) and (*B*) free peritoneal spillage of contrast which surrounds the ovary (*arrowhead*). OV, ovary; U, uterus.

Table 2
Mimics of fallopian tube diseases

Conditions	Etiologies	MR Imaging Findings	Distinguishing Features from FT Diseases
Mimics of FT Diseases			
Peritoneal inclusion cyst	Develops in females of childbearing age with functioning ovaries and pelvic adhesions that impair absorption of peritoneal fluid (PID, endometriosis, prior pelvic surgeries)	Unilocular or multilocular cyst demonstrating T2 hyperintensity, T1 hypointensity, ± smooth enhancement of wall and septations Commonly associated with normal appearing ovary, which may be suspended centrally or eccentrically located	Conformation of the cyst to peritoneal contours helps differentiate PIC from hydrosalpinx
Lymphocele	Commonly seen after lymphadenectomy, 3–8 wk after radical pelvic surgeries	Well-marginated simple cyst with thin wall without enhancement or restricted diffusion	Within the extraperitoneal space commonly along the iliac vessels and inguinal chains and away from the ovaries (FT diseases are in the intraperitoneal space and adjacent to the ovary)
Acute appendicitis	Acute inflammation of appendix due to lumen obstruction Most common cause of right lower quadrant pain, commonly presenting with fever and leukocytosis	Dilated blind-ending tubular structure with thickened and hyperenhancing wall Associated periappendiceal edema, fluid, and appendicolith	Identification of the tubular structure continuous with the cecum

to be the sites of origin for high-grade serous ovarian carcinoma. Therefore, the prevalence of PFTC may have been underestimated.[29]

Clinical and imaging findings can help diagnose PFTC and attempt differentiation from ovarian cancer. Although most patients present with nonspecific and insidious symptoms, approximately 15% of patients present with intermittent profuse serosanguineous vaginal discharge, colicky pelvic pain relieved by vaginal discharge and adnexal mass. A separate normal ovary can be seen in initial stages.[1] MR imaging findings show a dilated FT with nodular or papillary solid components, which demonstrate T2 iso- or hyperintensity, T1 hypointensity, and contrast enhancement (**Fig. 14**).[3] Associated hydrosalpinx is due to tubal distension from serous fluid secreted by the tumor. Unlike hydrosalpinx caused by PID, the FTs in PFTC are patent and the fluid secreted by the tumor can decompress into the

uterine cavity via the isthmus of the FT or into the peritoneal cavity via the fimbriae.[1,3] As a result, PFTC can change in shape on serial imaging depending on the degree of tubal distention from fluid decompression.[30] In contrast, ovarian tumors are usually not associated with hydrosalpinx or intrauterine fluid accumulation. The surgical staging and medical management are similar for both tumors, except for pelvic lymph node dissection, which is routinely performed in PFTC but not in ovarian tumors.[31]

Role of MR Imaging in Infertility Workup

Infertility is defined as failure to achieve pregnancy after 1 year of unprotected intercourse. FT disorders are a common cause of infertility from peritubal adhesions and tubal obstruction. HSG and HyCoSy (**Fig. 15**) are used for assessing tubal patency. Hysteroscopy is the gold standard for evaluation of peritubal environment in infertility workup. MR imaging has been helpful in challenging cases and provides noninvasive assessment of Mullerian anomalies, hydrosalpinx and hematosalpinx (see **Figs. 8** and **9**), salpingitis, pyosalpinx, TOA (see **Figs. 3–5**), SIN (see **Figs. 6** and **7**), and deep infiltrating endometriosis.[31]

Mimics of Fallopian Tube Diseases

Most cystic pelvic masses arise from the ovaries or FTs. When evaluating these cystic masses, it is crucial to consider nonovarian or non-FT disease processes. To reduce the risk of misinterpretation, delayed management, and unnecessary surgery, it is important to understand the anatomic location of the cyst, identify normal ovaries, and correlate with patient's clinical symptoms. Common mimics of FT disease include peritoneal inclusion cyst (see **Fig. 3**), lymphocele, and acute appendicitis. These conditions are described in **Table 2**.

SUMMARY

The increasing use of female pelvic MR imaging necessitates radiologists to be familiar with FT-related diseases, which range from congenital and benign-to-malignant conditions. Although rare, FT-related conditions should always be considered as a possibility in women with pelvic pain and careful evaluation of the FTs should be performed in every case. PID and endometriosis are some common disease processes affecting the tubes. Tubal pathology is a common cause for infertility, and FT assessment is critical for subfertility evaluation. Familiarity and knowledge of the wide spectrum of pathophysiology, clinical manifestations, and radiologic findings of FT-related diseases is important for the radiologist to make the timely and accurate diagnosis and thereby ensure prompt initiation of clinical treatment.

CLINICS CARE POINTS

- When a complex multiloculated pelvic mass is seen, it is important to differentiate an ovarian mass from pyosalpinx resulting from distended ampullary segments and fimbriae. Look for a dilated tubular structure arising from the uterine cornua extending to the ipsilateral ovary. A normal ovary should be seen.
- If normal ovaries with hydrosalpinx in a patient with acute lower abdominal pain are seen, consider isolated fallopian tube (FT) as one of the differential diagnoses.

- Clinical suspicion of ectopic pregnancy (EP) should be high in asymptomatic patients with an adnexal mass on US and elevated β-hCG level.
- The presence of hematosalpinx with a positive pregnancy test and no intrauterine pregnancy is highly suspicious for EP, even if an extrauterine gestational sac is not identified.
- If a patient presents with intermittent profuse serosanguineous vaginal discharge, colicky pelvic pain relieved by vaginal discharge, and an adnexal mass with hydrosalpinx, consider primary FT carcinoma as one of the differential diagnoses.
- If a pelvic cyst is seen, look for a normal ovary. Identification of the cyst adjacent to but separate from the ovary is the key feature of the paratubal cyst. The normal ovary centrally or eccentrically located within the cyst and the conformation of the cyst to the peritoneal contours is the key features of the peritoneal inclusion cyst. If cyst is seen in the extraperitoneal space along the iliac vessels or inguinal chains, consider lymphocele.
- When a tubular structure is found in the pelvis, find the origin of the structure. Tubular structure continuous with the cecum is most likely appendix and the structure arising from the uterine cornua is most likely FT.

DISCLOSURE

The authors have nothing to disclose.

REFERENCES

1. Rezvani M, Shaaban AM. Fallopian tube disease in the nonpregnant patient. RadioGraphics 2011;31: 527–48.
2. Simpson WL, Beitia LG, Mester J. RadioGraphics 2006;26:419–31.
3. Revzin MV, Moshiri M, Katz DS, et al. Imaging evaluation of fallopian tubes and related disease: a primer for radiologists. RadioGraphics 2020;40: 1473–501.
4. Pereira N, Kligman I. Clinical implications of accessory fallopian tube ostium in endometriosis and primary infertility. Women's Health 2016;12(4):404–6.
5. Sugi M, Penna R, Jha P, et al. Mullerian duct anomalies: role in fertility and pregnancy. RadioGraphics 2021;41:1857–75.
6. Revzin MV, Mathur M, Dave HB, et al. Pelvic inflammatory disease: multimodality imaging approach with clinical-pathologic correlation. RadioGraphics 2016;36:1579–96.
7. Soper DE. Pelvic inflammatory disease. Obstet Gynecol 2010;116(2):419–28.

8. Sam JW, Jacobs JE, Birnbaum BA. Spectrum of CT findings in acute pyogenic pelvic inflammatory disease. RadioGraphics 2002;22:1327–34.

9. Yitta S, Hecht EM, Slywotzky CM, et al. Added value of multiplanar reformation in the multidetector CT evaluation of the female pelvis: a pictorial review. RadioGraphics 2009;29:1987–2005.

10. Benjamiov O, Atri M. Sonography of the abnormal fallopian tube. AJR 2004;183:737–42.

11. Kim MY, Rha SE, Oh SN, et al. MR imaging findings of hydrosalpinx: a comprehensive review. RadioGraphics 2009;29:495–507.

12. Imaoka I, Wada A, Matsuo M, et al. MR imaging disorders associated with female infertility: use in diagnosis, treatment, and management. RadioGraphics 2003;23:1401–21.

13. Siegelman ES, Oliver ER. MR imaging of endometriosis: ten imaging pearls. RadioGraphics 2012;32:1675–91.

14. Giudice L, Kao LC. Endometriosis. Lancet 2004;364:1789–99.

15. Lorusso F, Scioscia M, Rubini D, et al. Magnetic resonance imaging for deep infiltrating endometriosis: current concept, imaging technique and key findings. Insights Imaging 2021;12(1):105.

16. Jha P, Sakala M, Chamie LP, et al. Endometriosis MRI lexicon: consensus statement from the society of abdominal radiology endometriosis disease-focused panel. Abdom Radiol 2020;45(6):1552–68.

17. Iraha Y, Okada M, Iraha R, et al. CT and MR imaging of gynecologic emergencies. RadioGraphics 2017;37(5):1569–86.

18. Pedrosa I, Zeikus EA, Levine D, et al. MR imaging of acute right lower quadrant pain in pregnant and nonpregnant patients. RadioGraphics 2007;27:721–53.

19. Creanga AA, Shapiro-Mendoza CK, Bish CL, et al. Trends in ectopic pregnancy mortality in the United States. Obstet Gynecol 2011;117(4):837–43.

20. Lin EP, Bhatt S, Dogra VS. Diagnostic clues to ectopic pregnancy. RadioGraphics 2008;28:1661–71.

21. Bouyer J, Coste J, Fernandez H, et al. Sites of ectopic pregnancy: a 10 year population-based study of 1800 cases. Hum Reprod 2002;17(12):3224–30.

22. Walker JJ. Ectopic pregnancy. Clin Obstet Gynecol 2007;50(1):89–99.

23. Tamai K, Koyama T, Togashi K. MR features of ectopic pregnancy. Eur Radiol 2007;17:3236–46.

24. Mol F, Mol BW, Ankum WM, et al. Current evidence on surgery, systemic methotrexate and expectant management in the treatment of tubal ectopic pregnancy: a systemic review and meta-analysis. Hum Reprod 2008;14(4):309–19.

25. Kishimoto K, Ito K, Awaya H, et al. Paraovarian cyst: MR imaging features. Abdom Imaging 2002;27:685–9.

26. Bohiltea RE, Cirstoiu MM, Turcan N, et al. Ultrasound diagnostic of mesonephric paraovarian cyst – case report. J Med Life 2016;9(3):280–3.

27. Moyle PL, Kataoka MY, Nakai A, et al. Nonovarian cystic lesions of the pelvis. RadioGraphics 2010;30:921–38.

28. Singh N, Gilks CB, WilkinsonN, et al. Assignment of primary site in high-grade serous tubal, ovarian and peritoneal carcinoma: a proposal. Histopathology 2014;65:149–54.

29. Kurman RJ, Shih IM. The origin and pathogenesis of epithelial ovarian cancer-a proposed unifying theory. Am J Surg Pathol 2010;34(3):433–43.

30. Shaaban AM, Rezvani M. Imaging of primary fallopian tube carcinoma. Abdom Imaging 2013;38:608–18.

31. Ma FH, Cai SQ, Qiang JW, et al. MRI for differentiating primary fallopian tube carcinoma from epithelial ovarian cancer. J Magn Reson Imaging 2015;42:42–7.

MR Imaging of Epithelial Ovarian Neoplasms Part I: Benign and Borderline

Shaun A. Wahab, MD*, Juliana J. Tobler, MD

KEYWORDS

• Ovarian tumor • Ovarian cyst • MR imaging • Epithelial ovarian tumors • Borderline

KEY POINTS

- Epithelial ovarian neoplasms are the most common type of ovarian tumors, and MR imaging plays a vital role in the characterization of lesions as benign, borderline, or malignant.
- Serous borderline ovarian tumors typically contain papillary projections and can have associated peritoneal implants, which are more common in micropapillary serous variant.
- Mucinous tumors tend to be larger and more complex than serous tumors.
- The identification of benign and borderline imaging features can help guide treatment, particularly those who may be candidates for fertility-sparing treatment.

INTRODUCTION

Incidentally detected adnexal lesions on imaging are common and there is an approximately 5% to 10% lifetime risk of women undergoing surgery for this indication.[1,2] Epithelial tumors represent approximately two-thirds of all ovarian tumors, thus representing a substantial proportion of the incidental lesions. Epithelial tumors are generally less common in younger patients and their prevalence increases with age, peaking in the sixth and seventh decades of life.[3] The World Health Organization (WHO) classifies epithelial ovarian tumors into six main types: serous, mucinous, Brenner tumors, clear cell, seromucinous, and endometrioid.[4,5] Epithelial ovarian tumors can be further classified as benign, borderline, or malignant according to their histologic features and clinical behavior. Although ultrasound is the primary modality for evaluating ovarian lesions, MR imaging is the preferred modality for characterization of indeterminant ovarian lesions given its superior soft tissue resolution and higher specificity for characterizing lesions as either benign or at increased risk of malignancy.[6]

This article covers the demographics, histology, and MR imaging characteristics of benign and borderline epithelial ovarian neoplasms followed by brief discussion of treatment and follow-up. Normal ovarian anatomy and MR imaging protocols are discussed in separate articles in this issue.

SEROUS TUMORS

Serous tumors are the most common epithelial ovarian neoplasm and the most common subtype of all ovarian neoplasms. They can be classified as benign (60%), borderline (15%), or malignant (25%).[7] Serous tumors are thought to represent distinct histologic subtypes rather than a continuum of tumorigenesis as seen in mucinous neoplasms.[8]

Benign: Serous Cystadenoma

Serous cystadenomas (SCAs) are the most common benign epithelial neoplasms and represent approximately 60% of all serous ovarian tumors.[9] Although, they can occur at any age, SCAs have a peak incidence in the fourth and fifth decades and are one of the most common simple cystic ovarian lesions found in postmenopausal women

Department of Radiology, University of Cincinnati, 234 Goodman Street, Cincinnati, OH 45267-0761, USA
* Corresponding author.
E-mail address: shaun.wahab@uc.edu

Magn Reson Imaging Clin N Am 31 (2023) 43–52
https://doi.org/10.1016/j.mric.2022.06.003
1064-9689/23/© 2022 Elsevier Inc. All rights reserved.

at surgery.[10,11] SCAs are smaller and more often bilateral than mucinous cystadenomas (MCAs).[5]

Histologically, SCAs are cysts lined by a single layer of tubal-type epithelium consisting of ciliated and secretary cells. Lesions with a borderline component comprising less than 10% of the tumor are classified as SCAs with focal proliferation.[12]

On MR imaging, SCAs are typically unilocular cysts with a thin wall without internal septations, papillary projections, or solid components and can be indistinguishable from follicular cysts. Unlike follicular cysts, which should regress spontaneously, SCA will remain unchanged or mildly increase in size over multiple menstruation cycles.[10] The serous fluid within these cysts is typically low signal on T1-weighted imaging (T1WI) and high signal on T2-weighted imaging (T2WI), with no diffusion restriction (**Fig. 1**). In addition, they can contain small nodules due to fibrosis or calcifications and papillary projections are generally very small when present.[9,10] Thin, smooth enhancement is typically seen along the cyst wall and septations when present.

Benign: Serous Cystadenofibroma

Serous cystadenofibromas are uncommon benign epithelial ovarian tumors containing both epithelial and fibrous stromal elements. They are rare and represent less than 2% of all ovarian neoplasms with a peak incidence in the fifth and sixth decades.[13] Most patients are asymptomatic, but symptoms can include lower abdominal pain and a palpable mass. Histologically, the cyst walls are lined by a single layer of epithelium without nuclear atypia overlying fibrous stroma.[8]

The MR imaging appearance of serous cystadenofibromas is variable depending on the amount of cystic and fibrous components. They may be purely cystic or have a complex cystic appearance with septations and solid components. Foci of solid or nodular fibrous stroma have low signal intensity on T2WI (**Fig. 2**).[14,15] The so-called "dark–dark" appearance of the solid fibrous tissue component is related to low signal on T2WI and diffusion-weighted imaging (DWI); however, this feature may be shared with other fibrous tumors such as fibromas/fibrothecomas or Brenner tumors.[16] The septations and fibrous components typically demonstrate slow progressive enhancement.

Serous Borderline

Serous borderline ovarian tumors (SBOTs) represent 65% of all borderline tumors and are the most common histologic subtype.[17] Approximately 15% of all serous tumors are borderline, and up to one-third of borderline tumor patients are less than 40 year old, with a mean age at diagnosis of approximately 50 years of age.[5] BRAF mutations are seen in up to 30% of SBOTs, and KRAS mutations are seen in up to 20%.[18] No specific risk factors have been linked to borderline ovarian tumors.[5] Typically, SBOTs demonstrate slow growth and overall excellent prognosis.[17]

SBOTs are divided into typical serous borderline tumors (90%) and borderline tumors with micropapillary pattern (5%–10%). Histologically, these tumors demonstrate epithelial proliferation with hierarchical branching papillae (typical) or a micropapillary/cribriform pattern (micropapillary), mild to moderate nuclear atypia, and no stromal invasion. By definition, SBOTs demonstrate epithelial growth and stratification in more than 10% of the tumor.[5]

On MR imaging, SBOTs are often bilateral and can be predominantly cystic, solid, or mixed solid/cystic. The cystic variety is usually unilocular and contains low T1, high T2 signal serous fluid. However, high T1 signal fluid can occur.[2,19] Papillary projections are common and can be exophytic, endophytic, or mixed (**Fig. 3**).[19] In addition, they can also involve septations when present. When the papillary projections occur on the surface of the ovary with no associated cystic component, they are commonly referred to as surface papillary borderline ovary tumors and have been likened to a sea anemone.[7] Papillary projections have low signal fibrous architecture centrally and intermediate to high signal along the periphery related to edema. Papillary projections may demonstrate diffusion restriction, but less so than solid elements of malignant tumors, and may also demonstrate enhancement (see **Fig. 3**; and Fig. 4).[2,19]

On dynamic contrast enhancement, SBOTs typically have a type 2 time intensity curve with early enhancement, but less than myometrium, followed by a plateau. This contrasts with early contrast uptake and washout seen with malignant lesions (type 3 curve) or gradual uptake of benign lesions (type 1 curve).[20]

Extraovarian spread in the form of peritoneal implants may be present in approximately 10% of SBOTs.[17] Most implants are noninvasive; however, invasive implants can be found in 20% to 25% of cases and can progress to invasive carcinoma.[21] Noninvasive implants will remain stable or regress after removal of the primary ovarian tumor.[22] The micropapillary variant has the highest risk of peritoneal implants. Ascites is an equivocal finding and can be seen in up to 43% of patients with borderline tumors.[17]

Cancer antigen-125 (CA-125) is an important tumor marker often used to distinguish between benign and malignant adnexal masses. However, serum CA-125 is elevated in approximately half of

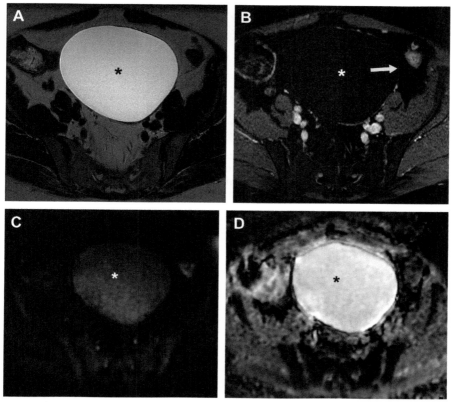

Fig. 1. Serous cystadenoma in a 60-year-old patient presenting with abdominal fullness. Axial T2WI (*A*) and axial post-contrast T1WI (*B*) demonstrating a unilocular simple cyst in the left pelvis (*asterisk*) with a thin rim of enhancement along the periphery (*yellow arrow*). DWI (*C*) and apparent diffusion coefficient (ADC) (*D*) demonstrating high signal and no diffusion restriction.

the patients with SBOT, especially stage 1 patients, with values overlapping with serous carcinoma.[2]

MUCINOUS

Mucinous epithelial ovarian tumors are the second most common epithelial subtype and account for approximately 10% to 15% of all ovarian tumors. They tend to occur in younger patients than serous neoplasms and generally have an excellent prognosis as most are benign or borderline.[23] Mucinous neoplasms are thought to progress sequentially from cystadenomas to borderline tumors to invasive carcinoma. This is due to the

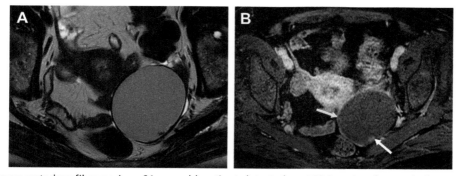

Fig. 2. Serous cystadenofibroma in a 64-year-old patient detected on MR imaging for cervical cancer staging. Axial T2WI (*A*) demonstrating a thin-walled cystic lesion hypointense peripheral mural nodule (*white arrow*). Axial post-contrast T1WI (*B*) demonstrating mild enhancement of the thin cyst wall (*yellow arrow*) and peripheral nodule (*white arrow*).

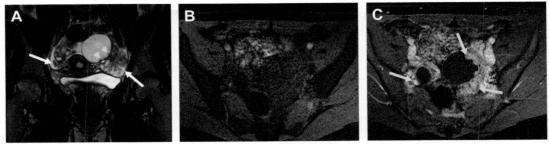

Fig. 3. Bilateral serous borderline tumors in a 29-year-old patient incidentally discovered on pelvic ultrasound. Coronal T2WI (*A*) demonstrating bilateral SBOT with exophytic papillary projections on the right and left (*white arrows*) and endophytic papillary projections on the left (*yellow arrowheads*). Axial pre-contrast (*B*) and post-contrast (*C*) T1WI demonstrating contrast enhancement of the papillary components (*yellow arrows*).

presence of benign, borderline, and invasive components in mucinous carcinomas with KRAS mutations in each.[24] It is important to note that metastasis should be considered in mucinous ovarian tumors. A large percentage of mucinous tumors are metastasis from other primary sites, particularly the gastrointestinal tract, and this distinction is important both from prognostic and treatment standpoints.[25]

Benign: Mucinous Cystadenoma and Cystadenofibroma

MCAs are the second most common benign epithelial tumor and are typically unilateral.[10] MCAs tend to be smaller in size than borderline mucinous tumors (10 cm compared with 21.5 cm), and approximately 5% to 10% of MCAs may present with other ovarian tumors such as Brenner tumors or mature teratomas.[26]

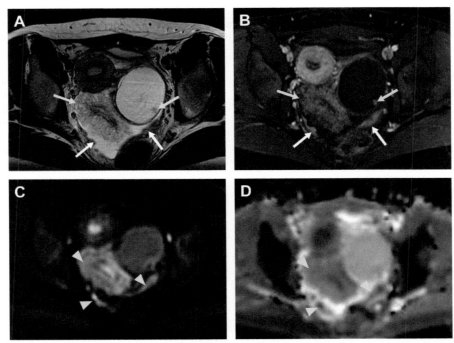

Fig. 4. Serous borderline tumor with micropapillary features in a 22-year-old patient with pelvic pain. Axial T2WI (*A*) and post-contrast T1WI (*B*) with a mixed cystic and solid left ovarian mass with exophytic and endophytic papillary projections (*yellow arrows*) and peritoneal implants (*white arrows*) that demonstrate enhancement. DWI (*C*) and ADC (*D*) demonstrating mild diffusion restriction of the papillary components and peritoneal nodules (*yellow arrowheads*).

Histologically, MCAs are lined by columnar epithelium in a simple non-stratified pattern with basal nuclei secreting mucin. Some epithelial cells may resemble gastric or intestinal mucosa with papillary or pseudopapillary infoldings.[4] The stroma found in MCAs is typically fibrous, and when found in abundance, the tumor is called a mucinous cystadenofibroma.[27]

On MR imaging, MCAs appear as unilateral, multiloculated cystic ovarian lesions with multiple thin septations (**Fig. 5**). The cystic components have variable T1 signal intensity due to the variable concentrations of mucin, giving a stained-glass appearance. MCAs may have papillary projections, but they are less common than with serous neoplasms. Owing to the highly viscous mucinous contents, these neoplasms can demonstrate mild diffusion restriction.[28] The cyst wall and septations may demonstrate mild progressive enhancement.

Mucinous Borderline

Mucinous borderline ovarian tumors (MBOTs) represent approximately 10% of mucinous tumors and are the second most common subtype of borderline tumor.[4] MBOTs may be present with Brenner tumors and mature teratomas.[26] KRAS mutations are seen up to 50% of MBOTs, and BRAF mutations are rare.[18]

Histologically, MBOTs were previously categorized as either intestinal-type or endocervical-type. However, the endocervical-type MBOT has been reclassified by the WHO as seromucinous borderline tumors and will be described separately.[4,5] Microscopically, MBOTs are lined by proliferating mucin secreting intestinal-type epithelium with mild to moderate nuclear atypia and typically no stromal invasion. They can have microinvasion which is defined as stromal invasion less than 5 mm.[4]

On MR imaging, MBOTs present as large, cystic, multiloculated lesions with multiple septations that may be irregular and thickened. Mural nodules or papillary projections can be present but are less common than in SBOT.[29] The contents of the cystic components are variable on T1WI and T2WI due to variable concentrations of mucin, with a similar stained glass appearance (**Fig. 6**). The viscous contents and mural nodules may demonstrate mild diffusion restriction, but to a lesser degree than malignant lesions.[30] The presence of densely aggregated loculi measuring approximately 5 to 10 mm is another characteristic feature that can be seen with MBOTs, also called "honeycomb loculi."[19] Unfortunately, the imaging appearance of MBOT can overlap with benign and malignant mucinous tumors.

Extraovarian spread is much less common in MBOT compared with SBOT and is seen in only 10% to 15% of cases.[22] Extra-ovarian spread is typically in the form of pseudomyxoma peritonei, which can occur in any type of intra-abdominal mucinous neoplasm. No unequivocal peritoneal implants associated with mucinous BOT have been reported in the literature.[4] If peritoneal implants, pseudomyxoma peritonei, or small bilateral mucinous tumors (less than 13 cm) are observed, it is essential to recognize the possibility of metastases from another primary site, most commonly from low-grade appendiceal mucinous neoplasms.[4,31,32]

BRENNER TUMOR

Brenner tumors are uncommon ovarian epithelial tumors and make up less than 3% of all ovarian tumors.[33] They are typically benign, with malignant and borderline types making up 2% to 5% of Brenner tumors. Extra-ovarian locations have rarely been reported in the testis and epididymis.[34] Up to 36% of Brenner tumors are associated with mucinous tumors including benign and borderline forms.[35]

Histologically, Brenner tumors are made up of fibrous tissue with areas of transitional/urothelial-type epithelial cells.[36] Therefore, the MR appearance of benign Brenner tumors is similar to that of other fibrous lesions such as ovarian fibromas/thecomas with mostly low T1 and T2 signal (**Fig. 7**). They demonstrate mild progressive enhancement without diffusion restriction. Calcifications are common though difficult to detect by MR imaging.[35]

Borderline Brenner tumors are mostly diagnosed in postmenopausal patients, unlike other borderline tumors, which are found in premenopausal patients.[37] Borderline Brenner tumors will have a similar appearance to other borderline epithelial ovarian neoplasms with papillary projections extending into a cystic component, which differentiates them from the predominantly solid, low-signal, benign Brenner tumors.

CLEAR CELL

Clear cell ovarian epithelial neoplasms are associated with endometriosis and are usually malignant. Benign clear cell cystadenoma and adenofibroma are uncommon and borderline forms are exceedingly rare.[38]

Case reports of benign clear cell adenofibromas describe very low T2 signal tumor with numerous

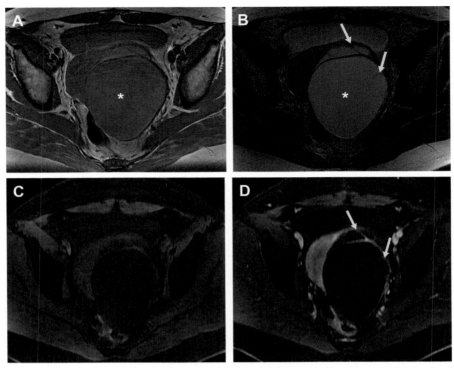

Fig. 5. Mucinous cystadenoma incidentally discovered on a pelvic ultrasound performed for ovarian torsion in a 30-year-old patient. Axial T1WI (*A*) demonstrating a mildly T1 hyperintense cystic mass arising from the left ovary (*asterisk*) with thin septations (*yellow arrows*) on T2WI (*B*). Axial pre-contrast (*C*) and post-contrast (*D*) axial T1WI with fat saturation demonstrate mild enhancement of the cyst wall and septations.

tiny cystic spaces for a "sponge-like" appearance. This rare tumor may be considered in the differential if there are adjacent/associated findings of endometriosis. Areas of high DWI signal should raise suspicion for malignancy.[39]

Less than 100 cases of clear cell borderline tumors are reported in the literature with the majority demonstrating adenofibromatous histology.[40] Unlike other borderline tumors, most of the reported cases were diagnosed in postmenopausal patients.

SEROMUCINOUS

Seromucinous tumor is a relatively new classification defined by the WHO in 2014.[26] Despite the name, seromucinous tumors are not composed of serous and MCA or mucinous borderline tumor. In fact, the presence of gastrointestinal differentiation as seen in MCA or mucinous borderline tumor exclude seromucinous designation.[41] This group now combines the previously separate, endocervical-like mucinous, Mullerian mixed

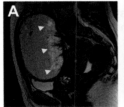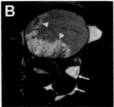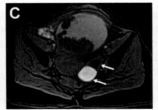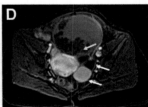

Fig. 6. Right mucinous ovarian borderline tumor and left benign mucinous cystadenoma in a 52-year-old woman with abdominal distention. Sagittal (*A*) and axial (*B*) T2WI with a large right MBOT containing endophytic papillary projections, a multiloculated left ovarian mucinous cystadenoma with variable T2 signal (*white arrows*) and small ascites. Axial pre-contrast (*C*) and post-contrast (*D*) T1-weighted images with fat saturation demonstrating mild enhancement of the fibrous center of the papillary projections (*yellow arrow*). Benign mucinous cystadenoma on the left (*white arrows*) demonstrates mild enhancement of the wall only.

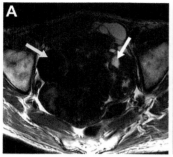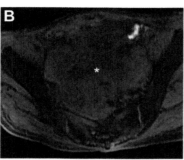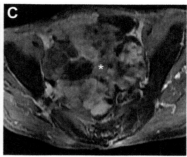

Fig. 7. Brenner tumor in a 68-year-old with lower abdominal pain. Axial T2WI (*A*) demonstrating predominantly hypointense signal (yellow arrow) with a few small cystic foci (white arrow). Axial fat-saturated pre- (*B*) and post-contrast (*C*) T1WI demonstrating heterogenous delayed enhancement of the Brenner tumor.

epithelial, and Mullerian mucinous tumors. Most seromucinous tumors are the borderline form with a strong association with endometriosis.[26]

Owing to the presence of mucin, a key imaging feature of seromucinous borderline tumor differentiating from serous borderline tumor is higher T1 and lower T2 signal of cyst contents (**Fig. 8**).[42] Papillary projections have a similar appearance to other borderline tumors and may demonstrate enhancement and mild diffusion restriction.

ENDOMETRIOID

Endometrioid epithelial tumors are rare, representing only 2% to 4% of all ovarian tumors, occurring commonly in the fourth and fifth decades.[43] Similar to clear cell epithelial ovarian tumors, they are associated with endometriosis and are usually malignant. Benign endometrioid cystadenomas/cystadenofibromas and endometrioid borderline ovarian tumors are much less common than endometrioid carcinoma.[44] Histologically, the benign endometrioid tumors are similar to endometriotic cysts but lack endometrial stroma, hemosiderin-laden macrophages, and a myofibroblastic wall. Borderline endometrioid tumors consist of atypical endometrioid epithelium without stromal invasion.[45] The imaging features of endometrioid tumors are nonspecific, and the diagnosis is often an incidental finding. Reported cases of benign and borderline endometrioid tumors have been confined to the ovary and are associated with a good prognosis.[46]

TREATMENT CONSIDERATIONS AND FOLLOW-UP

Benign epithelial ovarian tumors have an excellent prognosis and are typically treated surgically with resection/cystectomy or unilateral salpingo-oophorectomy (USO) in the absence of suspicion or malignancy.[47–49] Conservative management

and surveillance are also considerations when appropriate but are beyond the scope of this article.

Epithelial borderline ovarian tumors are usually confined to the ovaries at presentation, with 75% diagnosed at stage 1 and only 25% at stage 2 or greater. The prognosis is good with a 5-year survival of 95% with all stages combined, which only decreases to 90% at 10 years.[50,51] Adjuvant chemotherapy or radiation do not improve prognosis, and surgery is the mainstay of treatment.[17,52]

The type of surgery for borderline tumors depends on the need for fertility sparing. If there are no invasive implants, fertility sparing surgery is a viable option for young women with borderline ovarian tumors regardless of stage. Unilateral SBOT can be treated with either cystectomy or USO. On the contrary, MBOTs tend to be large and require a USO.[53–55] When SBOTs are bilateral, they are treated with bilateral cystectomy or USO combined with contralateral cystectomy.[53] Routine hysterectomy is generally not recommended because it is not associated with improved recurrence-free survival. In patients who do not desire fertility preservation, optimal treatment is total abdominal hysterectomy and bilateral salpingo-oophorectomy.[2,56–59] For mucinous tumors, an appendectomy may be concurrently performed, particularly if the appendix is grossly abnormal.[17,60–62].

Peritoneal staging is often performed to exclude low grade ovarian cancer, a contraindication to fertility sparing surgery.[63] A detailed description of the number, size and location of implants is recommended for optimal preoperative planning.[64] Lymphadenectomy does not have an impact on overall survival and is not routinely recommended.[65]

Patients treated for epithelial borderline ovarian tumors require long-term follow-up due to the risk of recurrence. Patients with fertility sparing surgery are particularly at risk. Thankfully, most recurrences are of the borderline type, having no effect on the overall survival rate.[51] National

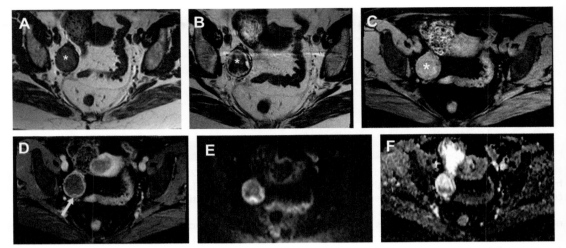

Fig. 8. Seromucinous borderline tumor in a 62-year-old patient. Axial T1WI (*A*), axial T2WI, axial fat-saturated pre-contrast (*C*) and post-contrast (*D*) T1WI demonstrating intrinsic high T1 signal and heterogenous T2 signal within the tumor (*asterisk*). There is also enhancement of the thickened cyst wall and nodular components (*yellow arrow*). DWI (*E*) and ADC (*F*) demonstrating mild diffusion restriction of the highly viscous cyst contents.

Comprehensive Cancer Network guidelines recommend patients follow-up every 3 to 6 months for the first 5 years and annually thereafter. Serial tumor markers are also recommended during follow-up, particularly if elevated at the time of initial diagnosis. If fertility sparing surgery was performed and the ovary or contralateral ovary has been retained, annual sonographic follow-up is generally recommended. CT, MR imaging, or PET/CT may be reserved for patients in whom there is a high level of suspicion for recurrence or malignancy.[66]

SUMMARY

Benign and borderline epithelial ovarian tumors represent a large proportion of incidental adnexal lesions and familiarity with the typical imaging features on MR imaging can aid in their diagnosis and management. Clinical information such as menstrual status, age, and associated conditions are also important considerations when evaluating an adnexal lesion. Radiologists play an integral role in the preoperative evaluation process and can help guide treatment, particularly in those with lesions demonstrating benign or borderline features and those who may be candidates for fertility sparing surgery.

CLINICS CARE POINTS

- CA-125 can be elevated in up to half of patients with borderline ovarian tumors and the range overlaps with malignancy.

- Papillary projections of borderline ovarian tumors can be exophytic, endophytic, or mixed.

- Peritoneal involvement is not a marker of malignancy and can be seen with serous borderline epithelial ovarian neoplasms, particularly the micropapillary serous variant.

- Mucinous tumors tend to be more complex than serous tumors and there can be similar imaging features in benign, borderline, and malignant subtypes.

- Detecting fibrous elements in an ovarian tumor can help to narrow the differential.

- Patient history of endometriosis or findings of concurrent endometriosis can aid in the diagnosis of endometriosis-associated tumors (ie, clear cell, seromucinous, endometrioid).

DISCLOSURE

The authors declare no relevant conflicts of interest or funding sources.

REFERENCES

1. McDonald JM, Modesitt SC. The incidental postmenopausal adnexal mass. Clin Obstet Gynecol 2006;49(3):506–16.
2. Naqvi J, Nagaraju E, Ahmad S. MRI appearances of pure epithelial papillary serous borderline ovarian tumours. Clin Radiol 2015;70(4):424–32.
3. Koonings PP, Campbell K, Mishell DR Jr, et al. Relative frequency of primary ovarian neoplasms: a 10-year review. Obstet Gynecol 1989;74(6):921–6.

4. Hauptmann S, Friedrich K, Redline R, et al. Ovarian borderline tumors in the 2014 WHO classification: evolving concepts and diagnostic criteria. Virchows Arch 2017;470(2):125–42.

5. Cheung A, Ellenson LH, Gilks CB. WHO classification of tumours: female genital tumours. 5th edition. International Agency for Research on Cancer; 2020.

6. Iyer VR, Lee SI. MRI, CT, and PET/CT for ovarian cancer detection and adnexal lesion characterization. AJR Am J Roentgenol 2010;194(2):311–21.

7. Tanaka YO, Okada S, Satoh T, et al. Ovarian serous surface papillary borderline tumors form sea anemone-like masses. J Magn Reson Imaging 2011;33(3):633–40.

8. Kurman RJ, Shih Ie M. Pathogenesis of ovarian cancer: lessons from morphology and molecular biology and their clinical implications. Int J Gynecol Pathol 2008;27(2):151–60.

9. Jung SE, Lee JM, Rha SE, et al. CT and MR imaging of ovarian tumors with emphasis on differential diagnosis. Radiographics 2002;22(6):1305–25.

10. Vargas HA, Barrett T, Sala E. MRI of ovarian masses. J Magn Reson Imaging 2013;37(2):265–81.

11. Griffin N, Grant LA, Sala E. Adnexal masses: characterization and imaging strategies. Semin Ultrasound CT MR 2010;31(5):330–46.

12. Folkins AK, Longacre TA. Low-grade Serous Neoplasia of the Female Genital Tract. Surg Pathol Clin 2019;12(2):481–513.

13. Khati NJ, Kim T, Riess J. Imaging of Benign Adnexal Disease. Radiol Clin North Am 2020;58(2):257–73.

14. Tang YZ, Liyanage S, Narayanan P, et al. The MRI features of histologically proven ovarian cystadenofibromas-an assessment of the morphological and enhancement patterns. Eur Radiol 2013;23(1):48–56.

15. Shimizu S, Okano H, Ishitani K, et al. Ovarian cystadenofibroma with solid nodular components masqueraded as ovarian cancer. Arch Gynecol Obstet 2009;279(5):709–11.

16. Khashper A, Addley HC, Abourokbah N, et al. T2-hypointense adnexal lesions: an imaging algorithm. Radiographics 2012;32(4):1047–64.

17. Flicek KT, VanBuren W, Dudiak K, et al. Borderline epithelial ovarian tumors: what the radiologist should know. Abdom Radiol (Ny) 2021;46(6):2350–66.

18. Mayr D, Hirschmann A, Löhrs U, et al. KRAS and BRAF mutations in ovarian tumors: a comprehensive study of invasive carcinomas, borderline tumors and extraovarian implants. Gynecol Oncol 2006;103(3):883–7.

19. Zhao SH, Qiang JW, Zhang GF, et al. MRI appearances of ovarian serous borderline tumor: pathological correlation. J Magn Reson Imaging 2014;40(1):151–6.

20. Thomassin-Naggara I, Balvay D, Aubert E, et al. Quantitative dynamic contrast-enhanced MR imaging analysis of complex adnexal masses: a preliminary study. Eur Radiol 2012;22(4):738–45.

21. Seidman JD, Horkayne-Szakaly I, Haiba M, et al. The histologic type and stage distribution of ovarian carcinomas of surface epithelial origin. Int J Gynecol Pathol 2004;23(1):41–4.

22. Tropé CG, Kaern J, Davidson B. Borderline ovarian tumours. Best Pract Res Clin Obstet Gynaecol 2012;26(3):325–36.

23. Prat J, D'Angelo E, Espinosa I. Ovarian carcinomas: at least five different diseases with distinct histological features and molecular genetics. Hum Pathol 2018;80:11–27.

24. Garrett AP, Lee KR, Colitti CR, et al. k-ras mutation may be an early event in mucinous ovarian tumorigenesis. Int J Gynecol Pathol 2001;20(3):244–51.

25. Duska LR, Kohn EC. The new classifications of ovarian, fallopian tube, and primary peritoneal cancer and their clinical implications. Ann Oncol 2017;28(suppl_8). viii8-viii12.

26. Kurman RJ CM, Herrington CS, Young RH. WHO classification of Tumours of Female Reproductive Organs. 4th edition. France: Lyon: International Agency for Research on Cancer; 2014.

27. Mills AM, Shanes ED. Mucinous Ovarian Tumors. Surg Pathol Clin 2019;12(2):565–85.

28. Dhanda S, Thakur M, Kerkar R, et al. Diffusion-weighted imaging of gynecologic tumors: diagnostic pearls and potential pitfalls. Radiographics 2014;34(5):1393–416.

29. Taylor EC, Irshaid L, Mathur M. Multimodality Imaging Approach to Ovarian Neoplasms with Pathologic Correlation. Radiographics 2021;41(1):289–315.

30. Ohya A, Ichinohe F, Matoba H, et al. Useful preoperative examination findings to classify the grade of ovarian primary mucinous tumor. Abdom Radiol (Ny) 2021;46(6):2393–402.

31. Abdel Wahab C, Rousset P, Bolze PA, et al. [Borderline Ovarian Tumours: CNGOF Guidelines for Clinical Practice - Imaging]. Gynecol Obstet Fertil Senol 2020;48(3):260–76.

32. Peng Y, Lin J, Guan J, et al. Ovarian collision tumors: imaging findings, pathological characteristics, diagnosis, and differential diagnosis. Abdom Radiol (Ny) 2018;43(8):2156–68.

33. Dimova J, Zlatareva D, Bakalova R, et al. Adnexal masses characterized on 3 tesla magnetic resonance imaging - added value of diffusion techniques. Radiol Oncol 2020;54(4):419–28.

34. Woodruff JD, Dietrich D, Genadry R, et al. Proliferative and malignant Brenner tumors. Review of 47 cases. Am J Obstet Gynecol 1981;141(2):118–25.

35. Montoriol PF, Hordonneau C, Boudinaud C, et al. Benign Brenner tumour of the ovary: CT and MRI features. Clin Radiol 2021;76(8):593–8.

36. Takahama J, Ascher SM, Hirohashi S, et al. Borderline Brenner tumor of the ovary: MRI findings. Abdom Imaging 2004;29(4):528–30.

37. Ricotta G, Maulard A, Genestie C, et al. Brenner Borderline Ovarian Tumor: A Case Series and Literature Review. Ann Surg Oncol 2021;28(11):6714–20.

38. Yin Z, Peters S, Chokshi R, et al. Ovarian Clear Cell Adenofibroma of Low Malignant Potential Developing Into Clear Cell Adenocarcinoma. Int J Surg Pathol 2018;26(6):578–80.

39. Takeuchi M, Matsuzaki K, Uehara H, et al. Clear cell adenocarcinoma arising from clear cell adenofibroma of the ovary: value of DWI and DCE-MRI. Magn Reson Med Sci 2013;12(4):305–8.

40. Ricotta G, Maulard A, Candiani M, et al. Clear Cell Borderline Ovarian Tumor: Clinical Characteristics, Prognosis, and Management. Ann Surg Oncol 2022;29(2):1165–70.

41. Nagamine M, Mikami Y. Ovarian Seromucinous Tumors: Pathogenesis, Morphologic Spectrum, and Clinical Issues. Diagnostics (Basel) 2020;10(2).

42. Kurata Y, Kido A, Moribata Y, et al. Differentiation of Seromucinous Borderline Tumor from Serous Borderline Tumor on MR Imaging. Magn Reson Med Sci 2018;17(3):211–7.

43. Bell DA, Scully RE. Atypical and borderline endometrioid adenofibromas of the ovary. A report of 27 cases. Am J Surg Pathol 1985;9(3):205–14.

44. Matias-Guiu X, Stewart CJR. Endometriosis-associated ovarian neoplasia. Pathology 2018;50(2):190–204.

45. Nakagawa E, Abiko K, Kido A, et al. Four cases of endometrioid borderline ovarian tumour: case reports and literature review. BJR Case Rep 2018;4(1):20170062.

46. Kommoss F, Gilks CB. Pathology of Ovarian Cancer: Recent Insights Unveiling Opportunities in Prevention. Clin Obstet Gynecol 2017;60(4):686–96.

47. Brun JL, Fritel X, Aubard Y, et al. Management of presumed benign ovarian tumors: updated French guidelines. Eur J Obstet Gynecol Reprod Biol 2014;183:52–8.

48. Beroukhim G, Ozgediz D, Cohen PJ, et al. Progression of Cystadenoma to Mucinous Borderline Ovarian Tumor in Young Females: Case Series and Literature Review. J Pediatr Adolesc Gynecol 2021;35(3):359–67.

49. Brown J, Frumovitz M. Mucinous tumors of the ovary: current thoughts on diagnosis and management. Curr Oncol Rep 2014;16(6):389.

50. Bourdel N, Huchon C, Abdel Wahab C, et al. Borderline ovarian tumors: Guidelines from the French national college of obstetricians and gynecologists (CNGOF). Eur J Obstet Gynecol Reprod Biol 2021;256:492–501.

51. Chevrot A, Pouget N, Bats AS, et al. Fertility and prognosis of borderline ovarian tumor after conservative management: Results of the multicentric OPTIBOT study by the GINECO & TMRG group. Gynecol Oncol 2020;157(1):29–35.

52. Patrono MG, Minig L, Diaz-Padilla I, et al. Borderline tumours of the ovary, current controversies regarding their diagnosis and treatment. Ecancermedicalscience 2013;7:379.

53. Vasconcelos I, de Sousa Mendes M. Conservative surgery in ovarian borderline tumours: a meta-analysis with emphasis on recurrence risk. Eur J Cancer 2015;51(5):620–31.

54. Daraï E, Fauvet R, Uzan C, et al. Fertility and borderline ovarian tumor: a systematic review of conservative management, risk of recurrence and alternative options. Hum Reprod Update 2013;19(2):151–66.

55. Palomba S, Falbo A, Del Negro S, et al. Ultra-conservative fertility-sparing strategy for bilateral borderline ovarian tumours: an 11-year follow-up. Hum Reprod 2010;25(8):1966–72.

56. deSouza NM, O'Neill R, McIndoe GA, et al. Borderline tumors of the ovary: CT and MRI features and tumor markers in differentiation from stage I disease. AJR Am J Roentgenol 2005;184(3):999–1003.

57. Acs G. Serous and mucinous borderline (low malignant potential) tumors of the ovary. Am J Clin Pathol 2005;123(Suppl):S13–57.

58. Chen VW, Ruiz B, Killeen JL, et al. Pathology and classification of ovarian tumors. Cancer 2003;97(10 Suppl):2631–42.

59. Cadron I, Leunen K, Van Gorp T, et al. Management of borderline ovarian neoplasms. J Clin Oncol 2007;25(20):2928–37.

60. Alvarez RM, Vazquez-Vicente D. Fertility sparing treatment in borderline ovarian tumours. Ecancermedicalscience 2015;9:507.

61. Lenhard MS, Mitterer S, Kümper C, et al. Long-term follow-up after ovarian borderline tumor: relapse and survival in a large patient cohort. Eur J Obstet Gynecol Reprod Biol 2009;145(2):189–94.

62. Feigenberg T, Covens A, Ghorab Z, et al. Is routine appendectomy at the time of primary surgery for mucinous ovarian neoplasms beneficial? Int J Gynecol Cancer 2013;23(7):1205–9.

63. McEvoy SH, Nougaret S, Abu-Rustum NR, et al. Fertility-sparing for young patients with gynecologic cancer: How MRI can guide patient selection prior to conservative management. Abdom Radiol (Ny) 2017;42(10):2488–512.

64. Alves AS, Félix A, Cunha TM. Clues to the diagnosis of borderline ovarian tumours: An imaging guide. Eur J Radiol 2021;143:109904.

65. Lesieur B, Kane A, Duvillard P, et al. Prognostic value of lymph node involvement in ovarian serous borderline tumors. Am J Obstet Gynecol 2011;204(5). 438.e431-437.

66. NCCN Guideline for Patients Ovarian Cancer. 2021. Available at: https://www.nccn.org/patients/guidelines/content/PDF/ovarian-patient.pdf. Accessed March 25 2022.

MR Imaging of Epithelial Ovarian Neoplasms Part II
Malignant

Limin Xu, MD[a],*, Susanna I. Lee, MD, PhD[b], Aoife Kilcoyne, MB BCh, BAO[b]

KEYWORDS

- MR imaging • Epithelial ovarian neoplasm • Serous • Mucinous • Endometrioid • Clear cell

KEY POINTS

- Advanced MR imaging techniques improve the discrimination of malignant ovarian lesions from benign and guide cancer management.
- Features of epithelial ovarian neoplasms include irregular wall thickening, papillary projections, solid components, large size, and necrosis.
- MR imaging features can characterize lesions to aid in the accurate diagnosis of subtypes of epithelial ovarian neoplasms.
- Standardized lesion evaluation and morphologic imaging descriptors are available to improve MR imaging findings communication.

INTRODUCTION

Ovarian cancer is the leading cause of mortality among gynecologic malignancies and the fifth leading cause of cancer death in women in the United States. Epithelial ovarian tumors comprise the most common type of ovarian neoplasm, representing up to 95% of malignant ovarian neoplasms.[1–4]

Ovarian cancer screening trials have demonstrated rapid progression of ovarian cancer from early-stage lesions, detectable sonographically, to spread outside the ovaries within weeks to months; thus, early diagnosis and subsequent triage are essential.[5] In the case of lesions suspicious of malignancy, MR imaging helps to guide ovarian cancer management, which ranges from lesion characterization to extent of disease assessment for staging and assessment of treatment response.[4,6,7]

MR imaging shows high sensitivity and specificity for characterizing benign and malignant lesions. Because of the superior soft tissue resolution of MR imaging, it is particularly useful in the accurate characterization of benign ovarian lesions (such as endometriomas, hemorrhagic cysts, and hydro- or hematosalpinx), previously indeterminate on either ultrasound or computed tomography (CT). Conversely, it also allows for lesions that remain indeterminate or demonstrate suspicious imaging features to be rapidly triaged to surgery.

The International Federation of Gynecology and Obstetrics (FIGO) staging system for ovarian cancer was most recently revised in 2014.[8,9] The FIGO staging system classifies ovarian malignancies into stages I through IV based on size and extent of the primary tumor; local invasion; and peritoneal, nodal, and distant organ involvement. An analogous tumor, node, and metastasis staging system also exists largely based on the same factors.[3] While CT is the more ubiquitous modality for staging, MR imaging has been shown to have equivalent accuracy to CT and is recommended

[a] Department of Radiology, Boston Children's Hospital, Harvard Medical School, Boston, MA 02115, USA;
[b] Department of Radiology, Massachusetts General Hospital, Harvard Medical School, 55 Fruit Street, Boston, MA 02114, USA
* Corresponding author.
E-mail address: liminMxu@gmail.com

Magn Reson Imaging Clin N Am 31 (2023) 53–64
https://doi.org/10.1016/j.mric.2022.07.002
1064-9689/23/

mri.theclinics.com

for patients for restaging in the setting of fertility preservation.[4,10]

ADVANCED TECHNIQUES

Evaluation of pelvic pathology often begins with ultrasound, which is readily available and widely utilized.[11] Frequently, CT may be ordered to evaluate nonspecific intra-abdominal pathology as well, which may also yield pelvic findings.

Once adnexal lesions are identified, further characterization is frequently required to differentiate benign from borderline and malignant pathologies and subsequently, to stage disease for the borderline and malignant lesions. Borderline neoplasms are those that do not demonstrate stromal invasion but may display low malignant potential with findings of cellular proliferation and moderate nuclear atypia on histology.[12,13]

Epithelial ovarian neoplasms are predominantly cystic and may be uni- or multilocular. Features, such as irregular wall thickening, papillary projections, and solid, echogenic foci are suspicious for malignancy on ultrasound.[3,14] If a lesion remains indeterminate by ultrasound, MR imaging is the imaging modality of choice and has been shown to demonstrate 97% sensitivity and 84% specificity for characterizing indeterminate lesions on ultrasound.[15]

MR imaging also allows for the assessment of dynamic contrast enhancement of the lesion, which can help to detect early enhancement and/or washout.[3] Lesion characterization is integral to treatment planning, which consists of surgery, chemotherapy, and, rarely, radiation. Because some tumors are more chemoresistant than others, accurate diagnosis is critical to avoid pursuing ineffective treatment strategies. MR imaging also has the advantage of assessing for tissue invasion of adjacent structures because of its excellent soft tissue contrast. The extent of disease assessment aids in surgical treatment planning and the feasibility of debulking/cytoreduction.[3]

MR IMAGING PROTOCOL: TIPS FOR TAILORING FOR TUMOR EVALUATION

MR imaging protocols for evaluation of ovarian lesions should employ a small field-of-view with sequences optimized for increased signal-to-noise and soft tissue contrast.[5] Sequences acquired at the author's institution are summarized in **Table 1**.

- Three-dimensional sampling perfection with application-optimized contrasts using flip angle evolution sequences with multiplanar

post-processing can also be acquired where feasible in place of multiplanar fast spin echo T2-weighted images.
- If the necessary technology is available, in- and out-of-phase images are substituted with axial DIXON sequences.
- At our institution, contrast is administered as a dynamic bolus at 2 cc/s and imaging is acquired at 20, 70, and 180 seconds. Because dynamic contrast imaging is performed usually to evaluate the endometrial–myometrial interface, it is routinely acquired in the sagittal plane so that the interface is reliably orthogonal to the imaging plane. Nevertheless, the field of view is sufficiently large to include the ovaries and adnexa. Delayed axial and coronal post-contrast images are acquired after 3 minutes. Of note, contrast enhancement of the solid component of an endometrioma is particularly important in evaluating for potential malignant transformation.[16,17]
- Restricted diffusion should be evaluated using sequences with a high b value, for example, at least 600 s/mm^2. A study of qualitative diffusion-weighted imaging assessment of restricted diffusion using the uterine myometrium as an internal standard, or of small bowel wall in patients after hysterectomy, for diagnosis of malignancy, demonstrated a 100% negative predictive value. Thus, lesions determined to show no restricted diffusion could confidently be diagnosed as benign with a diagnostic performance of 100% sensitivity for ovarian malignancy.[18] Benign lesions demonstrating restricted diffusion, such as endometrioma and teratoma can also be evaluated using the T1-weighted sequences.
- Lesions with a mean apparent diffusion coefficient value higher than a threshold of 1.039×10^{-3} mm^2/s indicated a borderline nature rather than malignant with a sensitivity of 97.0% and specificity of 92.2% in a 2014 study.[19] Furthermore, a threshold value of 1.55×10^{-3} mm^2/s was also shown to suggest a greater than 99.9% chance of benignity of a lesion.[18]

IMAGING FINDINGS/PATHOLOGY

Malignant imaging features of ovarian epithelial neoplasm on MR imaging are similar to those seen in both ultrasound and CT, including irregular wall thickening greater than 3 mm, papillary projections, the solid component of varying degrees, septations greater than 3 mm in thickness, large size, and necrosis.[3,16] In particular, papillary projections are unique to epithelial tumors and

Table 1
Pelvic MR imaging protocol for evaluation of ovarian tumor

Sequences	Imaging Planes	Key Points
T2-weighted fast spin echo or 3D T2-weighted SPACE	Axial, coronal, sagittal	• Rapid acquisition of sequences reduces motion artifact • Provides information on soft tissue contrast to differentiate cystic from solid elements[5] • Lesion localization, confirm location of lesion as ovarian vs extraovarian[5]
T1-weighted in-/out-of-phase spin echo or DIXON	Axial	• Obtained as a pair to determine the presence of microscopic fat not readily appreciated on the T1-weighted sequences alone
T1-weighted sequence with and without fat suppression or DIXON	Axial	• Enable detection of hemorrhage and endometriosis with greater sensitivity than gradient echo sequences • T1 weighting allows for characterization of hemorrhagic products and macroscopic fat, and therefore discrimination of endometriosis, hemorrhagic cysts, and fat-containing teratoma from malignant lesions which can restrict diffusion[5]
Gradient echo T1-weighted sequence with fat saturation pre- then post-contrast	Axial, coronal, sagittal	• Dynamic contrast enhancement allows for examination of the adnexal lesion's enhancement kinetics • "Early washout" pattern of contrast enhancement suggests pathologic vascularization with a sensitivity of 84.2% and specificity of 85.7% for predicting borderline/malignant lesions vs benign[50]
T1-weighted subtraction	Axial, coronal, sagittal	• Useful in cases of equivocal enhancement for detecting enhancement on a background of T1 hyperintensity in the setting of endometriosis[5,16,17,51]
High b-value DWI	Axial	• Characterize lesion as benign or malignant • Useful to detect lymph nodes, peritoneal and omental implants
ADC map	Axial	• Required for simultaneous evaluation with DWI sequence for evaluation of restricted diffusion • Mean ADC value of the solid component of a lesion can be quantitated to further differentiate borderline from malignant epithelial ovarian tumors[19]
T2-weighted large field-of-view	Axial	• Renal hilum to pubic symphysis • Evaluation for retroperitoneal lymphadenopathy and potential intraabdominal mimics of ovarian lesions, such as appendiceal mucocele

Abbreviations: ADC, apparent diffusion coefficient; DWI, diffusion-weighted imaging; SPACE, sampling perfection with application optimized contrasts using flip angle evolution.

suggest borderline or malignant characteristics when multifocal.[20] Papillary projections result from the folding of proliferating epithelium and seem hyperintense on T2-weighted MR images due to edema with an underlying fibrous core, which is hypointense on T2-weighted images.[20]

They typically enhance with the administration of gadolinium-based contrast agents.

Associated malignant findings, such as ascites, peritoneal implants, pelvic wall invasion, and adenopathy can also be assessed. In particular, the pouch of Douglas, greater omentum, and the subphrenic region should be carefully scrutinized.[21] The pelvic and retroperitoneal lymph nodes are preferentially involved.[21] Hematogenous metastases, while less common, can occur in the liver, lung, and bone.

Epithelial cancers are hypothesized to arise from malignant transformation of the ovarian surface, fallopian tubal, and peritoneal epithelium.[22] They may arise de novo or in the setting of genetic mutations, such as breast cancer types 1 and 2. Subtypes of epithelial ovarian tumors can be determined by imaging characteristics in addition to histology. Accurate subtyping is important because of the biological difference of the subtypes which influences patterns of spread, treatment response, and prognosis.[12,23] Neoplasms can further be classified as low-grade, high-grade, or borderline. For example, low-grade epithelial ovarian neoplasms tend to demonstrate a more indolent course relative to high-grade epithelial cancers and are usually diagnosed in younger patients.[23]

Borderline neoplasms account for approximately 15% of all primary ovarian neoplasms and are generally serous or mucinous, though they can occur in all of the subtypes of epithelial ovarian tumors.[13,19,24] While they may rarely be accompanied by invasive peritoneal implants, categorization depends on the primary ovarian tumor.[13] Because of the lack of unique features in imaging, preoperative diagnosis of borderline tumors is uncommon.

Serous

Serous carcinomas comprise the majority of malignant epithelial ovarian neoplasms, representing approximately 75%. They are further subdivided into high-grade versus low-grade tumors via the MD Anderson Cancer Center grading system, with later revisions of the FIGO staging classification and the World Health Organization (WHO) classification in 2014 adopting a similar two-tier grading system.[9,22,25–27] While high-grade (HGSC) and low-grade serous carcinomas (LGSC) are distinct pathologic entities, a common precursor originating from the fallopian tube has been proposed.[12,28]

On imaging, serous ovarian carcinomas seem as mixed solid and cystic masses and are frequently bilateral with associated peritoneal carcinomatosis.[20] The serous components show high signal intensity on T2-weighted images.

LGSC comprises 3% to 4% of ovarian carcinomas and less than 5% of epithelial ovarian tumors.[3,12,29] They are proposed to originate from "endosalpingiosis/Müllerian rests" in a background of ovarian benign or borderline serous tumors.[12,30] Because they are slow-growing and indolent, LGSCs are typically diagnosed at an advanced stage.[12,29] Complete surgical resection is key to optimal management as they tend to be chemoresistant.[23,31] On imaging, LGSCs are more often multilocular cysts with papillary projections in contrast to HGSCs, which are more likely to appear as nonpapillary solid masses with scattered cystic changes, hemorrhage, or necrosis (Figs. 1 and 2).[23] They can be associated with tumor calcification, even before therapy. Increased calcification may be linked with disease progression following therapy (Fig. 3).[23,32]

HGSC represents 68% of ovarian carcinomas and 70% to 80% of malignant epithelial ovarian tumors, with a peak incidence in patients between the ages of 45 and 65 years.[3,29,31] In contrast to LGSCs, HGSCs typically demonstrate a more aggressive course.[23] HGSC are rarely diagnosed while localized to the ovaries.[31] They are often staged III or IV at the time of diagnosis.[12,29] HGSCs originate from "serous tubal intraepithelial carcinoma" with the majority arising from the distal fimbrial end of the fallopian tube and secondarily involve the ovary.[12,31,33] On imaging, HGSCs tend to be solid and cystic masses with larger solid portions and components of hemorrhage or necrosis.[23]

Recent molecular and immunohistochemical data demonstrate the shared genetic mutations between transitional cell carcinoma and HGSC, suggesting that transitional cell carcinomas are distinct from malignant Brenner tumors, in contrast to previous understanding, and are rather subtypes of HGSC.[8,12,34]

Mucinous

Mucinous carcinomas comprise 3% to 4% of ovarian carcinomas.[3,12,29] They are most frequently metastases, most commonly from the gastrointestinal tract.[9] The peak incidence of mucinous carcinomas is in perimenopausal women in their fifth and sixth decades. They are more likely to be diagnosed at an early stage.[29] Because they are often seen concurrently with and adjacent to mucinous borderline neoplasms, ovarian mucinous carcinomas are believed to arise from these mucinous borderline neoplasms, which are consistently confined to the ovary.[12]

On imaging, mucinous carcinomas seem as mixed cystic and solid masses with the variable signal intensity of the cystic portion due to the concentration of the mucin (Fig. 4). Mucinous carcinomas can rupture resulting in pseudomyxoma peritonei.[20]

Endometrioid

Endometrioid carcinomas comprise approximately 11% of ovarian carcinomas and up to 10% of ovarian epithelial neoplasms with a peak

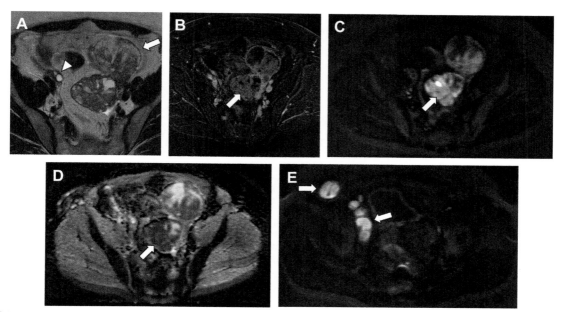

Fig. 1. A 54-year-old woman with an incidental pelvic mass noted on kidney and bladder ultrasound. Axial T2-weighted MR imaging (A) demonstrates a predominantly solid mass with areas of cystic change in the left adnexa (arrow) and normal right ovary (arrowhead). Axial T1-weighted pre-from post-contrast subtraction (B), axial DWI [b = 1000] (C), and axial ADC (D) images demonstrate enhancement and restricted diffusion of the solid component (arrows). Axial DWI [b = 1000] (E) demonstrates right pelvic and inguinal lymphadenopathy (arrows). High-grade serous carcinoma was diagnosed on biopsy of the right inguinal lymph node and confirmed on subsequent resection of the pelvic mass.

incidence in women in their fifth and sixth decades.[3,29,35] Patients have a better prognosis compared with serous carcinomas as they are typically diagnosed at earlier stages.[29,35]

There is an association with endometriosis, otherwise, imaging features are nonspecific.[36] The tumor seems as a large solid and cystic mass with bilateral involvement in up to 50% of cases (Fig. 5).[20] Because of its association with endometriosis, endometriomas should be carefully scrutinized for the presence of enhancing mural nodules. In the case of endometriosis-associated ovarian cancers, concurrent endometrial carcinoma is seen in up to one-third of cases.[35,36] An ovarian primary is favored if the tumor is unilateral and large without ovarian surface involvement or there is little to no myometrial invasion of the endometrial carcinoma, no

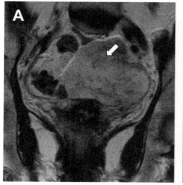
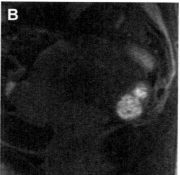
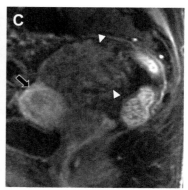

Fig. 2. A 65-year-old woman with bilateral pelvic masses seen on pelvic ultrasound. Coronal T2-weighted MR imaging (A) demonstrates a predominantly cystic left adnexal mass with T2-hypointense papillary projections (arrow). Sagittal T1-weighted fat saturated pre- (B) and post-contrast enhanced (C) images demonstrate heterogeneous enhancement of the papillary projections (arrowhead), which are hypoenhancing relative to the myometrium (black arrow). This mass was resected and demonstrated low-grade serous carcinoma.

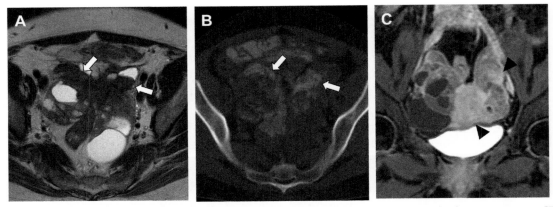

Fig. 3. A 48-year-old woman who underwent MR imaging for further characterization of pelvic mass seen on CT. Axial T2-weighted MR imaging pelvis (*A*) demonstrates areas of hypointense signal corresponding to foci of calcification seen on CT (*B*, *arrows*). Coronal T1-weighted contrast-enhanced image (*C*) demonstrates the enhancing solid components of the mass (*arrowheads*). Final pathology demonstrated low-grade serous carcinoma with psammomatous features.

lymphovascular invasion in the uterus, and background of endometriosis or endometrioid borderline neoplasm.[12]

Endometriosis-associated endometrioid carcinoma demonstrates distinct characteristics in contrast to endometrioid carcinoma without a background of endometriosis and tends to be diagnosed at an earlier FIGO stage and lower grade of the tumor.[36]

Seromucinous carcinoma was introduced as a new category of ovarian cancer in the fourth edition of the WHO classification revised in 2014 but is now recategorized as a subtype of endometrioid

carcinoma with mucinous differentiation in the fifth edition published in 2020, as they are similar to a molecular level.[27,30,33] Seromucinous tumors comprise the previous endocervical-type mucinous borderline ovarian tumors.[27]

Clear Cell

Clear cell carcinoma comprises 12% of ovarian carcinomas and up to 10% of ovarian epithelial neoplasms.[3,29,35] Peak incidence of clear cell carcinomas occur in perimenopausal women in their fifth and sixth decades.[12] Similar to endometrioid carcinoma, clear cell carcinoma demonstrates an

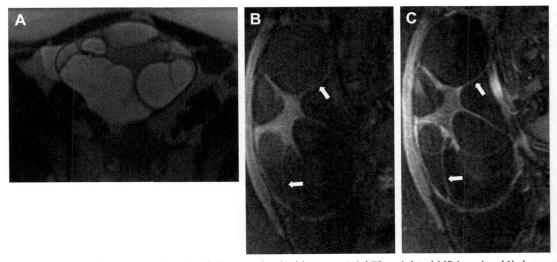

Fig. 4. A 24-year-old woman with pelvic fullness and palpable mass. Axial T2-weighted MR imaging (*A*) shows a multiloculated right adnexal cystic mass with heterogenous T2 signal intensity. Sagittal T1-weighted fat saturated pre- (*B*) and post-contrast enhanced (*C*) images demonstrate nonenhancement of the cystic components and mild enhancement of the septations (*arrows*). The mass was resected, demonstrating mucinous adenocarcinoma of the right ovary.

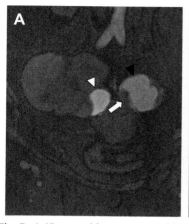
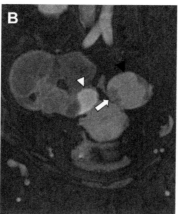
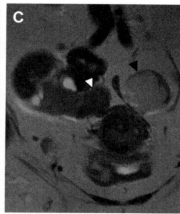

Fig. 5. A 45-year-old woman with bilateral ovarian and cervical masses (not shown). Coronal T1-weighted precontrast (*A*) and coronal T1-weighted contrast-enhanced (*B*) with fat saturation and coronal T2-weighted (*C*) MR images demonstrate bilateral solid and cystic masses. There are enhancing solid components (*arrows*). In addition, there are areas of intrinsic T1-hyperintense signal with associated T2-hypointensity, consistent with an underlying endometrioma of the right ovary (*white arrowheads*) and left ovarian endometrioma (*black arrowheads*). Endometrioid adenocarcinoma representing malignant degeneration of endometriosis was found on biopsy of the cervical mass and subsequent resection of the ovarian masses.

association with endometriosis.[35,36] While the majority of patients are diagnosed in the early stages, given its relative insensitivity to platinum-based chemotherapeutic agents, clear cell carcinoma has a worse prognosis than serous or endometrioid carcinomas and is essentially considered high grade.[3,12,35]

An important associated feature at presentation to evaluate for imaging is venous thromboemboli, which is statistically significantly associated with clear cell carcinoma of the ovary in contrast to the other subtypes of epithelial ovarian cancers.[37] Of the epithelial ovarian neoplasms, clear cell carcinoma is also the most commonly associated with paraneoplastic hypercalcemia.[35]

On imaging, clear cell carcinoma frequently presents as a large, smoothly marginated cystic structure with solid components with a variable signal on T1-weighted MR images (**Fig. 6**).[20]

Brenner

Malignant Brenner tumors are extremely rare low-grade ovarian carcinomas with a peak incidence in women between ages 45 and 60 years.[8,38] These tumors can range from mixed solid and multilocular cystic to predominantly solid.[16,38,39] Papillary projections into the cystic component are more commonly seen in the borderline and malignant tumors, which also tend to be larger in size compared with benign, ranging from 8 to 10 cm[38] The solid components of the malignant

tumors tend to demonstrate increased signal on T2-weighted images.[40]

Mesonephric-Like Adenocarcinoma

Introduced as a new category of epithelial ovarian tumors in the 2020 revision of the WHO classification, the mesonephric-like adenocarcinoma is proposed to arise from paraovarian mesonephric remnants or Müllerian carcinomas with possible associations with endometriosis, cystadenomas, adenofibromas, borderline tumors, and LGSC.[30,33] They are typically diagnosed in postmenopausal women at stage I and are unilateral.[30,33]

Undifferentiated and Dedifferentiated Carcinomas

As a group, these tumors are uncommon and comprise approximately 0.5% of ovarian carcinomas.[33] A new subtype as of 2020, dedifferentiated carcinoma is usually diagnosed at an advanced stage with nodal involvement.[30] Dedifferentiated carcinomas are composed of juxtaposed undifferentiated carcinoma and differentiated component on histology.[30,33] Undifferentiated carcinomas lack evidence of a specific line of differentiation.[33] While imaging features are nonspecific, tumors tend to be large solid masses with extensive necrosis.[33] Ancillary imaging findings include bulky pelvic and para-aortic lymph nodes because of typical presentation with advanced-stage disease.[33]

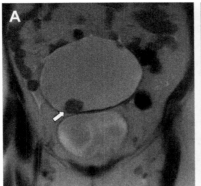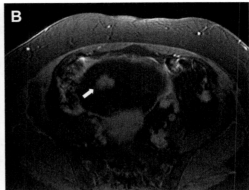

Fig. 6. A 49-year-old woman with a left ovarian mass seen on renal ultrasound. Coronal T2-weighted (*A*) and axial T1-weighted contrast-enhanced (*B*) images demonstrate a large, smoothly marginated cystic mass. There is a T2-hypointense nodule within which demonstrates enhancement (*arrows*). This mass was resected, demonstrating clear cell carcinoma.

Carcinosarcoma

Carcinosarcoma had previously been considered a mixed epithelial-mesenchymal tumor but is now considered a subtype of epithelial carcinoma consisting of high-grade carcinomatous and sarcomatous components.[30] These tumors typically present in postmenopausal women aged more than 60 years.[33] While imaging diagnosis is challenging because of lack of distinguishing features, when compared to HGSC, carcinosarcomas on MR imaging are more likely to demonstrate hemorrhage, necrosis, and "stained-glass appearance," defined as variable signal intensities of tumor components on both T1-and T2-weighted imaging.[41] The tumors are also characteristically large, with a mean size of 14 cm.

Mixed Carcinoma

Lastly, mixed carcinoma has also been introduced as a very uncommon subtype of epithelial ovarian tumor and is diagnosed when at least two distinct tumor types are present on histology.[30,33]

DIAGNOSTIC CRITERIA

Various systems exist for the classification of ovarian lesions. Imaging features of ovarian malignancy on MR imaging can be aggregated using the ADNEX MR scoring system, which categorizes the lesions into a 5-point system of benign, probably benign, indeterminate, or probably malignant with a sensitivity and specificity of up to 94.9% and 96.6% for malignancy, respectively.[42,43] Not only does the ADNEX MR scoring system standardize lesion evaluation, but it also serves to guide clinical recommendations. The ADNEX MR scoring system takes advantage of the imaging characteristics obtained from the protocol as outlined previously.

The American College of Radiology Ovarian-Adnexal Reporting and Data Systems (O-RADS) MRI standardized reporting system is a revision of the ADNEX MR system to parallel the other "RADS" reporting systems (eg, BI-RADS, LI-RADS) for radiologic reporting. It establishes a consistent lexicon in MR imaging descriptors of lesion morphology. The O-RADS MRI standardized reporting system aligned these morphologic descriptors with the risk stratifications system derived from the ADNEX MR data into seven major categories consisting of physiologic and nonphysiological observations based on size, lesion components, shape or contour of the solid component, and MR imaging signal characteristics and enhancement pattern as well as ancillary findings.[44] These systems were established with the goal of further assisting in lesion characterization and treatment planning by improving communication between radiologists and clinicians.[44,45]

DIFFERENTIAL DIAGNOSIS

There are many potential mimics of malignancy. Two notable examples include struma ovarii and polypoid endometriosis as their MR imaging appearance is often indistinguishable from malignancy.

In the case of struma ovarii, malignant elements may, in fact, be present in 5% to 10%.[46,47] Struma ovarii is a subtype of mature ovarian teratoma consisting of thyroid tissue and can appear as a mixed solid and cystic mass.[21] Some cystic areas demonstrate variable signal intensity on T1-and T2-weighted sequences and some may seem hypointense on both T1-and T2-weighted sequences

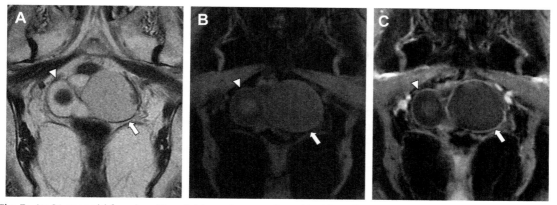

Fig. 7. An 81-year-old female with a right ovarian mass found incidentally on ultrasound for evaluation for right lower extremity swelling. Coronal T2-weighted (*A*) and coronal T1-weighted fat saturated precontrast (*B*) MR images demonstrate a predominantly cystic mass with intermediate signal intensity of the left cystic component (*arrows*) compared with the right (*arrowheads*) due to different concentrations of colloidal material. There was no enhancement of these cystic components on coronal T1-weighted contrast-enhanced image (*C*). Struma ovarii was found on pathology.

because of colloidal material (**Fig. 7**).[21,48] Patients may present with thyrotoxicosis.

Polypoid endometriosis is a distinct subtype of endometriosis with histologic features of an endometrial polyp.[49] In contrast to classic endometriosis which occurs in premenopausal women, polypoid endometriosis occurs in older women with exposure to hormone replacement therapy

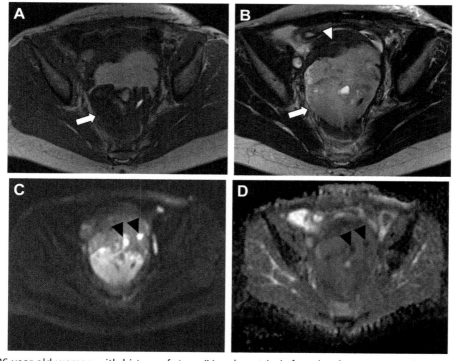

Fig. 8. A 36-year-old woman with history of stage IV endometriosis found to have a new pelvic mass. Axial T1-weighted MR image (*A*) demonstrates a T1-isointense polypoid mass (*arrows*) with T2-hyperintense signal similar to the uterine endometrium (*arrowhead*) on axial T2-weighted image (*B*). The adjacent homogeneously T1 hyperintense portion containing foci of restricted diffusion on DWI [b = 1000] (*C*) and ADC (*D*) sequences (*black arrowheads*) is favored to represent underlying endometriosis. The patient did not receive intravenous contrast due to renal impairment. The mass was resected, demonstrating polypoid endometriosis.

and tamoxifen.[49] On imaging, the polypoid mass demonstrates features similar to the uterine endometrium: hyperintense signal on T2-weighted imaging with a peripherally hypointense, fibrotic rim, and enhancement similar to the endometrium associated with a distinct lack of restricted diffusion (**Fig. 8**).[49] While the diagnosis is ultimately made histopathologically, the described imaging features should prompt consideration of this diagnosis, which could prevent unnecessary surgical intervention.

SUMMARY

MR imaging is a valuable tool to distinguish malignant ovarian lesions from benign and to further subtype malignant tumors, which has important implications for guiding treatment strategies. Communication of MR imaging findings and the clinical utility of MR imaging in guiding the treatment of ovarian malignancies is further enhanced by recent improvements in standardized reporting systems, such as the ADNEX MR scoring system and the O-RADS MRI standardized lexicon for morphologic descriptors and risk stratification. Appropriate performance of MR imaging examinations to incorporate sequences that provide the most clinically relevant information is foundational to these goals.

CLINICS CARE POINTS

- Advanced MR imaging techniques, such as diffusion-weighted and dynamic contrast imaging, improve accuracy in distinguishing benign from malignant ovarian lesions.

- Malignant epithelial ovarian tumors are commonly seen as mixed cystic and solid masses with enhancement and restricted diffusion of the solid components.

- Benign lesions with restricted diffusion are usually identified by careful examination of additional sequences.

DISCLOSURE

L. Xu has nothing to disclose. S.I. Lee receives royalties from Springer and Wolters Kluwer and editor honorarium from the Radiological Society of North America. A. Kilcoyne is an author on "Hysterosalpingography" for UpToDate, Wolters Kluwer and Panel Chair for Gynecologic and Obstetric Imaging, Panel 2, American College of Radiology Appropriateness Criteria.

REFERENCES

1. Siegel RL, Miller KD, Fuchs HE, et al. Cancer Statistics, 2021. CA: a Cancer J clinicians 2021;71(1):7–33.
2. Thomassin-Naggara I, Bazot M, Daraï E, et al. Epithelial ovarian tumors: value of dynamic contrast-enhanced mr imaging and correlation with tumor angiogenesis. Radiology 2008;248(1):148–59.
3. Javadi S, Ganeshan DM, Qayyum A, et al. Ovarian Cancer, the Revised FIGO Staging System, and the Role of Imaging. AJR Am J roentgenology 2016;206(6):1351–60.
4. Expert Panel on Women's I, Kang SK, Reinhold C, et al. Acr appropriateness criteria® staging and follow-up of ovarian cancer. J Am Coll Radiol 2018;15(5S):S198–207.
5. Masch WR, Daye D, Lee SI. MR Imaging for Incidental Adnexal Mass Characterization. Magn Reson Imaging Clin N Am 2017;25(3):521–43.
6. Chandrashekhara SH, Thulkar S, Srivastava DN, et al. Pre-operative evaluation of peritoneal deposits using multidetector computed tomography in ovarian cancer. Br J Radiol 2011;84(997):38–43.
7. Rettenmaier NB, Rettenmaier CR, Wojciechowski T, et al. The utility and cost of routine follow-up procedures in the surveillance of ovarian and primary peritoneal carcinoma: a 16-year institutional review. Br J Cancer 2010;103(11):1657–62.
8. Mutch DG, Prat J. 2014 FIGO staging for ovarian, fallopian tube and peritoneal cancer. Gynecol Oncol 2014;133(3):401–4.
9. Prat J. Staging classification for cancer of the ovary, fallopian tube, and peritoneum. Int J Gynaecol Obstet official Organ Int Fed Gynaecol Obstet 2014;124(1):1–5.
10. Tempany CM, Zou KH, Silverman SG, et al. Staging of advanced ovarian cancer: comparison of imaging modalities–report from the Radiological Diagnostic Oncology Group. Radiology 2000;215(3):761–7.
11. Atri M, Alabousi A, Reinhold C, et al. ACR Appropriateness Criteria(®) Clinically Suspected Adnexal Mass, No Acute Symptoms. J Am Coll Radiol 2019;16(5s):S77–93.
12. Rendi MH. Epithelial carcinoma of the ovary, fallopian tube, and peritoneum: histopathology. In: Post TW editor. UpToDate. UpToDate; 2021. Available at: https://www.uptodate.com/contents/epithelial-carcinoma-of-the-ovary-fallopian-tube-and-peritoneum-histopathology. Accessed July 3, 2021.
13. Bent CL, Sahdev A, Rockall AG, et al. MRI appearances of borderline ovarian tumours. Clin Radiol 2009;64(4):430–8.
14. Shetty M. Imaging and differential diagnosis of ovarian cancer. Semin Ultrasound CT MR 2019;40(4):302–18.

15. Sohaib SA, Mills TD, Sahdev A, et al. The role of magnetic resonance imaging and ultrasound in patients with adnexal masses. Clin Radiol 2005;60(3):340–8.

16. Iyer VR, Lee SI. MRI, CT, and PET/CT for ovarian cancer detection and adnexal lesion characterization. AJR Am J roentgenology 2010;194(2):311–21.

17. Tanaka YO, Yoshizako T, Nishida M, et al. Ovarian carcinoma in patients with endometriosis: MR imaging findings. AJR Am J roentgenology 2000;175(5): 1423–30.

18. Davarpanah AH, Kambadakone A, Holalkere NS, et al. Diffusion MRI of uterine and ovarian masses: identifying the benign lesions. Abdom Radiol 2016; 41(12):2466–75.

19. Zhao SH, Qiang JW, Zhang GF, et al. Diffusion-weighted MR imaging for differentiating borderline from malignant epithelial tumours of the ovary: pathological correlation. Eur Radiol 2014;24(9):2292–9.

20. Jung SE, Lee JM, Rha SE, et al. Ct and mr imaging of ovarian tumors with emphasis on differential diagnosis. RadioGraphics 2002;22(6):1305–25.

21. Foti PV, Attinà G, Spadola S, et al. MR imaging of ovarian masses: classification and differential diagnosis. Insights Imaging 2016;7(1):21–41.

22. Desai A, Xu J, Aysola K, et al. Epithelial ovarian cancer: An overview. World J Transl Med 2014;3(1):1–8.

23. Elsherif S, Javadi S, Viswanathan C, et al. Low-grade epithelial ovarian cancer: what a radiologist should know. BJR 2019;92(1095):20180571.

24. Skírnisdóttir I, Garmo H, Wilander E, et al. Borderline ovarian tumors in Sweden 1960-2005: trends in incidence and age at diagnosis compared to ovarian cancer. Int J Cancer 2008;123(8):1897–901.

25. Bodurka DC, Deavers MT, Tian C, et al. Reclassification of serous ovarian carcinoma by a 2-tier system: a Gynecologic Oncology Group Study. Cancer 2012;118(12):3087–94.

26. Zeppernick F, Meinhold-Heerlein I. The new FIGO staging system for ovarian, fallopian tube, and primary peritoneal cancer. Arch Gynecol Obstet 2014;290(5):839–42.

27. Meinhold-Heerlein I, Fotopoulou C, Harter P, et al. The new WHO classification of ovarian, fallopian tube, and primary peritoneal cancer and its clinical implications. Arch Gynecol Obstet 2016;293(4): 695–700.

28. Nik NN, Vang R, Shih Ie M, et al. Origin and pathogenesis of pelvic (ovarian, tubal, and primary peritoneal) serous carcinoma. Annu Rev Pathol 2014;9: 27–45.

29. Köbel M, Kalloger SE, Huntsman DG, et al. Differences in tumor type in low-stage versus high-stage ovarian carcinomas. Int J Gynecol Pathol : official J Int Soc Gynecol Pathol 2010;29(3):203–11.

30. Turashvili G, Lastra R. What's new in gynecologic pathology 2021: ovary and fallopian tube. J Pathol Translational Med 2021;55(5):366–7.

31. Kurman RJ. Origin and molecular pathogenesis of ovarian high-grade serous carcinoma. Ann Oncol : official J Eur Soc Med Oncol 2013;24(Suppl 10): x16–21.

32. Ganeshan D, Bhosale P, Wei W, et al. Increase in post-therapy tumor calcification on CT scan is not an indicator of response to therapy in low-grade serous ovarian cancer. Abdom Radiol 2016;41(8): 1589–95.

33. WHO Classification of Tumours Editorial Board. Female genital tumours. Lyon (France): International Agency for Research on Cancer; 2020. WHO classification of tumours series, 5th edition.; vol. 4).

34. Ali RH, Seidman JD, Luk M, et al. Transitional cell carcinoma of the ovary is related to high-grade serous carcinoma and is distinct from malignant brenner tumor. Int J Gynecol Pathol : official J Int Soc Gynecol Pathol 2012;31(6):499–506.

35. Seidman JD, Kurman RJ. Pathology of ovarian carcinoma. Hematology/Oncology Clin North America. 2003;17(4):909–25, vii.

36. Mangili G, Bergamini A, Taccagni G, et al. Unraveling the two entities of endometrioid ovarian cancer: a single center clinical experience. Gynecol Oncol 2012;126(3):403–7.

37. Duska LR, Garrett L, Henretta M, et al. When 'never-events' occur despite adherence to clinical guidelines: the case of venous thromboembolism in clear cell cancer of the ovary compared with other epithelial histologic subtypes. Gynecol Oncol 2010;116(3): 374–7.

38. Takahama J, Ascher SM, Hirohashi S, et al. Borderline Brenner tumor of the ovary: MRI findings. Abdom Imaging 2004;29(4):528–30.

39. Moon WJ, Koh BH, Kim SK, et al. Brenner tumor of the ovary: CT and MR findings. J Comput Assist tomography 2000;24(1):72–6.

40. Takeuchi M, Matsuzaki K, Sano N, et al. Malignant Brenner tumor with transition from benign to malignant components: computed tomographic and magnetic resonance imaging findings with pathological correlation. J Comput Assist tomography 2008;32(4):553–4.

41. Saida T, Mori K, Tanaka YO, et al. Carcinosarcoma of the ovary: MR and clinical findings compared with high-grade serous carcinoma. Jpn J Radiol 2021; 39(4):357–66.

42. Thomassin-Naggara I, Aubert E, Rockall A, et al. Adnexal masses: development and preliminary validation of an MR imaging scoring system. Radiology 2013;267(2):432–43.

43. Basha MAA, Abdelrahman HM, Metwally MI, et al. Validity and Reproducibility of the ADNEX MR Scoring System in the Diagnosis of Sonographically Indeterminate Adnexal Masses. J Magn Reson Imaging : JMRI 2021;53(1):292–304.

44. Reinhold C, Rockall A, Sadowski EA, et al. Ovarian-adnexal reporting lexicon for mri: a white paper of the acr ovarian-adnexal reporting and data systems mri committee. J Am Coll Radiol 2021;18(5):713–29.

45. Adusumilli S, Hussain HK, Caoili EM, et al. MRI of sonographically indeterminate adnexal masses. AJR Am J roentgenology 2006;187(3):732–40.

46. Robboy SJ, Scully RE. Strumal carcinoid of the ovary: an analysis of 50 cases of a distinctive tumor composed of thyroid tissue and carcinoid. Cancer 1980;46(9):2019–34.

47. Yamashita Y, Hatanaka Y, Takahashi M, et al. Struma ovarii: MR appearances. Abdom Imaging 1997; 22(1):100–2.

48. Park SB, Kim JK, Kim KR, et al. Imaging findings of complications and unusual manifestations of ovarian teratomas. RadioGraphics 2008;28(4):969–83.

49. Ghafoor S, Lakhman Y, Park KJ, et al. Polypoid endometriosis: a mimic of malignancy. Abdom Radiol 2020;45(6):1776–82.

50. Mansour SM, Saraya S, El-Faissal Y. Semi-quantitative contrast-enhanced MR analysis of indeterminate ovarian tumours: when to say malignancy? Br J Radiol 2015;88(1053):20150099.

51. McDermott S, Oei TN, Iyer VR, et al. MR imaging of malignancies arising in endometriomas and extraovarian endometriosis. RadioGraphics 2012;32(3): 845–63.

MR Imaging of Germ Cell and Sex Cord Stromal Tumors

Jacob R. Mitchell, MD, Evan S. Siegelman, MD,
Karthik M. Sundaram, MD, PhD*

KEYWORDS

- Germ cell • Sex cord stromal • Teratoma • Dysgerminoma • Granulosa • Fibroma • Thecoma

KEY POINTS

- Patient demographics, clinical findings, and hormonal laboratory values combined with MR imaging findings can suggest that an adnexal mass is a germ cell or sex cord stromal tumor.
- The use of fat-suppression techniques to detect bulk fat and chemical shift imaging to characterize microscopic fat is helpful for differentiation among sex cord stromal and germ cell tumors.
- The presence of low T2 signal intensity within a solid adnexal neoplasm can suggest a diagnosis of fibroma or fibrothecoma.

CLINICAL PEARLS

- The most common complication of mature cystic teratoma (MCT) is torsion, which affects up to 15% of lesions.
- Although small (<2 cm) enhancing foci are occasionally present in benign MCT, larger areas of enhancement suggest malignant transformation. Other risk factors for malignancy include age greater than 50 years, tumor size greater than 10 cm, and elevated CA125 levels.
- Although MCT and immature teratoma (IT) can contain bulk fat, the amount of fat within ITs tends to be more variable with some lesions having minimal to no fat. Intralesional hemorrhage is also commonly identified in IT, a feature rarely present in MCT.
- Systemically treated immature teratoma can undergo retroconversion, a phenomena whereby immature components differentiate into mature tissues resembling MCT on imaging, and remain stable for long periods of time.
- Up to 5% of women with struma ovarii present with signs and symptoms of hyperthyroidism.
- Granulosa cell tumors represent the most common estrogen-secreting ovarian neoplasm and the most common ovarian tumor to cause clinical hyperestrogenism.
- Sertoli-Leydig cell tumor is the most common androgen-producing ovarian tumor.
- Thecomas are usually hormonally active, commonly secreting estrogen. Consider thecoma/fibrothecoma when encountering a low T2 signal mass with concomitant widening of the endometrial complex.
- Although steroid cell tumor and Leydig cell tumors often secrete testosterone and cause virilization, stromal luteomas can secrete estrogen and cause clinical hyperestrogenism.

Department of Radiology, Hospital of the University of Pennsylvania, One Silverstein, 3400 Spruce Street, Philadelphia, PA 19104-4283, USA
* Corresponding author.
E-mail address: Karthik.Sundaram@pennmedicine.upenn.edu

Magn Reson Imaging Clin N Am 31 (2023) 65–78
https://doi.org/10.1016/j.mric.2022.07.003
1064-9689/23/© 2022 Elsevier Inc. All rights reserved.

Abbreviations	
MCT	Mature Cystic Teratoma
GCT	Germ Cell Tumor
IT	Immature Teratoma
GRCT	Granulosa Cell Tumor
SCST	Sex Cord Stromal Tumor

INTRODUCTION

Nonepithelial ovarian neoplasms including germ cell tumors (GCTs) and sex cord stromal tumors (SCSTs) represent a significant portion of benign and malignant ovarian neoplasms, usually affecting women younger than the age of 50 years. GCTs represent 15% to 20% of all ovarian neoplasms (second most common ovarian neoplasm), whereas SCSTs represent 5% to 10% of all ovarian neoplasms (**Table 1**).[1] Both tumor types share overlapping imaging and clinical features that can make diagnosis challenging. Pathologic overlap is also possible as gonadoblastoma and mixed GCT-SCST demonstrate germ and sex cord stromal cell derivatives. This review discusses more commonly encountered GCTs and SCSTs with notable MR imaging and clinical characteristics to aid differential diagnosis and help guide treatment.

GERM CELL TUMORS

GCTs originate from primordial germ cells. Histologically, GCTs include mature teratoma, immature teratoma (IT), dysgerminoma, endodermal sinus/yolk sac tumor, embryonal carcinoma, choriocarcinoma, and mixed tumors (**Box 1**). Benign mature cystic teratoma (MCT) is the most common subtype, representing approximately 70% of all GCTs.[2] The other nonteratomatous tumor subtypes are the malignant GCTs, accounting for 3% to 5% of malignant ovarian neoplasms.[3,4] Imaging findings are detailed below and summarized in **Table 2**.

Table 1
Most common ovarian tumors

Ovarian Tumor Type	Percent of All Ovarian Neoplasms	Percent of All Malignant Ovarian Neoplasms
Epithelial	60%–70%	85%–90%
Germ cell	15%–20%	2%–5%
Sex cord stromal	5%–10%	3%–8%
Metastases (eg, Krukenberg)	10%	5%

Box 1
WHO classification of germ cell tumors of the ovary

Dysgerminoma

Yolk sac tumor (endodermal sinus tumor)

Mature teratoma

Immature teratoma

Monodermal teratoma

   Struma ovarii

   Carcinoid

   Neuroectodermal tumors

Embryonal carcinoma

Choriocarcinoma

Mixed forms

WHO, World Health Organization.

Source. – WHO Classification of Tumors Editorial Board. Female Genital Tumors: WHO Classification of Tumors, 5th ed.; IARC: Lyon, France, 2020; Volume 4

Table 2
MR imaging characteristics of common GCTs of the ovary

GCTs of the Ovary	MR Imaging Characteristics
Mature teratoma	Encapsulated, unilocular/multilocular cystic mass containing bulk and microscopic fat; Rokitansky nodule containing calcifications
Immature teratoma	Large, heterogenous solid to cystic mass containing scattered foci of fat, hemorrhage, and calcification
Struma ovarii	Encapsulated, complex solid/multiloculated cystic mass containing fluids of variable signal characteristics (stained glass appearance)
Carcinoid	Heterogeneous, hypervascular solid mass
Dysgerminoma	Large, encapsulated, homogenous solid mass with low-signal enhancing fibrovascular septa and restricted diffusion

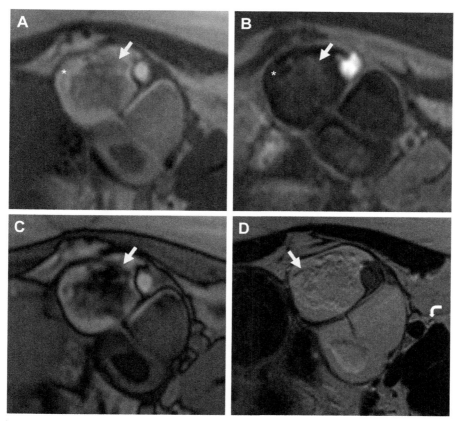

Fig. 1. MR imaging depiction of a benign MCT in a 37-year-old woman. (*A*) In-phase T1-weighted image shows a right ovarian mass containing low, intermediate (*arrow*), and high signal intensity (*asterisk*) components. (*B*) Fat-suppressed T1-weighted image shows marked loss of signal intensity in the portion of the MCT composed of bulk fat (*asterisk*) with less noticeable signal loss in those components that were of intermediate signal intensity (*arrows*) on the in-phase image. (*C*) Opposed-phase image shows greater loss of signal (*arrow*) within the intermediate signal intensity components in *A*. In- and opposed-phase imaging is the technique of choice for showing adipocytes and nonfatty tissue within the same voxel of MCTs. (*D*) T2-weighted image shows a chemical shift artifact in the frequency encoding direction (*straight arrow*) at the interface of the fatty and nonfatty elements in the MCT. Note a similar artifact at the interface of a vein coursing through the pelvic retroperitoneal fat (*curved arrow*).

Mature Cystic Teratoma

Mature cystic teratoma (MCT), also known as dermoid cyst, is the most common GCT (>95% of all ovarian teratomas).[2] Typically, ovarian MCTs are asymptomatic and incidentally diagnosed or when associated complications (eg, torsion, mass effect, rupture, infection) cause symptoms. They are usually encountered in younger women with an average age of 30.[5] MCTs are thought to arise from a single totipotent primordial germ cell after a defective first meiotic division.[6] Because these cells migrate from the allantois of the hindgut to the gonads during embryogenesis, GCTs can form in a variety of midline locations from the head to the sacrum; however, the gonads are the most common location.[7] MCTs are composed

exclusively of well-differentiated mature tissues from more than one of the three germ cell layers (ectoderm, mesoderm, and endoderm). Ectodermal derivatives, such as skin and glia, are usually present. Mesodermal tissues, such as fat, bone, and muscle, are present in up to 90% of lesions. Endodermal components, such as gastrointestinal and respiratory epithelium, are less frequent, identified in approximately one-quarter of lesions.[5,6,8] MCTs often contain a "dermoid plug" or "Rokitansky nodule," which is a raised protuberance along the inner surface of the lesion wall commonly containing teeth, bone, fat, and hair.

On imaging, MCTs most commonly present as an encapsulated unilocular cystic mass.[5,7] However, multilocular/multiseptated MCTs also occur.

MCTs are bilateral in 10% of cases.[6,7] Correlating with pathology, MCTs often contain bulk fat either within sebaceous fluid or adipose tissue, the most specific finding, reportedly seen in up to 93% of tumors.[5,7] On MR imaging, adipose tissue appears hyperintense on T1-weighted images (T1WI) and moderately hyperintense on non-fat-suppressed T2-weighted images (T2WI) (**Fig. 1**). Sebaceous fluid appears hyperintense on T1WI sequences with more variable appearance on T2WI, usually appearing close to that of adipose tissue, although occasionally T2 hypointense.[5,6] Those components comprised entirely of bulk fat show signal suppression on fat-suppressed T1WI (**Fig. 1B**), whereas components composed of admixed fat and water show signal loss on opposed-phase imaging (**Fig. 1C**) when compared with a corresponding in-phase image (**Fig. 1A**). Chemical shift artifact at the interfaces of intralesional fat and adjacent water containing tissue on T2WI is an additional specific sign denoting the presence of macroscopic fat and non-fat-containing tissue within a single lesion (see **Fig. 1D**). If immiscible sebum and aqueous fluids are present in a single space, a pathognomonic fat-fluid level is seen with intervening chemical shift artifact.[9] In addition to characteristic fatty components, MCTs often contain squamous material that appears T1 hypointense and T2 hyperintense.[6] Keratinoid substances when present display hyperintensity on T2WI; hypointensity on T1WI; and unlike serous fluid with similar imaging characteristics, show diffusion restriction.[7,9] Floating hair within the lesions usually appears T2 hypointense. Calcifications (bone and teeth), if present, are commonly localized within the Rokitansky nodule and are more accurately detected with radiography and sonography.[7]

Torsion, the most common complication of MCT, affects up to 16% of lesions.[6] Imaging findings include tumoral wall thickening, edema, hemorrhage, adnexal inflammatory changes, hemoperitoneum, twisting of the vascular pedicle, and uterine deviation toward the side of the torsion (**Fig. 2**).[5,6] Torsed MCTs are larger on average than uncomplicated lesions, with a mean diameter of 11 cm compared with 6 cm.[5] Although larger lesions are predisposed to torsion, this size disparity is possibly the result of torsion rather than the cause of it.[5] Rupture is a rare complication affecting up to 3.8% of cases.[6] Imaging findings include inflammatory stranding, hemoperitoneum, and dispersed fat within the peritoneal cavity.[6] Chronic rupture/long-standing leakage can incite granulomatous peritonitis, which can mimic peritoneal carcinomatosis or tuberculosis, with ascites and nodular peritoneal enhancement.[10] Malignant

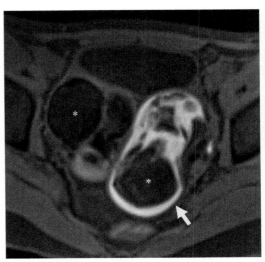

Fig. 2. MR imaging depiction of bilateral MCT with associated left ovarian torsion in a 28-year-old woman with left lower quadrant pain. Fat-suppressed T1-weighted image shows bilateral MCT containing suppressed bulk fat (*asterisks*). The left MCT also contains nonsuppressing intrinsically T1 hyperintense hemorrhage (*arrow*) representing acute ovarian torsion that was confirmed at subsequent laparoscopic resection.

transformation is a rare complication effecting between 0.5% and 3% of MCTs.[6,10,11] Squamous cell carcinoma is the most common type, representing more than 80% of malignant MCTs.[7,11] Risk factors for malignant transformation include age greater than 50 years, tumor size greater than 10 cm, and elevated CA125 levels.[10,11,12] Imaging findings include large tumor diameter, large irregular solid components, interval enlargement of solid portions or enlargement of the Rokitansky nodule, obscuration of intratumoral fat, gross invasion of surrounding tissues, and distant metastatic disease (**Fig. 3**).[6,10,12] Although small (<2 cm) benign enhancing foci are occasionally present, larger areas of enhancement can suggest malignancy (**Fig. 3B**).[13] Other complications include hormone excretion or autoimmune phenomena, such as anti-*N*-methyl-D-aspartate encephalitis.

MCTs have a growth rate of less than 2 mm per year.[7] Because MCTs are almost invariably benign, laparoscopic cystectomy with preservation of the ipsilateral ovary is the surgical treatment of choice and is usually curative. Although an arbitrary maximum diameter of 5 to 6 cm is sometimes used as the criteria for surgical resection, there is no evidence-based consensus on a specific lesion size at which surgery should be considered.[14]

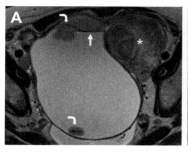 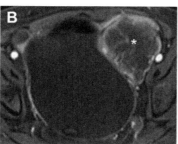 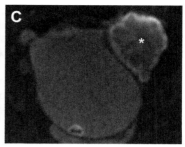

Fig. 3. MR imaging depiction of squamous cell carcinoma arising in an MCT from a 68-year-old woman. (A) T2-weighted image shows an encapsulated MCT containing pathognomonic fat-fluid level with intervening chemical shift (straight arrow), floating debris (curved arrows), and large heterogenous solid component along its left lateral border (asterisk). (B) Postcontrast fat-suppressed T1-weighted image demonstrates heterogenous enhancement of the solid malignant component. (C) High B value diffusion-weighted image shows peripheral diffusion restriction within the solid portion.

Immature Teratoma

IT is the third most common GCT (second to dysgerminoma), and second most common subtype of teratoma. ITs comprise 10% of encountered germ cell neoplasms usually affecting patients in the second decade of life.[5,6] Unlike most MCTs, IT is malignant constituting approximately 40% of all malignant GCTs.[5,6] Tumor markers (eg, β-human chorionic gonadotropin) may be elevated in IT.[6]

Histologically, ITs can contain tissues from all three germ layers similar to its mature counterpart. However, unlike MCT, they contain immature elements most frequently in the form of immature neuroepithelium. The amount present has been shown to have prognostic implications, and helps to determine the grade of tumor.[6]

The typical imaging appearance of IT is that of a large heterogenous solid to cystic mass, with an ill-defined/discontinuous capsule (Fig. 4A).[5] Bilaterality is seen in 10% to 20% of cases, and contralateral MCT is present in approximately 10% of cases.[5,6] Lesions are typically larger than MCTs, with sizes ranging from 14 to 25 cm on average compared with 7 cm.[5] Serous, mucinous, or sebaceous fluids usually comprise the nonsolid elements on the tumors.[5,6] The solid elements may contain small foci of bulk and/or admixed lipid, which is characterized with similar MR imaging techniques described in the MCT discussion (Fig. 4B, C).[5,6] The amount of fat within ITs tends to be more variable than what is typically seen in MCT, with some lesions having minimal to no fat.[6] Calcifications may also be present, usually appearing diffusely throughout the solid portions as compared with confined calcification in the Rokitansky nodules of MCTs.[6] Another feature of IT is the presence of intralesional hemorrhage, which is seen as hyperintense methemoglobin on T1WI.[5]

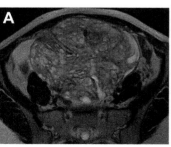 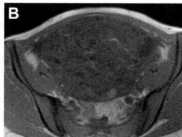 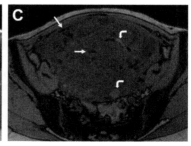

Fig. 4. MR imaging illustration of lipid within a mature and immature teratoma of the left ovary in a 33-year-old woman. The serum α-fetoprotein was 1200 IU/mL (normal <5). (A) T2-weighted image shows a heterogenous mass with cystic and solid components. (B) In-phase T1-weighted image exhibits intermediate and high signal intensity components, and low signal intensity components corresponding to cystic foci in A. (C) Opposed-phase image shows loss of signal in those regions of tumor that have admixed fat and water components (straight arrows) and residual high signal intensity components without adjacent etching artifact representing foci of intratumoral protein or hemorrhage (curved arrows). This lesion showed regions of restricted diffusion and solid enhancement (not shown).

An unusual complication of IT occurs when tumor cells implant throughout the peritoneal cavity and differentiate into mature glial tissue (gliomatosis peritonei), often indistinguishable from malignant carcinomatosis on imaging.[6,10]

Treatment of IT depends on tumor stage and grade, with low-grade disease requiring surgery alone, and higher-grade disease treated with surgery and systemic chemotherapy.[6] Systemically treated IT can occasionally undergo retroconversion, a phenomena whereby immature components differentiate into mature tissues resembling MCT on imaging, and remain stable for long periods of time.[5]

Monodermal Teratoma

Monodermal teratoma is the least common type of teratoma, containing tissues solely or predominately from a single germ cell layer. Common subtypes include struma ovarii and neuroendocrine/carcinoid tumors with the neuroectodermal subtype rarely seen. A rare composite tumor termed stromal carcinoid contains neuroendocrine/carcinoid and thyroid tissue.[10]

Struma Ovarii

Struma ovarii comprise 1% to 3% of ovarian teratomas.[5,6,10] They are lesions composed solely or predominantly of thyroid tissue, defined as mature teratoma containing at least 50% thyroid cells forming colloid-filled follicles of different sizes.[6] Although most lesions are benign, 5% to 10% of lesions are malignant accounting for approximately 0.5% of all malignant ovarian tumors.[6,10] Like native thyroid carcinoma, serum thyroglobulin is used as a tumor marker.[15] Struma ovarii is most commonly seen in women younger than 40 years of age.[6] Up to 5% of women present with signs and symptoms of hyperthyroidism.[6,10]

On imaging, struma ovarii typically presents as a smoothly marginated complex/multiloculated cystic and solid mass.[5,6,10] Although these lesions often cannot reliably be differentiated from other types of teratomas on imaging, they do not demonstrate intralesional fat, which distinguishes them from MCTs and ITs.[5,6] Prominent cystic spaces are also occasionally seen containing fluids of variable signal characteristics; the so-called "stained glass" appearance has been described (**Fig. 5**).[16] If these spaces contain colloid, they show variable degrees of T2 hypointensity relative to simple fluid based on the viscosity of the colloid.[5,6,10,16] If they contain condensed thyroglobulin and thyroid hormones, they can appear hyperintense on T1WI.[17]

Benign struma ovarii is treated with surgical resection alone. Malignant lesions, which is either

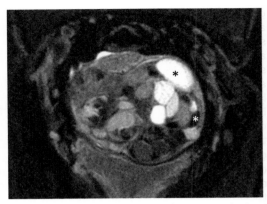

Fig. 5. MR imaging depiction of a "stained glass" appearance of struma ovarii in a 37-year-old woman. Coronal fat-suppressed T2-weighted imaging shows a multilocular mass of the left adnexa that contains locules that vary in signal intensity from isointense to fluid (*black asterisk*) to isointense to muscle (*white asterisk*).

follicular or papillary subtypes, are managed similar to native thyroid malignancy using a multidisciplinary approach including surgery with local excision and thyroidectomy, thyroid-stimulating hormone inhibiting therapy, and radioactive iodine ablation.[15] Surgical removal is curative in the rare cases of struma ovarii–induced hyperthyroidism.[10]

Carcinoid

Differentiated neuroendocrine tumor or carcinoid tumor represents 0.1% of ovarian neoplasms and 1% of all carcinoid tumors.[18] Histologically they are divided into insular, trabecular, stromal, mucinous, and mixed subtypes, with insular being the most common and associated with hormonal production and carcinoid syndrome.[19,20] They usually present in postmenopausal women as heterogeneous, solid, hypervascular masses on imaging.[5,6,19,20] Necrosis is uncommon, although they can show T2 hyperintense mucinous components.[5,19] Lesions are almost always unilateral, although if metastatic disease is present, contralateral ovarian involvement is common.[19] Nuclear medicine somatostatin receptor imaging can also aide in establishing this diagnosis.

Dysgerminoma

Dysgerminoma is the second most common GCT accounting for 1% to 2% of all primary ovarian neoplasms, and most common malignant GCT accounting for approximately one-third of all malignant GCTs.[21,22] Histologically they are identical to testicular seminoma, being composed of undifferentiated germ cell resembling primordial germ cells.[22,23] They can arise at any age, although are most commonly encountered in the second and third decades of life.[22,23] They are associated with gonadal dysgenesis and chromosomal abnormalities.[22,23] Although commonly asymptomatic, they can cause pelvic pain, bloating, menstrual irregularities, and infertility.[21,22] Dysgerminomas commonly produce lactate dehydrogenase and mixed lesions containing syncytiotrophoblasts can also produce β-human chorionic gonadotropin, both which are used as tumor markers if present.[1,21–23] Approximately 75% of tumors are discovered at an early stage.[23] Surgery is typically curative and the prognosis is excellent, with a 5-year survivability approaching 100%.[21,23]

On imaging, dysgerminomas most commonly appear as purely solid, well marginated/encapsulated, multilobulated masses with fibrovascular septa (Fig. 6).[1,21–23] They have a mean diameter of 11.9 cm and are bilateral in 10% to 15% of cases.[1,21] On T1WI, they commonly appear homogenously isointense to hypointense. On T2WI, they display homogenous isointense to hyperintense cellular lobules, with intervening low signal fibrous septa.[1,21–23] The lobules also typically show restricted diffusion because of increased cellularity.[21] Intralesional hemorrhage, necrosis, and cystic change is uncommonly encountered.[21–23] Calcification is also uncommon, although when seen appears in a speckled pattern.[1,21–23] On postcontrast sequences, the septa and the lobules typically show progressive enhancement, with a greater degree of septal enhancement (see Fig. 6B).[1,21–23]

SEX CORD STROMAL TUMORS

SCSTs of the ovary comprise a heterogeneous group of benign and malignant tumors, which represent 5% to 10% of all ovarian neoplasms.[24,25] This class of tumors originate from the specialized cells that surround and support oocytes, comprising the follicles (sex cord) and connective tissues (stroma) of the ovary. The sex cord cells include granulosa and Sertoli cells, and the stromal cells include fibroblasts, Leydig, and theca cells. These cells also contribute to normal ovarian endocrine functions, with granulosa and theca cells producing estrogen, and Leydig and Sertoli cells producing testosterone. Thus, SCSTs form most of the hormone-producing ovarian neoplasms. However, many SCSTs are hormonally inactive and asymptomatic, only diagnosed at the time of imaging or at pathologic examination.

In 2014, the World Health Organizations revised their former classification organizing SCST into three categories based around this histologic grouping (Box 2): pure stromal tumors, pure sex-cord tumors, and mixed SCST.[24] Although these tumors can present at any age, they most commonly occur in women younger than 50 years of age, with a higher incidence in African American women compared with Caucasians.[24,25] Some report 80% of fibromas, thecomas, adult granulosa cell tumors (GRCTs), and sclerosing stromal tumors (SSTs) occur in women younger than 30 years of age.[24] The malignant SCSTs tend to present earlier and follow a less aggressive clinical course with a better overall prognosis as

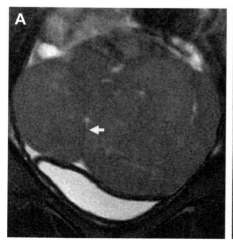
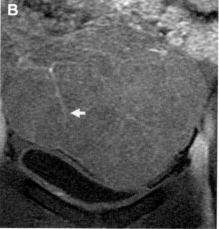

Fig. 6. MR imaging depiction of ovarian dysgerminoma in a 24-year-old woman. (A) Coronal T2-weighted image shows a large encapsulated multilobulated mass anterior to the uterus. The lobules appear hyperintense relative to skeletal muscle, with hypointense septations (arrow). (B) Postcontrast fat-suppressed T1-weighted image shows enhancement of the mass, with the septal enhancement (arrow) greater than the lobular enhancement.

Box 2
WHO classification of sex cord stromal tumors of the ovary

Pure sex cord tumors

  Fibroma

  Cellular Fibroma

  Fibrosarcoma

  Thecoma

  Sclerosing stromal tumor

  Signet-ring stromal tumor

  Microcystic stromal tumor

  Leydig cell tumor

  Steroid cell tumor (benign and malignant)

Pure stromal tumors

  Granulosa cell tumor (Adult and Juvenile)

  Sertoli cell tumors

  Sex cord tumor with annular tubules

Mixed group

  Sertoli-Leydig cell tumors

WHO, World Health Organization.

Adapted from Horta M, Cunha TM. Sex cord-stromal tumors of the ovary: a comprehensive review and update for radiologists. Diagn Interv Radiol. 2015;21(4):277–286. doi:10.5152/dir.2015.34414.

Table 3
MR imaging characteristics of common SCSTs of the ovary

SCSTs of the Ovary	MR Imaging Characteristics
Granulosa cell tumor	Large, complex mixed multiseptated cystic/solid hemorrhagic mass; "sponge-like" appearance, associated uterine changes
Fibroma/ thecoma	Encapsulated, homogenous solid low-signal mass with low-level enhancement
Sclerosing stromal tumor	Encapsulated, heterogenous solid mass with cystic changes; "spoke-wheel" appearance, avid centripetal enhancement
Leydig cell tumor	Small, solid mass containing intracellular lipid with delayed enhancement
Steroid cell tumor	Large, solid mass with/ without cystic spaces, significant intracellular lipid, avid enhancement

compared with the more common, epithelial ovarian malignancies.[24,25] Imaging findings are detailed below and summarized in **Table 3**.

Pure Sex Cord Tumors

Granulosa cell tumor group

GRCTs are the most common malignant SCST accounting for 90% of malignant lesions[25] and represent only 2% to 5% of all ovarian cancers.[24–27] There are two subtypes, adult and juvenile, with the adult type representing approximately 95% of encountered lesions.[24,25] The juvenile subtype affects children and women younger than the age of 30 years while the adult subtype affects early postmenopausal women around the age of 50 years.[24,25] The juvenile subtype is associated with Ollier disease and Maffucci syndrome.[25]

GRCTs represent the most common estrogen secreting ovarian tumor and the most common ovarian tumor to cause clinical hyperestrogenism.[24,26] However, only a minority of lesions (~20%) are symptomatic.[25] Clinical presentation of increased estrogen production vary from amenorrhea to altered menstrual patterns to excessive uterine bleeding with endometrial hyperplasia

reported in 32% to 85% of women and endometrial cancer in 3% to 22% of cases.[24] The presence of increased estrogen also increases the risk of breast cancer.[24] Many GRCTs secrete inhibin B and the unregulated production can lead to infertility. This hormone also represents a tumor marker that is used to assess tumor burden, treatment response, or posttreatment disease recurrence.[24,28] A small subset of GRCTs have also been reported to secrete androgens, which may result in virilization.[24,29]

Both adult and juvenile subtypes have similar imaging characteristics. They are almost invariably unilateral with a mean tumor size of 10 cm for adult subtypes, and 12.5 cm for juvenile subtypes.[25] They most commonly appear as complex multiseptated cystic, mixed multicystic and solid, or heterogenous solid masses, only rarely presenting as unilocular cystic or homogenous solid masses.[24,25,30] They have classically been described as having a "sponge-like" appearance because of their multicystic appearance (**Fig. 7**A). On T2WI, the cystic components can appear hyperintense, with the septations usually appearing hypointense (fibrous), and solid components appearing isointense.[24,25] Intralesional hemorrhage is commonly seen, with the cystic components frequently displaying intrinsic T1 hyperintensity, and fluid-fluid levels (**Fig. 7**).[24,25,30] Solid components enhance

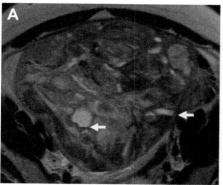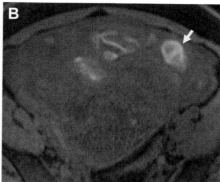

Fig. 7. MR imaging depiction of granulosa cell tumor arising from the right ovary in a 50-year-old woman presenting with abnormal uterine bleeding. Serum inhibin B value was elevated at 820 pg/mL (normal <5). (*A*) T2-weighted image shows a complex "sponge-like" multilocular cystic mass posterior to the uterus, with hypointense septations and fluid-fluid levels (*arrows*). (*B*) Fat-suppressed T1-weighted image shows hyperintense component (*arrow*) representing intralesional hemorrhage.

heterogeneously after contrast administration.[24,25] Because of the hyperestrogenic effects of these lesions, endometrial changes are commonly observed at the time of imaging.

GCTs tend to present at an early stage because of their hormonal activity and have a good overall prognosis. Some 74% to 95% of patients present with stage 1 disease, which has a 10-year survival rate of 82% to 95%.[25,31] Treatment of stage 1 disease usually consists of early surgical resection, with unclear benefit of adjuvant chemotherapy.[25] Less than 40% of patients with stage 1 disease develop recurrence, which tends to happen in a late, unpredictable fashion with intraperitoneal disease.[24,25,31]

Pure Stromal Tumors

Fibroma thecoma group

Fibroma, fibrothecoma, and thecoma represent a spectrum of tumors that arise from the ovarian stroma. Although these lesions are uncommon they constitute most asymptomatic solid ovarian neoplasms.[32] Fibroma, being the most common SCST, accounts for approximately 4% of all ovarian neoplasms.[24–26]

Pure fibromas arise from collagen-producing spindle cells of the ovarian stroma, typically presenting during the fourth decade of life.[24–26,32] They are most often benign, although the rare hypercellular subtypes have malignant potential. These subtypes include the low malignant potential cellular fibroma, which accounts for 10% of lesions, histologically characterized by mild nuclear atypia and increased mitotic activity with four or more mitotic figures per 10 high power field.[24,25] Lesions that display significantly increased cellularity, high mitotic activity, and moderate to severe

nuclear atypia are classified as malignant fibrosarcoma.[24,25]

Thecomas, like fibromas, are also composed of ovarian stromal cells, which typically display lipid-laden cytoplasm and resemble theca cells. These lesions typically occur in postmenopausal women and are less common than fibromas accounting for 0.5% to 1% of ovarian neoplasms.[24,25] Unlike fibromas, they are usually hormonally active, commonly secreting estrogen and rarely androgens.[24,25] Fibrothecoma refers to tumors with intermediate features between fibromas and thecomas. Although fibrothecomas are commonly discussed, they are not part of the World Health Organization classification of stromal tumors.

These pure stromal lesions are usually asymptomatic and discovered incidentally at the time of imaging. That said, larger lesions may cause ovarian torsion, whereas hormonally active thecoma/fibrothecoma can cause symptoms of hyperestrogenism, and more rarely hyperandrogenism. Hyperestrogenism associated with thecoma and fibrothecoma can result in endometrial hyperplasia and carcinoma in 15% and 20-25% of cases, respectively.[25] Lesions can also be associated with various degrees of benign ascites, termed Meigs syndrome. Fibromas/fibrothecoma/thecoma are characteristically benign tumors; if clinically warranted, they are treated with surgical resection. Ascites caused by Meigs syndrome typically resolves after tumor resection.[25]

On imaging, ovarian fibromas typically appear as encapsulated, predominantly solid masses of homogenous low signal on T2WI and T1WI.[25,26,32] Lesions are typically unilateral, although bilateral lesions are seen in Gorlin syndrome, a predisposing condition (**Fig. 8**).[24,32] Larger lesions (>6 cm in one study[32]) are more

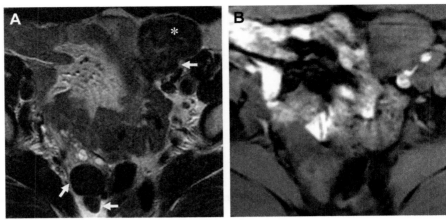

Fig. 8. MR imaging depiction of multiple fibromas in a 25-year-old woman with Gorlin syndrome. (*A*) T2-weighted image shows multiple bilateral well-marginated masses isointense to skeletal muscle suggesting fibrous tissue (*arrows*), all of which are homogenous except for the largest lesion (*asterisk*). (*B*) Contrast-enhanced fat-suppressed T1-weighted image shows low-level mass enhancement.

likely to appear heterogenous because of cystic degeneration, edema, necrosis, and occasionally hemorrhage.[25,26,30] Rarely, lesions can present as mixed solid and cystic (11%), or predominantly cystic lesions (5%).[25] In these atypical cases, the correct identification of low T2 signal intensity components narrows the differential diagnosis to lesions composed of fibrous tissue. Brenner tumor of the ovary is an uncommon, predominantly benign epithelial ovarian neoplasm composed of transitional cells surrounded by fibrosis and can have similar MR imaging appearances to solid ovarian fibroma. Fibromas typically display low-level homogenous delayed enhancement (see **Fig. 8**B), with larger lesions more commonly displaying heterogenous enhancement. Lesions also tend to have low signal intensity on ADC maps, lower on average compared with other SCSTs of the ovary, possibly because of their low intrinsic T2 signal and subsequent "blackout" effect.[25,33] Functional thecomas and fibromas may show diffusion restriction because of their increased cellularity.[33] In cases of Meigs syndrome, tumor size correlates with the presence of ascites.[24]

Thecomas have similar appearance to fibromas on imaging, typically appearing as a homogenous, solid, unilateral ovarian mass. However, they tend to be of higher signal intensity on T2WI, and display higher levels of enhancement, as compared with fibroma.[25,32,33] Larger lesions also tend to have a more heterogeneous appearance, more likely to show cystic changes, and more frequently associated with ascites.[25] Intracellular lipid, a rare histologic feature, is detected on chemical shift imaging if present.[34] Thecomas tend to have similar diffusion-weighted imaging

and ADC values as leiomyomas, although larger lesions can display more heterogenous signal.[24,25] If the tumor is hormonally active, concomitant thickening of the endometrial complex is seen from polyps and/or hyperplasia (**Fig. 9**).

In cases of torsion, lesions demonstrate increased signal intensity on T1WI and T2WI because of congestion and edema, with peripheral areas of high T1 signal because of hemorrhagic infarction and necrosis.[24–26] Additionally, nonspecific findings of torsion are seen such as fallopian tube thickening and hemorrhage, ascites, deviation of the lesion to the twisted side, and a vascular pedicle torsion knot.[26]

Sclerosing stromal tumor

SST of the ovary represents less than 5% of all ovarian sex cord neoplasms.[24,25] SSTs occur most commonly in young, premenopausal women and rarely premenarchal young girls.[24–26] They are clinically benign lesions, occasionally discovered incidentally on imaging as well as in the setting of pelvic pain. They are rarely associated with menstrual irregularities (due to secreted estrogens and/or androgens) or associated with ascites.[24] Surgical resection is curative.[24,25]

Histologically SSTs are characterized by ill-defined pseudolobular cellular architecture separated by edematous stroma, termed by pathologists who described collagenous sclerosis in cellular regions.[24,35] On imaging, these lesions usually present as encapsulated unilateral, heterogenous solid masses with cystic changes.[24,25] The histologic architecture is occasionally reflected on imaging with some lesions displaying a heterogenous spoke-wheel appearance on T2WI, with

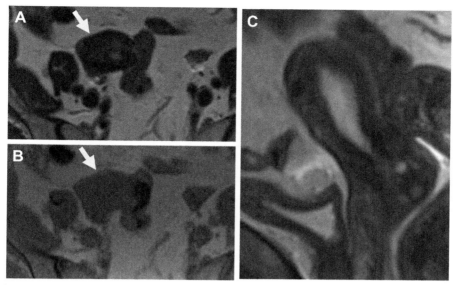

Fig. 9. MR imaging depiction of presumed right ovarian fibrothecoma and endometrial hyperplasia in a 74-year-old woman. (A, B) T2-weighted and in-phase T1-weighted images show a right ovarian mass (arrow) that is iso-intense to psoas muscle. Solid components within an adnexa mass that are T2 isointense to muscle are suggestive of fibrous tissue. (C) Corresponding sagittal T2-weighted image shows a widened endometrial complex suggestive of hyperplasia. The combination of a T2 hypointense adnexa mass and a widened endometrial complex in a postmenopausal woman is suggestive if a fibrothecoma. After discussion with the patient and her gynecologist, the patient opted to undergo therapeutic and diagnostic uterine dilation and curettage and forego the surgical removal of the ovary.

isointense-hypointense pseudolobules separated by hyperintense edematous septa (**Fig. 10**A). A thick capsule usually appears T2 hypointense and is comprised of compressed ovarian stroma, which reflects the slow growing/nonaggressive nature of these lesions.[24,25] Avid, early peripheral enhancement with centripetal filling is seen after contrast administration, reflecting the high vascularity of these lesions (**Fig. 10**B, C).[24,25,36]

Steroid cell tumor group

Steroid cell tumors (SCT) are rare accounting for 0.1% of all ovarian tumors.[24,25,37] SCTs are divided into three subtypes based on their cell of origin: (1) stromal luteomas, (2) Leydig cell tumor, and (3) SCT not otherwise specified (NOS).[37] SCT NOS accounts for most lesions (60%–80%),[24,37] with the other subtypes each accounting for an additional 20% to 25% of lesions.[38] Histologically, they are highly vascular tumors composed of cells resembling typical steroid-secreting cells such as Leydig or adrenocortical cells and contain varying amounts of internal lipid (**Fig. 11**D). The Leydig subtype displays intracellular Reinke crystals, whereas the stromal luteoma and NOS subtypes do not.[24,37]

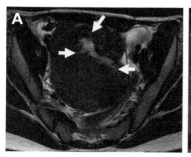
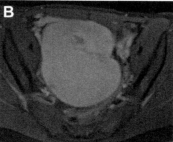
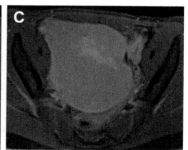

Fig. 10. MR imaging depiction of a sclerosing stromal tumor in an 18-year-old woman. (A) T2-weighted image shows an encapsulated intermediate signal intensity mass with hyperintense edematous septa radiating in a "spoke wheel" appearance (arrows). Dynamic enhanced fat-suppressed T1-weighted images show (B) early mass enhancement with (C) centripetal fill-in on more delayed sequence .

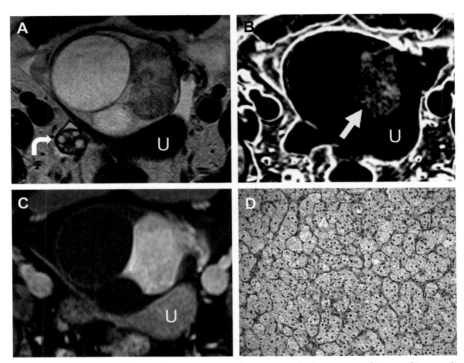

Fig. 11. MR imaging illustration of a lipid-containing androgen-producing sex cord stromal tumor in a 22-year-old woman with hirsutism, oligomenorrhea, and elevated testosterone. (*A*) Axial T2-weighted image shows a solid and cystic left adnexal mass. The right ovary (*curved arrow*) and uterus (U) have a normal appearance. (*B*) Image created by subtracting the opposed-phase image from the in-phase image highlights those voxels that contain both lipid and water protons. The lipid-containing solid components of the mass are shown as high signal intensity (*arrow*). (*C*) Fat-suppressed enhanced T1-weighted image shows enhancement of the solid component of the lesion. (*D*) Hematoxylin-eosin stain (original magnification ×20) shows significant cytoplasmic lipid within the tumor cells. (Image courtesy of Lauren E. Schwartz, MD., Associate Professor of Clinical Pathology and Laboratory Medicine at Penn Medicine).

SCT NOS can present at any age, although with a predilection for younger women with a mean age of 43 years.[24,37] One-third of lesions are clinically malignant, and 50% to 75% of lesions are hormonally active. SCT NOS most commonly secrete testosterone (causing virilization) and rarely secrete estrogen or cortisol.[24,25,37] These lesions are associated with von Hippel-Lindau disease.[25] On imaging, they typically appear as unilateral solid masses with or without small cysts, or occasionally as multilocular cystic masses with mural nodules (**Fig. 11**A).[24,25,36] They are typically larger, with a mean size of 8.4 cm.[24] They show isointensity on T2WI, may demonstrate increased intrinsic T1 signal with out-of-phase signal dropout on dual phase chemical shift imaging because of significant intracellular lipid, and typically show avid enhancement on postcontrast sequences (**Fig. 11**B, C).[24,25]

Leydig and stromal luteoma, as opposed to SCT NOS, are almost invariably benign lesions typically presenting in older postmenopausal females in the fifth to sixth decades of life.[24,25,39] Whereas Leydig cell tumors most commonly present with hyperandrogenic symptoms because of androgen production, stromal luteomas tend to present with hyperestrogenism.[24,25,39] These lesions are typically small, with an average size of 2.4 cm for the Leydig subtype and 1.3 cm for the stromal luteoma subtype.[24,25,39] They both tend to present as unilateral, solid masses. On MR imaging, Leydig cell tumors show variable T2 signal depending on the amount of fibrous stroma present. They occasionally display intrinsic T1 hyperintensity, with out-of-phase signal dropout on dual-phase chemical shift imaging because of intracellular lipid. On postcontrast sequences they exhibit gradual delayed enhancement, and can demonstrate increased signal on diffusion-weighted imaging sequence.[24,25] The MR imaging appearance of stromal luteomas is not well described because of its rarity and small size. Because these lesions are benign, they are treated with surgical excision.

Mixed Sex Cord Stromal Tumors

Sertoli-Leydig cell tumor

Sertoli-Leydig is a rare mixed SCST that is the most common androgen-producing ovarian tumor, usually occurring in women younger than 30 years of age.[25,26] These tumors have variable gross appearance including solid, partially cystic, or completely cystic. On MR imaging, they have a nonspecific appearance with solid components showing variable T2 signal depending on the amount of fibrous tissue present.[25,26] Most lesions are benign (82%–90%) or diagnosed at a low grade/stage and therefore have good prognosis.[25,26,40]

SUMMARY

We present clinical, histologic, and MR imaging features of two less common categories of ovarian neoplasm: the GCT and the SCST. The detection and characterization of lipid on MR imaging can aid in diagnosing some of the germ cell tumors of the ovary. Additional imaging features and clinical findings can also aid radiologists in constructing a differential for mixed solid and cystic adnexal neoplasms. The ability to differentiate benign tumors from possible malignancy can aid in patient management.

DISCLOSURES

- Funding: No funding or research support for this article
- Conflicts of interest/Competing interest: No conflict of interest or competing interests
- Availability of data and material: Not applicable
- Code availability: Not applicable
- Authors' contributions: All authors made substantial contributions to the conception or design of the work; drafted the work or revised it critically for important intellectual content; approved the version to be published; and agree to be accountable for all aspects of the work in ensuring that questions related to the accuracy or integrity of any part of the work are appropriately investigated and resolved.
- Ethics approval: Not applicable
- Consent to participate: Not applicable
- Consent for publication: Not applicable

REFERENCES

1. Jung SE, Lee JM, Sung M, et al. Education exhibit CT and MR imaging of ovarian tumors with emphasis on differential diagnosis. RadioGraphics 2002;22: 1305–25.
2. Evers M, Rechnitzer C, Graem N, et al. Epidemiological study of paediatric germ cell tumours revealed the incidence and distribution that was expected, but a low mortality rate. Acta Paediatr 2017;106(5): 779–85.
3. Smith HO, Berwick M, Verschraegen CF, et al. Incidence and survival rates for female malignant germ cell tumors. Obstet Gynecol 2006;107(5). Available at: https://journals.lww.com/greenjournal/Fulltext/2 006/05000/Incidence_and_Survival_Rates_for_Fem ale_Malignant.19.aspx.
4. Brammer HM 3rd, Buck JL, Hayes WS, et al. From the archives of the AFIP. Malignant germ cell tumors of the ovary: radiologic-pathologic correlation. Radiographics 1990;10(4):715–24.
5. Outwater EK, Siegelman ES, Hunt JL. Ovarian teratomas: tumor types and imaging characteristics. Radiographics 2001;21(2):475–90.
6. Saleh M, Bhosale P, Menias CO, et al. Ovarian teratomas: clinical features, imaging findings and management. Abdom Radiol 2021;46(6):2293–307.
7. Bernot JM, Haeusler KA, Lisanti CJ, et al. Mature cystic teratoma: AIRP Best Cases in Radiologic-Pathologic Correlation. RadioGraphics 2017;37(5): 1401–7.
8. Caruso PA, Marsh MR, Minkowitz S, et al. An intense clinicopathologic study of 305 teratomas of the ovary. Cancer 1971;27(2):343–8.
9. Sahin H, Abdullazade S, Sanci M. Mature cystic teratoma of the ovary: a cutting edge overview on imaging features. Insights Imaging 2017;8(2): 227–41.
10. Magudia K, Menias CO, Bhalla S, et al. Unusual imaging findings associated with germ cell tumors. Radiographics 2019;39(4):1019–35.
11. Li C, Zhang Q, Zhang S, et al. Squamous cell carcinoma transformation in mature cystic teratoma of the ovary: a systematic review. BMC Cancer 2019;19(1): 217.
12. Goudeli C, Varytimiadi A, Koufopoulos N, et al. An ovarian mature cystic teratoma evolving in squamous cell carcinoma: a case report and review of the literature. Gynecol Oncol Rep 2017;19:27–30.
13. Shin HJ, Kim KA, Kim B, et al. Benign enhancing components of mature ovarian teratoma: magnetic resonance imaging features and pathologic correlation. Clin Imaging 2016;40(6):1156–61.
14. Sinha A, Ewies AAA. Ovarian mature cystic teratoma: challenges of surgical management. Obstet Gynecol Int 2016;2016:2390178. https://doi.org/10.1155/2016/2390178.
15. Cui Y, Yao J, Wang S, et al. The clinical and pathological characteristics of malignant struma ovarii: an analysis of 144 published patients. Front Oncol 2021;11:645156.

16. Leite I, Cunha TM, Figueiredo JP, et al. Papillary carcinoma arising in struma ovarii versus ovarian metastasis from primary thyroid carcinoma: a case report and review of the literature. J Radiol Case Rep 2013;7(10):24–33.

17. Joja I, Asakawa T, Mitsumori A, et al. Struma ovarii: appearance on MR images. Abdom Imaging 1998; 23(6):652–6.

18. Zhai L-R, Zhang X-W, Yu T, et al. Primary ovarian carcinoid: two cases report and review of literature. Medicine (Baltimore) 2020;99(40). Available at: https://journals.lww.com/md-journal/Fulltext/2020/10020/Primary_ovarian_carcinoid__Two_cases_report_and.2.aspx.

19. Talerman A. Carcinoid tumors of the ovary. J Cancer Res Clin Oncol 1984;107(2):125–35.

20. Georgescu TA, Bohiltea RE, Varlas V, et al. A 15-year comprehensive literature review of 99 primary ovarian carcinoid tumors. Clin Exp Obstet Gynecol 2022; 49(1). https://doi.org/10.31083/j.ceog4901016.

21. Cacioppa LM, Crusco F, Marchetti F, et al. Magnetic resonance imaging of pure ovarian dysgerminoma: a series of eight cases. Cancer Imaging 2021; 21(1):1–7.

22. Shaaban AM, Rezvani M, Elsayes KM, et al. Ovarian malignant germ cell tumors: cellular classification and clinical and imaging features. Radiographics 2014;34(3):777–801.

23. Heo SH, Kim JW, Shin SS, et al. Review of ovarian tumors in children and adolescents: radiologic-pathologic correlation. Radiographics 2014;34(7): 2039–55.

24. Horta M, Cunha TM. Sex cord-stromal tumors of the ovary: a comprehensive review and update for radiologists. Diagn Interv Radiol 2015;21(4):277–86.

25. Javadi S, Ganeshan DM, Jensen CT, et al. Comprehensive review of imaging features of sex cord-stromal tumors of the ovary. Abdom Radiol 2021; 46(4):1519–29.

26. Jung SE, Rha SE, Lee JM, et al. CT and MRI findings of sex cord-stromal tumor of the ovary. AJR Am J Roentgenol 2005;185(1):207–15.

27. Koukourakis GV, Kouloulias VE, Koukourakis MJ, et al. Granulosa cell tumor of the ovary: tumor review. Integr Cancer Ther 2008;7(3):204–15.

28. Zhang H, Zhang H, Gu S, et al. MR findings of primary ovarian granulosa cell tumor with focus on the differentiation with other ovarian sex cord-stromal tumors. J Ovarian Res 2018;11.

29. Adefris M, Fekadu E. Postmenopausal mild hirsutism and hyperandrogenemia due to granulosa cell tumor of the ovary: a case report. J Med Case Rep 2017;11(1):242.

30. Montoriol P-F, Mons A, Da Ines D, et al. Fibrous tumours of the ovary: aetiologies and MRI features. Clin Radiol 2013;68(12):1276–83.

31. Matsuki M, Numoto I, Suzuki A, et al. Magnetic resonance imaging of recurrent adult granulosa cell tumor of the ovary: a retrospective analysis of 11 cases. J Comput Assist Tomogr 2020;44(6):887–92.

32. Shinagare AB, Meylaerts LJ, Laury AR, et al. MRI features of ovarian fibroma and fibrothecoma with histopathologic correlation. Am J Roentgenol 2012; 198(3). https://doi.org/10.2214/AJR.11.7221.

33. Agostinho L, Horta M, Salvador JC, et al. Benign ovarian lesions with restricted diffusion. Radiol Bras 2019;52:106–11.

34. Okajima Y, Matsuo Y, Tamura A, et al. Intracellular lipid in ovarian thecomas detected by dual-echo chemical shift magnetic resonance imaging: report of 2 cases. J Comput Assist Tomogr 2010;34(2): 223–5.

35. Chalvardjian A, Scully RE. Sclerosing stromal tumors of the ovary. Cancer 1973;31(3):664–70.

36. Tanaka YO, Tsunoda H, Kitagawa Y, et al. Functioning ovarian tumors: direct and indirect findings at MR imaging. Radiographics 2004;24:147–66.

37. Sood N, Desai K, Chindris AM, et al. Symptomatic ovarian steroid cell tumor not otherwise specified in a post-menopausal woman. Rare Tumors 2016; 8(2):69–72.

38. Numanoglu C, Guler S, Ozaydin I, et al. Stromal luteoma of the ovary: a rare ovarian pathology. J Obstet Gynaecol (Lahore) 2015;35(4):420–1.

39. Akhtar K, Saeed N, Alam S, et al. Stromal luteoma of the ovary: a rare case presentation. J Pathol Infect Dis 2020;3. https://doi.org/10.33309/2639-8893.030101.

40. Outwater EK, Wagner BJ, Mannion C, et al. Sex cord-stromal and steroid cell tumors of the ovary. RadioGraphics 1998;18(6):1523–46.

Ovarian-Adnexal Reporting and Data Systems MR Imaging Nuts and Bolts

Kira Melamud, MD[a],*, Nicole Hindman, MD[b], Elizabeth Sadowski, MD[c]

KEYWORDS

• Adnexal • O-RADS MR imaging score • Lexicon • Risk stratification • Ovary

KEY POINTS

- MR imaging plays a primary role in the characterization of sonographically indeterminate adnexal lesions as either benign or malignant.
- The O-RADS MRI risk stratification system has been recently developed, validated, and found to be highly accurate for risk assessment of malignancy of an adnexal lesion.
- The O-RADS MRI risk score incorporates a codified lexicon and a 5-point scoring system based on the MR imaging features of an adnexal lesion.
- Widespread utilization of standardized O-RADS MRI risk stratification and management system can enhance communication between radiologists and referrers, and thus facilitate the optimal management algorithm depending on the determined risk of malignancy.

INTRODUCTION

Adnexal masses are common, with an estimated prevalence of 15% in the general population detected using ultrasound (US).[1–3] US is a powerful tool in the characterization of adnexal lesions and aids in appropriately guiding the management algorithm, either by avoiding unnecessary surgery when a lesion is clearly sonographically benign (ie, when classic imaging features of a simple or hemorrhagic cyst, dermoid or endometrioma are present) or by helping triage the patient to gynecologic oncology, if the lesion is found to have malignant features. However, literature indicates that up to 30% of sonographically detected adnexal masses remain indeterminate and cannot be classified as clearly benign or malignant based on US findings alone.[4–7] To avoid mischaracterizations and unnecessary interventions, further interrogation of such indeterminate lesions can be achieved with MR imaging. In fact, MR imaging can increase the positive predictive value (PPV) for malignancy to 71%, compared with a wide range of 7% to 50%, reported with US.[7–12] Furthermore, MR imaging can virtually exclude the possibility of malignancy in sonographically indeterminate lesions, with a reported negative predictive value of 98%.[11]

Due to its superior soft tissue resolution and ability to assess tissue composition, the greatest contribution of MR imaging to evaluation of adnexal masses is its high specificity, facilitating confident diagnosis of many benign adnexal lesions.[11] The absence of enhancing solid tissue in a lesion is a reliable sign of benignity.[1,13–15] Furthermore, the larger field of view and multiplanar capabilities of

[a] Department of Radiology, New York University Grossman School of Medicine, 660 First Avenue, 3rd Floor, New York, NY 100016, USA; [b] Department of Radiology and Surgery, New York University Grossman School of Medicine, 660 First Avenue, 3rd Floor, New York, NY 10016, USA; [c] Department of Radiology and Obstetrics and Gynecology, University of Wisconsin School of Medicine, 600 Highland Avenue, E3/372, Madison, WI 53792-3252, USA
* Corresponding author.
E-mail address: kira.melamud@nyulangone.org

Magn Reson Imaging Clin N Am 31 (2023) 79–91
https://doi.org/10.1016/j.mric.2022.06.004
1064-9689/23/© 2022 Elsevier Inc. All rights reserved.

MR imaging, compared with ultrasonography, can facilitate interrogation of large adnexal lesions, identify extra-adnexal findings such as peritoneal disease, and more accurately pinpoint the origin of an adnexal mass in cases that may be uncertain.[8] Finally, MR imaging can help classify and diagnose specific adnexal lesion types, allowing for optimization and tailoring of treatment options for patients. The last point is not insignificant in the current clinical milieu, when a variety of treatment options are available, including determining the feasibility of fertility preserving surgery versus oncologic cytoreductive surgery.[16–19] Radiologists play a critical role in these decision-making processes.

To improve accuracy of lesion characterization, interpretation agreement, and to optimize communication between radiologists and referrers, efforts have been undertaken to standardize reporting with use of MR imaging-related morphologic imaging descriptors and definitions. Most recently, the American College of Radiology (ACR) Ovarian-Adnexal Reporting and Data System (O-RADS) MRI lexicon and scoring system was developed to aid in the risk stratification of sonographically indeterminate adnexal masses. The lexicon includes standardized terms and definitions for evaluating and reporting adnexal lesions, while the risk stratification scoring system allows for evidence-based means of assigning the probability of malignancy, using a validated scoring rubric from 1 to 5 to reflect the likelihood of malignancy, with higher score portending higher risk[8,11,20] (**Fig. 1**). The benefit of using a codified lexicon is to improve the quality of communication between radiologists and referring physicians, to optimally and appropriately guide patient management, and to support best practices. Furthermore, similar to previously established and widely used reporting systems, such as the ACR Breast Imaging Reporting and Data System, an established lexicon can facilitate impactful multicenter research endeavors to ultimately improve patient outcomes. The goal of this article is to review the nuts and bolts nuances of the O-RADS MRI lexicon and scoring system to streamline adoption into daily clinical practice.

DEVELOPMENT AND UTILIZATION OF OVARIAN-ADNEXAL REPORTING AND DATA SYSTEMS MR IMAGING STANDARDIZED REPORTING SYSTEM: WHEN IS IT HELPFUL?

To understand when and how the O-RADS MRI standardized reporting system is helpful, it is beneficial to understand its development. The first steps in the process of developing the system took place in 2015, when the ACR O-RADS committee was first established. The committee was a multidisciplinary international consortium of experts, divided into an US arm and an MR imaging arm. The committee's initial goal was to compile evidence-based, standardized MR imaging-based lexicon, using universally accepted terms.[4,21] The details of the lexicon will be reviewed in a later discussion in the article. The second step was to establish the MRI risk stratification system. This was founded on a previously developed and validated European 5-point rubric called ADNEX MR scoring system.[13] This system, similar to the current O-RADS MRI risk stratification system, assigned a score with a corresponding PPV for malignancy based on MR imaging features. On its development, the O-RADS MRI risk stratification system was validated in a large prospective, multicenter European study, demonstrating high accuracy (91%) for stratifying the risks of malignancy in adnexal masses.[11]

The O-RADS MRI risk stratification system can be applied to most adnexal lesions referred to MR imaging, when US is not able to classify the finding as clearly benign or malignant. There are, however, several governing principles provided by the ACR O-RADS MRI committee for appropriate application of the system. First, the risk assessment system can only be applied to patients of average risk for malignancy because the performance of this system in a high-risk population has not been studied. Second, the system should not be used in patients with acute symptoms. This minimizes the chance of risk stratifying lesions that are inflammatory, such as an adnexal abscess or of upgrading a lesion due to transient alterations of imaging findings, such as from superinfection, torsion, or recent rupture. Third, the management decision of an adnexal lesion should rely on the synergistic contributions of clinical history, laboratory findings, and the risk score, and not solely on the imaging findings. Finally, when imaging findings are classic for a particular diagnosis (eg, dermoid, papillary serous tumor, and so forth) this can be reported in addition to the O-RADS MRI risk score, because this information can aid in more precise tailoring of the treatment options, which has been shown to improve clinical outcomes.[22–28]

MR IMAGING TECHNIQUE AND PROTOCOL

MR imaging evaluation of an adnexal lesion can be achieved using a 1.5T or 3T scanner. Patient preparation to optimize images may include fasting (4–6 hours), emptying the bladder, and administration of antiperistaltic agents before the examination.

O-RADS MRI Risk Stratification and Management System

O-RADS MRI Score	Risk Category	Positive Predictive Value for Malignancy[a]	Lexicon Description
0	Incomplete Evaluation	N/A	N/A
1	Normal Ovaries	N/A	No ovarian lesion
			Follicle defined as simple cyst ≤3 cm in a premenopausal woman
			Hemorrhagic cyst ≤3 cm in a premenopausal woman
			Corpus luteum +/- hemorrhage ≤3 cm in a premenopausal woman
2	Almost Certainly Benign	<0.5%[a]	Cyst: Unilocular- any type of fluid content • No wall enhancement • No enhancing solid tissue[b]
			Cyst: Unilocular – simple or endometriotic fluid content • Smooth enhancing wall • No enhancing solid tissue
			Lesion with lipid content[c] • No enhancing solid tissue
			Lesion with "dark T2/dark DWI" solid tissue • Homogeneously hypointense on T2 and DWI
			Dilated fallopian tube - simple fluid content • Thin, smooth wall/endosalpingeal folds with enhancement • No enhancing solid tissue
			Para-ovarian cyst – any type of fluid • Thin, smooth wall +/- enhancement • No enhancing solid tissue
3	Low Risk	~5%[a]	Cyst: Unilocular – proteinaceous, hemorrhagic or mucinous fluid content[d] • Smooth enhancing wall • No enhancing solid tissue
			Cyst: Multilocular - Any type of fluid, no lipid content • Smooth septae and wall with enhancement • No enhancing solid tissue
			Lesion with solid tissue (excluding T2 dark/DWI dark) • Low risk time intensity curve on DCE MRI
			Dilated fallopian tube – • Non-simple fluid: Thin wall /folds • Simple fluid: Thick, smooth wall/ folds • No enhancing solid tissue
4	Intermediate Risk	~50%[a]	Lesion with solid tissue (excluding T2 dark/DWI dark) • Intermediate risk time intensity curve on DCE MRI • If DCE MRI is not feasible, score 4 is any lesion with solid tissue (excluding T2 dark/DWI dark) that is enhancing ≤ myometrium at 30-40s on non-DCE MRI
			Lesion with lipid content • Large volume enhancing solid tissue
5	High Risk	~90%[a]	Lesion with solid tissue (excluding T2 dark/DWI dark) • High risk time intensity curve on DCE MRI • If DCE MRI is not feasible, score 5 is any lesion with solid tissue (excluding T2 dark/DWI dark) that is enhancing > myometrium at 30-40s on non-DCE MRI
			Peritoneal, mesenteric or omental nodularity or irregular thickening with or without ascites

Fig. 1. Reprinted, with permission from the American College of Radiology. Image shows Ovarian-Adnexal Reporting and Data System (O-RADS) MRI risk stratification system. DCE, dynamic contrast enhancement with a time resolution of 15 seconds or less; DWI, diffusion weighted images; MRI, Magnetic resonance imaging. [a]Approximate PPV based on data from Thomassin Naggara, et al, O-RADS MRI Score for risk Stratification of sonographically indeterminate adnexal masses. JAMA Network Open. 2023;3(1):e1919896. Please note that the PPV provided applies to the score catagory overall and not to individual characteristics. Definitive PPV are not currently available for individual characteristics. The PPV values for malignancy include both borderline tumors and invasive cancers. [b]Solid tissues is defined as a lesion component that enhances and conforms to one of these morphologies papillary projection, papillary projection, mural nodule, irregular septation/wall or other larger solid portions. [c]Minimal enhancement of Rokitansky nodules in lesions containing lipid does not change to O-RADS MRI-4. [d]Hemorrhagic cyst ≤3 cm in pre-menopausal woman is O-RADS MRI 1.

The field of view should be adjusted for each patient to ensure coverage of the whole adnexal lesion. The imaging protocol should include precontrast axial T1-weighted imaging (T_1WI) series, T2-weighted imaging (T_2WI) series (in at least 2 planes), diffusion-weighted imaging (DWI) series (b-value ≥ 1000 s/mm^2) and postcontrast T_1WI series. It is essential to include fat-saturated and nonfat-saturated set of either T_1WI or T_2WI to detect the presence of macroscopic fat. Similarly, in-phase and out-of-phase T_1WI should be included for the assessment of intravoxel fat. Use of dynamic contrast-enhanced (DCE) MR imaging technique with 15-second temporal resolution along with time-intensity curve (TIC) analysis is the preferred methodology for the identification and assessment of enhancing solid tissue in an adnexal lesion. The advantage of this technique is the ability to stratify between low-risk, intermediate-risk, or high-risk patterns of enhancement. Details of TIC analysis will be discussed in a later section. If DCE imaging is not feasible, a postcontrast T_1WI series obtained 30 to 40 seconds after injection can be obtained; however, this technique has narrower scope in discriminating patterns of enhancement, limiting the scores to O-RADS MRI 4 or 5, resulting in potential upstaging of lesions that may have been classified as O-RADS MRI 3 based on DCE analysis. See **Table 1** for details of a suggested MR imaging protocol.

AMERICAN COLLEGE OF RADIOLOGY OVARIAN-ADNEXAL REPORTING AND DATA SYSTEMS MRI LEXICON: OVERVIEW

To fully understand the O-RADS MRI risk stratification system, it is imperative to understand the lexicon, which comprises it. There are 7 major O-RADS MRI lexicon categories: (1) major categories which help define physiologic adnexal observations from nonphysiologic observations (aka "lesions"), (2) size (stipulates that maximum diameter of a lesion and/or solid component; can be measured in any imaging plane), (3) shape or contour of solid lesion or tissue (which can be described as smooth or irregular), (4) signal intensity, (5) lesion components (cystic, solid, nonenhancing solid components), (6) enhancement, and (7) extraovarian findings (such as physiologic fluid, ascites, and peritoneal thickening). A consolidated summary of the major themes and terms will be provided here. For a complete list of all lexicon terms, please refer to the ACR O-RADS MRI lexicon table (https://www.acr.org/-/media/ACR/Files/RADS/O-RADS/O-RADS-MRI-Lexicon-Terms-Table.pdf).

Physiologic Observations Versus Adnexal Lesions

The first category in the O-RADS MRI Lexicon makes a fundamental distinction between physiologic and nonphysiologic observations. *Physiologic observations* include (1) a follicle, defined as a unilocular simple cyst 3 cm or lesser in premenopausal women and a (2) corpus luteum defined as a cyst 3 cm or lesser, with a thick, enhancing wall, and can be simple or contain hemorrhagic products. These latter physiologic hormone-producing structures arise at the site of a follicle after the release of an ovum and frequently demonstrate crenulated appearance from infolding. A *lesion* is defined as an adnexal structure, which is not considered physiologic. This is subdivided further into cystic lesion, lesion with solid component, and solid lesion. Cystic lesions can be unilocular or multilocular. Solid lesions are defined as having less than 20% cystic component.

Fluid Descriptors

The O-RADS MRI lexicon includes several descriptors for cystic and solid components of an adnexal observation. *Simple fluid* follows signal intensity of CSF on all sequences. *Nonsimple fluid* can be described with the following lexicon descriptors:

- *Hemorrhagic fluid* can demonstrate variable signal depending on the age of blood products. For example, subacute hemorrhage would be hyperintense on T_1WI and T_2WI sequences.
- *Endometriotic fluid* is typically hyperintense on T_1WI, with corresponding hypointensity on T_2WI. This is classically referred to as "T2 shading." Ancillary findings of endometriotic cysts including multiplicity and the presence of "T2 dark spots," can further support diagnosis and differentiate from hemorrhagic fluid.
- *Proteinaceous fluid*, such as fluid composed of mucin, colloid, or purulent material, can also demonstrate variable signal characteristics.
- *Fat-containing or lipid-containing fluid* is expected to be hyperintense on both T1W and T2W images, with signal loss on fat-saturated sequences. Of note, an ovarian observation with the presence of intravoxel fat as detected on chemical shift T1W out-of-phase sequences, without detectable macroscopic fat, still represents "lipid-containing fluid" (ie, dermoid cyst).

Solid Component Descriptors

Nonfluid parts of an adnexal lesion are considered solid components. The lexicon makes a distinction between solid tissue and other solid components not considered solid tissue. *Solid tissue* is strictly defined as enhancing components, which exhibits at least one of the following morphologic features:

- *Papillary projection:* An enhancing arborizing protrusion on a stalk, with an acute angle to the cyst wall or septation.

Table 1
Suggested MR imaging protocol for adnexal lesion characterization at 1.5T or 3T MR imaging

Sequence	Detail
Sagittal T_2WI without fat sat	• Slice thickness: $\leq$ 4 mm
Axial T_2WI without fat sat	• Slice thickness: $\leq$ 3 mm
Axial T_1WI in-phase and out-of-phase	• Slice thickness: $\leq$ 4 mm
Axial DWI	• Slice thickness: $\leq$ 3 mm • b-value $\geq$ 1000 s/mm^2
DCE MR imaging: 3D T_1WI with fat sat	• Injection occurs 30 s *after* initiating scanning • Total duration of imaging is 4 min • Slice thickness: $\leq$ 3 mm • Minimal temporal resolution $\leq$ 15 s
Nondynamic 3D T_1WI with fat sat	• Precontrast series and then begin scanning 30–40 s after the end of injection • Slice thickness: $\leq$ 3 mm

- *Mural nodule:* A solid tissue, enhancing nodular protrusion, with a convex margin and obtuse angle to the cyst wall or septation, measuring 3 mm or greater in height.
- *Irregular septation:* A complete enhancing linear strand, which runs from one internal surface of a cyst wall to another, demonstrating uneven and variable thickness.
- *Irregular wall:* Enhancing cyst wall with jagged, uneven margin.
- *Larger solid portion:* This is a descriptive term for enhancing solid tissue that does not meet criteria for other morphologic descriptors.

Other solid components that do not meet criteria for solid tissue defined above includes fat, blood clot and nonenhancing debris, smooth walls or septations, and fibrin stranding. Hair, calcification, and Rokitansky nodules are components of dermoid cysts and are also not considered solid tissue.

Enhancement

It is essential to meticulously assess enhancement characteristics of an adnexal lesion. Enhancement in an adnexal lesion may be confined to the wall, septation, or solid tissue. A lesion that does not demonstrate any enhancement is almost certainly benign. Subtraction images are especially useful to assess for subtle foci of enhancement, especially in lesions that are intrinsically hyperintense on T1-weighted images.

Dynamic contrast enhancement (DCE) technique is recommended for optimal assessment of enhancement characteristics of adnexal lesions. This involves a 3D T_1WI fat-saturated sequence with a spatial resolution of 3 mm and temporal resolution of 15 seconds. DCE acquisition can allow for the generation of a TIC, by placing a region of interest on the earliest enhancing region of the solid tissue component and a second region of interest, to act as a reference standard, on the outer myometrium (making sure to avoid the arcuate vessels). Three types of TICs have been defined (**Fig. 2**). A low-risk or Type 1 curve demonstrates low level but gradually increasing enhancement over time without a shoulder or plateau. An intermediate-risk or Type 2 curve demonstrates a moderate level of enhancement within the adnexal lesion with an initial slope, followed by a shoulder and a plateau that is less than or equal to the myometrium. Finally, a high-risk or Type 3 curve demonstrates an initial slope that is steeper than the myometrium, followed by a shoulder and a plateau.

If DCE is not available, nondynamic MR imaging sequences may be acquired, including precontrast sequences followed by acquisition at 30 to 40 seconds after contrast injection, with the assessment of relative enhancement in the adnexal mass compared with outer myometrium. As previously noted, this technique limits the classification of a lesion with enhancing solid tissue (not believed to be O-RADS MRI 2) to O-RADS MRI scores of 4 and 5.

If the uterus is absent, intermediate-risk and high-risk TICs cannot be discerned but a low-risk TIC can be recognized by its progressive enhancement without a plateau.

OVARIAN-ADNEXAL REPORTING AND DATA SYSTEMS MR IMAGING STRATIFICATION SCORE: THE NUTS AND BOLTS

The O-RADS MR imaging risk stratification and management system table, along with supporting documents and links to O-RADS MRI calculator can be found on the ACR website (https://www.acr.org/Clinical-Resources/Reporting-and-Data-Systems/O-Rads). The management system is composed of 4 major columns: the O-RADS MR imaging score, risk category, PPV for malignancy (based on the validation article from Thomassin-Naggara and colleagues), and associated lexicon descriptors that apply to each score.

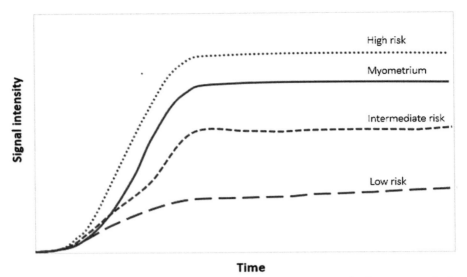

Fig. 2. Line graph representation depicting different TICs comparing pattern of enhancement of adnexal lesions to enhancement of myometrium. The low-risk or "type 1" curve demonstrates gradual increase in enhancement over time, although slower than myometrium, without a shoulder or plateau. Intermediate-risk or "type 2" TIC has a shoulder and an initial rate (slope) of enhancement less than or equal to myometrium. High-risk or "type 3" TIC has a slope greater than myometrium, with a shoulder and a plateau.

Ovarian-Adnexal Reporting and Data Systems MRI Score 0—Incomplete Evaluation

Adnexal lesions are classified as O-RADS MRI 0 when the lesion is incompletely assessed at MR imaging. This may be the result of exclusion of a portion of a lesion due to large size or technical limitations such as large artifacts or missing sequences.

Ovarian-Adnexal Reporting and Data Systems MRI Score 1—Normal Ovaries

This score can be assigned when ovaries seem normal. In premenopausal women (assumed younger than 50 years if status is unknown), normal physiologic observations include follicles, hemorrhagic cysts, or corpus luteum cysts 3 cm or lesser (**Fig. 3**). In postmenopausal women, small residual follicles can be observed, and if the radiologist subjectively evaluates the ovaries as normal, O-RADS MRI 1 classification can be assigned.

Ovarian-Adnexal Reporting and Data Systems MRI Score 2—Almost Certainly Benign

O-RADS MRI score 2 is assigned to adnexal lesions that are almost certainly benign, with a PPV for malignancy of less than 0.5%. This category can be applied readily to unilocular cystic

lesions with simple or clearly endometriotic fluid. If the presence of proteinaceous or hemorrhagic fluid content is observed within a unilocular cyst, it is the presence of wall enhancement that dictates the scoring assignment. If no wall enhancement is observed, O-RADS MRI score of 2 is appropriate. However, a proteinaceous or hemorrhagic cyst with an enhancing wall should be scored O-RADS MRI 3.

Lipid-containing lesions (dermoids or mature teratomas) are also classified as O-RADS MRI 2. It is important to note that Rokitansky nodules found in dermoid cysts may demonstrate nodular enhancement and should not deter from appropriate classification as an almost certainly benign lesion (**Fig. 4**). Malignant transformation of these lesions is markedly rare, with incidence of 1% of dermoid cysts, and such concern should be raised only when there is subjectively large enhancing soft tissue within a lipid-containing lesion. In such a case, O-RADS MRI 4 should be assigned.

Adnexal lesions with homogeneously hypointense signal on both T2-weighted and high-b-value DWI sequences related to internal fibrous component can be assigned O-RADS MRI 2. These are referred to as "dark T2/dark DWI" lesions in the stratification system (**Fig. 5**). At pathology, these lesions are usually found to be benign fibromas and fibrothecomas. Of note, the

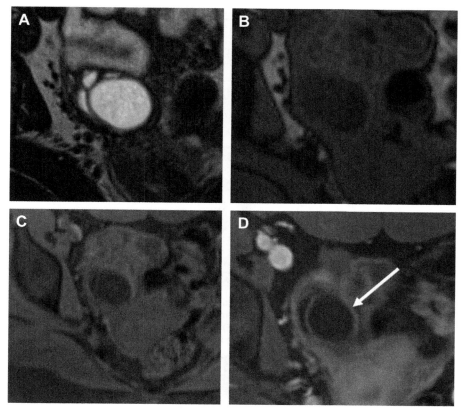

Fig. 3. Example of O-RADS MRI score 1, "normal ovaries." Axial T_2WI (*A*), T_1WI out-of-phase (*B*), fat-saturated T_1WI (*C*), and postcontrast T_1WI (*D*) images demonstrate a 2.5-cm unilocular physiologic follicle with smooth wall enhancement (*arrow*) in a premenopausal woman.

enhancement characteristics of these lesions do not influence the scoring assignment.

Finally, dilated fallopian tubes containing simple fluid and paraovarian cysts without solid tissue can be scored as O-RADS MRI 2. Paraovarian cysts may contain any type of fluid and may demonstrate a thin enhancing wall. Dilated fallopian tubes, or hydrosalpinges, can be recognized by their characteristic serpiginous morphology and the presence of enhancing endosalpingeal folds.

Ovarian-Adnexal Reporting and Data Systems MRI Score 3—Low Risk

Adnexal lesions classified as O-RADS MRI 3 are almost certainly benign with PPV of approximately 5% for malignancy. Included in this category are unilocular cysts with proteinaceous or hemorrhagic contents with enhancing walls and multilocular cysts with smooth enhancing walls and septations. Multiloculated endometriomas, if recognized as such, should still be classified as O-RADS MRI 2.

Adnexal lesions with solid tissue, which is not homogeneously hypointense on T2W and DWI sequences, can be classified as O-RADS MRI 3 if the enhancement pattern follows the low-risk TIC (**Fig. 6**). These lesions carry an approximately 7% risk of malignancy and most are found to be borderline tumors.[8,11]

Dilated fallopian tubes with nonsimple fluid or with thickened walls or endosalpingeal folds are also classified as O-RADS MRI 3. This designation reflects the concern that high-grade serous carcinomas arise from fallopian tubes, and this appearance may represent early-stage disease, although supporting literature is limited.

Ovarian-Adnexal Reporting and Data Systems MRI Score 4—Intermediate Risk

Adnexal lesions with O-RADS MRI score 4 are deemed intermediate risk with PPV of approximately 50% for malignancy . By definition, these lesions contain solid tissue that follows intermediate-risk TICs (**Fig. 7**). If DCE MR imaging sequences are not available, lesions containing

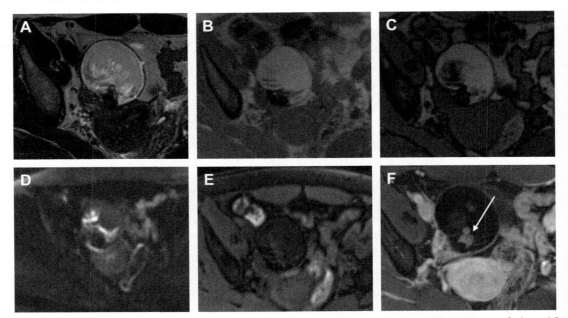

Fig. 4. Example of O-RADS MRI score 2, dermoid cyst. Axial T_2WI (*A*), T_1WI in-phase (*B*), T_1WI out-of-phase (*C*), DWI (b-value of 1000 s/mm^2) (*D*), fat-saturated T_1WI (*E*), and contrast-enhanced T_1WI (*F*) demonstrating nodular enhancement related to a Rokitansky nodule (*arrow in F*). Notice also increased diffusion signal (D) within the dermoid cyst related to its fat content, which should not be mistaken for a sign of malignancy.

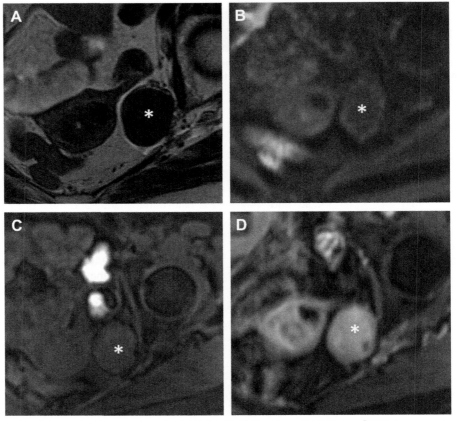

Fig. 5. Example of O-RADS MRI score 2. Axial T_2WI (*A*), DWI (b-value of 1000 s/mm^2) (*B*), fat-saturated T_1WI (*C*), and contrast-enhanced T_1WI (*D*) demonstrating a classic "dark T2/dark DWI" lesion marked with an asterisk, confirmed as a fibroma.

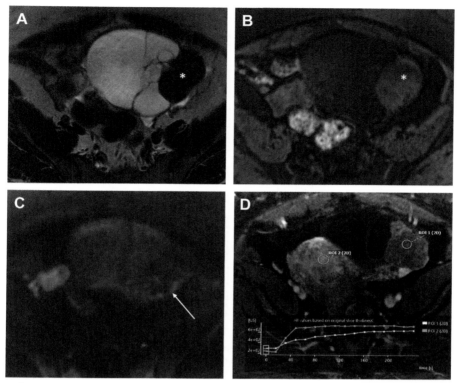

Fig. 6. Example of O-RADS MRI score 3. Axial T_2WI (*A*), fat-saturated T_1WI (*B*), and DWI (b-value of 1000 s/mm^2) (*C*) demonstrate the presence of a left adnexal multiloculated cystic mass with smooth septa and solid tissue (*asterisk*). Notice that the solid tissue demonstrated heterogeneously hyperintense signal on DWI (*arrow*). DCE acquisition (*D*) allows for plotting of TIC curves, with the solid tissue (*ROI 1 in white*) demonstrating a low-risk curve without a shoulder or plateau, compared with TIC of the uterine myometrium (*ROI 2 in green*). At pathology, this was shown to be a benign Brenner tumor associated with mucinous cystadenoma. Note, that if DCE was not available, this lesion would be classified as O-RADS MRI score 4.

solid tissue (with notable exception of solid tissue which is homogeneously T2W and DWI hypointense, which are O-RADS MRI 2) that enhances less than or equal to the myometrium at 30 to 40 seconds after contrast injection on non-DCE MR imaging, satisfy criteria. Lipid-containing lesions with subjectively large soft tissue component should also be assigned O-RADS MRI 4.

Ovarian-Adnexal Reporting and Data Systems MRI 5—High Risk

Adnexal lesions classified as O-RADS MRI score 5 are high risk and carry a PPV of approximately 90% for malignancy. High-risk stigmata include the presence of peritoneal implants and/or the presence of adnexal lesions that demonstrate high-risk intensity curve dynamics (**Fig. 8**). In the event of absence of DCE MR imaging, lesions that enhance greater than myometrium 30 to 40 seconds after contrast injection can be assigned this category.

PRACTICAL APPROACH TO THE OVARIAN-ADNEXAL REPORTING AND DATA SYSTEMS MRI SCORING SYSTEM

An online calculator is available for quick classification of an adnexal lesion (https://oradsmricalc. com/). **Fig. 9** represents a stepwise approach to the O-RADS MRI scoring system, which walks through some of the considerations built into the calculator. First, consider if the finding is truly adnexal. If it is not, application of O-RADS MRI scoring system is inappropriate. Once recognized as adnexal, evaluate for advanced signs of malignancy, specifically for the presence of peritoneal implants. If present, this satisfies criteria for O-RADS MRI 5. If no implants are seen, the next step is to assess if the finding is physiologic (eg, follicle, hemorrhagic or corpus luteum cyst $\leq$ 3 cm) in a premenopausal woman or if normal ovaries are present (premenopausal or postmenopausal). If there is a physiologic finding or the ovaries are normal in appearance, O-RADS

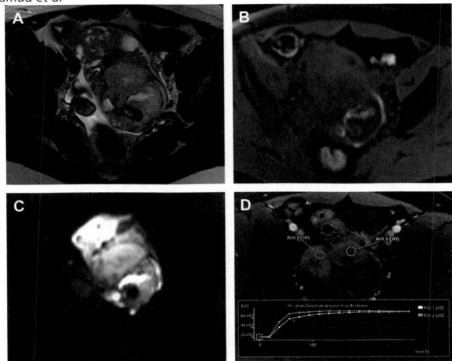

Fig. 7. Example of O-RADS MRI score 4. Axial T_2WI (*A*), fat-saturated T_1WI (*B*), and DWI (b-value of 1000 s/mm^2) (*C*) demonstrate a large, partially hemorrhagic, diffusion restricting left adnexal mass. The enhancing solid tissue (*ROI 1 in white*) exhibits an intermediate risk TIC at DCE acquisition (*D*), which follows the TIC of the uterine myometrium (*ROI 2 in green*), with presence of a shoulder and a plateau. At pathology this was confirmed to be a granulosa cell tumor.

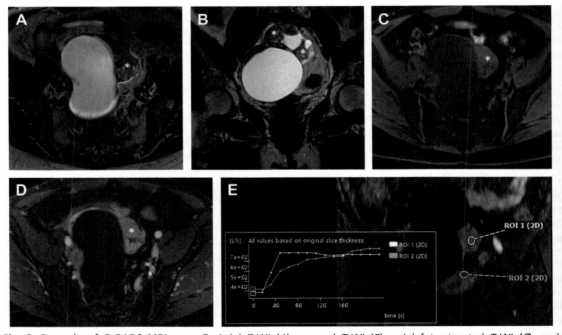

Fig. 8. Example of O-RADS MRI score 5. Axial T_2WI (*A*), coronal T_2WI (*B*), axial fat-saturated T_1WI (*C*), and contrast-enhanced T_1WI (*D*) demonstrate a right adnexal cystic lesion with solid tissue (astrisks). Evaluation of coronal reformat of DCE acquisition (*E*) indicates that the solid tissue exhibits a high-risk TIC (*ROI 1 in white*), with a steeper slope compared with the uterine myometrium (*ROI 2 in green*). Based on these findings the patient is currently awaiting total abdominal hysterectomy with bilateral salpingo-oophorectomy and exploratory laparotomy for staging with gynecology–oncology.

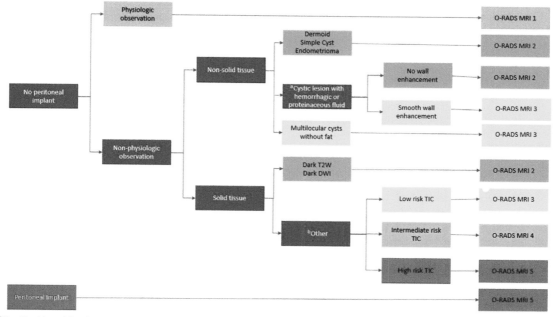

Fig. 9. Algorithmic approach to assessment of adnexal lesions with O-RADS MRI scoring system. Key: [a]Hemorrhagic cysts less than 3 cm in premenopausal women are excluded as they are considered physiologic. [b]Notable exception of lesions with solid tissue is dermoid cysts that should be classified as O-RADS MRI 2, unless there is a substantial solid component.

MRI 1 score is assigned. If there is a nonphysiologic finding, assess for the presence of simple cyst (excluding follicles), dermoid or endometrioma, which can be classified as O-RADS MRI 2. If there is a cystic lesion with hemorrhagic or proteinaceous fluid (excluding hemorrhagic cysts ≤3 cm in premenopausal women), then the score depends on wall enhancement: if there is no wall enhancement, the lesion is scored as O-RADS MRI 2 and if there is smooth wall enhancement, it is scored as O-RADS MRI 3. Nonfatty multilocular cysts are scored as O-RADS MRI 3.

If the lesion still does not meet any of the above criteria, the next step is to evaluate for the presence of enhancing solid tissue. If there is homogenously dark signal solid tissue on T_2WI and the high b-value DWI, then the lesion is score as O-RADS MRI 2. If the solid tissue within the lesion is at least partially intermediate or high signal, then the pattern of enhancement will determine the score, with low-risk TIC resulting in O-RADS MRI score 3, intermediate-risk TIC in O-RADS MRI score 4, and high-risk TIC yielding O-RADS MRI score 5. A notable exception to this basic stepwise approach are lipid-containing lesions with large solid tissue concerning for malignant degeneration. These lesions are scored as O-RADS MRI 4 regardless of the type of enhancement.

SUMMARY

MR imaging plays a preeminent role in the characterization of indeterminate adnexal lesions found at ultrasonography. Risk stratifying adnexal lesions with MR imaging helps to expedite appropriate care when the risk of malignancy is high and avoid overtreatment if such a risk is low. Noncontributory but frequently encountered descriptors such as "complex lesion" should be replaced with standardized evidence-based lexicon as presented here, thus enhancing the utility and applicability of radiologic reporting in this clinical context. Ongoing research will continue to update the role of imaging and radiologists in ovarian cancer management algorithm.

CLINICS CARE POINTS

- O-RADS MRI score can be used to risk stratify sonographically indeterminate adnexal lesions in women of average risk for malignancy.
- O-RADS MR imaging score should not be applied to patients with acute symptoms.
- DCE MR imaging is preferred for O-RADS MRI scoring because it allows for greater stratification of adnexal lesions with solid tissue as low, intermediate, or high risk based on TICs.

- Non-DCE imaging can only discern lesions with solid tissue as intermediate (O-RADS MRI 4) or high (O-RADS MRI 5) risk.
- Lipid-containing lesions (dermoid cysts) are almost certainly benign (O-RADS MRI 2) and can demonstrate enhancement related to Rokitansky nodules; however, if the solid component is subjectively large, a score of O-RADS MRI 4 is appropriate for the risk of mature teratoma or malignant conversion.

DISCLOSURE

K. Melamud—Nothing to disclose. N. Hindman—Nothing to disclose. E. Sadowski—Nothing to disclose.

REFERENCES

1. Sadowski EA, et al. Ovary: MRI characterisation and O-RADS MRI. Br J Radiol 2021;94(1125):20210157.
2. Greenlee RT, et al. Prevalence, incidence, and natural history of simple ovarian cysts among women >55 years old in a large cancer screening trial. Am J Obstet Gynecol 2010;202(4):373. e1-9.
3. Sharma A, et al. Risk of epithelial ovarian cancer in asymptomatic women with ultrasound-detected ovarian masses: a prospective cohort study within the UK collaborative trial of ovarian cancer screening (UKCTOCS). Ultrasound Obstet Gynecol 2012;40(3):338–44.
4. Reinhold C, et al. Ovarian-Adnexal Reporting Lexicon for MRI: A White Paper of the ACR Ovarian-Adnexal Reporting and Data Systems MRI Committee. J Am Coll Radiol 2021;18(5):713–29.
5. Timmerman D, et al. Predicting the risk of malignancy in adnexal masses based on the Simple Rules from the International Ovarian Tumor Analysis group. Am J Obstet Gynecol 2016;214(4):424–37.
6. Van Calster B, et al. Evaluating the risk of ovarian cancer before surgery using the ADNEX model to differentiate between benign, borderline, early and advanced stage invasive, and secondary metastatic tumours: prospective multicentre diagnostic study. BMJ 2014;349:g5920.
7. Sadowski EA, et al. Indeterminate Adnexal Cysts at US: Prevalence and Characteristics of Ovarian Cancer. Radiology 2018;287(3):1041–9.
8. Sadowski EA, et al. O-RADS MRI Risk Stratification System: Guide for Assessing Adnexal Lesions from the ACR O-RADS Committee. Radiology 2022;303(1):35–47.
9. Andreotti RF, et al. O-RADS US Risk Stratification and Management System: A Consensus Guideline from the ACR Ovarian-Adnexal Reporting and Data System Committee. Radiology 2020;294(1):168–85.
10. Timmerman D, et al. Simple ultrasound rules to distinguish between benign and malignant adnexal masses before surgery: prospective validation by IOTA group. BMJ 2010;341:c6839.
11. Thomassin-Naggara I, et al. Ovarian-Adnexal Reporting Data System Magnetic Resonance Imaging (O-RADS MRI) Score for Risk Stratification of Sonographically Indeterminate Adnexal Masses. JAMA Netw Open 2020;3(1):e1919896.
12. Patel-Lippmann KK, et al. Comparison of International Ovarian Tumor Analysis Simple Rules to Society of Radiologists in Ultrasound Guidelines for Detection of Malignancy in Adnexal Cysts. AJR Am J Roentgenol 2020;214(3):694–700.
13. Thomassin-Naggara I, et al. Adnexal masses: development and preliminary validation of an MR imaging scoring system. Radiology 2013;267(2):432–43.
14. Bernardin L, et al. Effectiveness of semi-quantitative multiphase dynamic contrast-enhanced MRI as a predictor of malignancy in complex adnexal masses: radiological and pathological correlation. Eur Radiol 2012;22(4):880–90.
15. Pereira PN, et al. Accuracy of the ADNEX MR scoring system based on a simplified MRI protocol for the assessment of adnexal masses. Diagn Interv Radiol 2018;24(2):63–71.
16. McEvoy SH, et al. Fertility-sparing for young patients with gynecologic cancer: How MRI can guide patient selection prior to conservative management. Abdom Radiol (Ny) 2017;42(10):2488–512.
17. Morice P, et al. Recommendations of the Fertility Task Force of the European Society of Gynecologic Oncology about the conservative management of ovarian malignant tumors. Int J Gynecol Cancer 2011;21(5):951–63.
18. Rockall AG, et al. Role of Imaging in Fertility-sparing Treatment of Gynecologic Malignancies. Radiographics 2016;36(7):2214–33.
19. Stein EB, Hansen JM, Maturen KE. Fertility-Sparing Approaches in Gynecologic Oncology: Role of Imaging in Treatment Planning. Radiol Clin North Am 2020;58(2):401–12.
20. ACR O-RADS-MR-risk-stratification-system-table https://www.acr.org/-/media/ACR/Files/RADS/O-RADS/O-RADS-MR-Risk-Stratification-System-Table-September-2020.pdf. Accessed February 2022.
21. Andreotti RF, et al. Ovarian-Adnexal Reporting Lexicon for Ultrasound: A White Paper of the ACR Ovarian-Adnexal Reporting and Data System Committee. J Am Coll Radiol 2018;15(10):1415–29.
22. Shim SH, et al. Impact of surgical staging on prognosis in patients with borderline ovarian tumours: A meta-analysis. Eur J Cancer 2016;54:84–95.

23. Zhou J, et al. The Effect of Histological Subtypes on Outcomes of Stage IV Epithelial Ovarian Cancer. Front Oncol 2018;8:577.
24. Trimbos JB. Surgical treatment of early-stage ovarian cancer. Best Pract Res Clin Obstet Gynaecol 2017;41:60–70.
25. Anthoulakis C, Nikoloudis N. Pelvic MRI as the "gold standard" in the subsequent evaluation of ultrasound-indeterminate adnexal lesions: a systematic review. Gynecol Oncol 2014;132(3):661–8.
26. Hricak H, et al. Complex adnexal masses: detection and characterization with MR imaging–multivariate analysis. Radiology 2000;214(1):39–46.
27. Forstner R, et al. ESUR recommendations for MR imaging of the sonographically indeterminate adnexal mass: an update. Eur Radiol 2017;27(6):2248–57.
28. Spencer JA, et al. ESUR guidelines for MR imaging of the sonographically indeterminate adnexal mass: an algorithmic approach. Eur Radiol 2010;20(1):25–35.

Imaging of Metastatic Disease to the Ovary/ Adnexa

Molly E. Roseland, MD[a], John D. Millet, MD, MHS[a], Ashish P. Wasnik, MD[a],*

KEYWORDS

- Ovarian metastases • Secondary ovarian malignancy • Krukenberg tumor
- Adnexal mass characterization • MR imaging

KEY POINTS

- Ovarian metastases may be caused by any malignancy but are usually due to primary colorectal, gastric, breast, and gynecologic carcinomas.
- In a patient with an incidental, malignant-appearing adnexal mass, consider ovarian metastasis if known (advanced) malignancy, young age, bilateral tumors, and tumors with hyper-enhancing, irregular, heterogeneous solid components.
- Stomach and breast cancer metastases tend to be solid, whereas colorectal cancer metastases tend to be mixed solid-cystic.
- Compared with primary mucinous ovarian tumors, metastatic mucinous tumors (usually GI origin) are smaller, frequently bilateral, and more often associated with peritoneal metastatic disease.

INTRODUCTION

Adnexal metastases may occur in the setting of various solid and hematologic malignancies and may develop at any time during the course of a patient's disease. Although such metastases are relatively uncommon (in comparison to liver or lungs),[1] certain cancers have a unique predilection to involve the ovaries, where they may mimic a primary ovarian neoplasm.[2] Accurate diagnosis has significant clinical implications because adnexal mass(es) may be the initial manifestation of an extraovarian malignancy, and both treatment and prognosis differ based on tumor origin and disease extent.[3] Familiarity with potential imaging appearances of ovarian metastases is therefore essential for radiologists, who play a critical role in cancer staging and adnexal mass characterization. Even when imaging cannot provide a definitive diagnosis, radiologists may be the first to propose secondary ovarian malignancy as a differential consideration, helping to guide additional workup.

In this article, we first review the epidemiology and pathophysiology of adnexal metastases. We then provide a comprehensive summary of the radiologic appearances of secondary ovarian malignancies, with an emphasis on distinguishing MR imaging characteristics by cancer subtype. We briefly discuss the role of biopsy and pathologic diagnosis. Finally, we conclude with a discussion of treatment implications and outcomes.

BACKGROUND AND EPIDEMIOLOGY

Metastases are estimated to comprise 5% to 30% of all malignant ovarian tumors worldwide[4–10] with fluctuating rates related to diverse populations and study designs.[11] Numerous analyses recognize cancers of the gastrointestinal (GI) tract (colon, rectum, and stomach) as the most common primary malignancies to involve the ovaries,[2,4–7,9,10,12–14] followed by breast and gynecologic cancers (endometrium, cervix).[2] The distribution of ovarian metastases is likely

a Department of Radiology, Division of Abdomnal Imaging, Michigan Medicine, University of Michigan, UH B1D502D, 1500 East Medical Center Drive, Ann Arbor, MI 48109, USA
* Corresponding author:
E-mail address: ashishw@med.umich.edu

Magn Reson Imaging Clin N Am 31 (2023) 93–107
https://doi.org/10.1016/j.mric.2022.06.005
1064-9689/23/© 2022 Elsevier Inc. All rights reserved.

influenced by variable rates of baseline cancer incidence. For example, colorectal cancer is the second-most common cancer among adult women globally,[15] with increasing incidence throughout the developing world.[16] Accordingly, it is also the most common cause of ovarian metastases in various studies from Europe and North America,[2,5,6,12,13,17] as well as newer studies from Asia and Africa.[4,9,14,18]

Patients with secondary ovarian malignancies typically present at younger ages (30–55 years) compared with those with primary ovarian neoplasms.[4,8,10,14,18] Similarly, among women with similar primary malignancies, those with ovarian metastases tend to be younger than those without, suggesting premenopausal status may increase the risk of ovarian involvement.[11] Because these ages overlap with typical childbearing years, ovarian metastases may be diagnosed in pregnancy.[19,20]

Primary malignancies are unreliably detected before ovarian metastases. Only 44% to 58% of adult patients with confirmed ovarian metastases have a preexisting cancer diagnosis at the time of adnexal mass detection.[5,6] Hence, nearly half of all patients will present with ovarian masses as the first (and possibly only) manifestation of an occult malignancy, highlighting inherent diagnostic challenges. Synchronous metastases to the ovaries are more likely to occur in GI cancers, whereas late, metachronous ovarian metastases occur more frequently in breast and endometrial cancers.[2]

In contrast to ovarian metastases, little is known about the frequency of metastatic disease involving the fallopian tubes. Diagnosis is usually established pathologically. A histologic analysis of a small cohort of adult patients with nongynecologic metastases to the ovaries finds that 65% have concurrent tubal metastases, most frequently from GI cancers.[21] Variable microscopic patterns of tumor growth are observed, many of which cannot be appreciated on gross specimens. These findings suggest the fallopian tube may be an underestimated site of disease, where metastases are potentially challenging to diagnose prospectively.[2,21] However, given lack of published studies regarding the imaging of fallopian tube metastases, our review of adnexal metastatic disease will henceforth focus only on the ovaries.

PATHOPHYSIOLOGY AND MECHANISMS OF METASTATIC SPREAD

Of the female reproductive organs, the ovaries are most frequently involved by distant metastases from nongynecologic cancers.[1] In contrast, the vagina, cervix, and uterus are more likely to be affected by local spread of gynecologic malignancies.[2] These trends likely relate to underlying differences in tumor affinity for secondary sites (known as the "seed and soil" hypothesis), as well as variable pathways of metastatic tumor dissemination.[22]

Certain pathologic cancer subtypes have a particular "organ tropism" for the ovaries. The so-called Krukenberg tumor (KT) was first identified in 1896, precisely defined as a metastatic carcinoma of the ovary composed of signet-ring cells (tumor cells with abundant intracellular mucin that eccentrically displaces cellular nuclei) and sarcoma-like stromal proliferation.[22] Although this name is a potential source of confusion in the literature—often misapplied to any ovarian metastases or to all ovarian metastases from gastric cancer—it remains useful to illustrate the association of tumor histology with patterns of metastatic disease. Signet-ring histology is often present in diffuse and scirrhous-type gastric cancers (classically causing "linitis plastic") and is rarely present in colorectal, appendiceal, and breast cancers. Regardless of their organ of origin, signet-ring carcinomas have a high likelihood of early, bilateral ovarian involvement in young women, potentially related to their affinity for ovarian stoma. Although disease may not always be evident clinically, nearly half of patients with gastric signet-ring carcinoma may have microscopic ovarian metastases, compared with 60% to 100% of patients with colorectal signet-ring carcinomas.[19,22,23]

Metastatic tumors are hypothesized to reach the ovaries via several key routes of spread: lymphatic, peritoneal, hematogenous, and/or direct extension.[11,22] Abdominal malignancies (such as those of GI origin) may cause lymphatic obstruction and metastatic lymphadenopathy, which can result in "lymphatic backflow" of tumor into the ovaries. Any disseminated tumor cells in the peritoneal cavity may settle dependently in the pelvis and can become trapped along the ovarian surface due to local inflammation from ovulation. The ovaries also receive increased blood flow in premenopausal women, which may increase their likelihood of exposure to circulating tumor cells (particularly from distant cancers, such as breast). Finally, the ovaries may become secondarily involved by large or infiltrative pelvic malignancies through local tumor extension.[11,22]

SYMPTOMS AND PRESENTATION

Patients with metastatic ovarian tumors present with variable signs and symptoms, rarely related to their primary malignancy. Smaller tumors are unlikely to be symptomatic and are often detected incidentally on imaging. Larger masses may cause nonspecific symptoms, such as abdominal or pelvic pain, bloating, dyspareunia, bladder-bowel dysfunction, distension, or weight changes.[7,19,22,24] Ascites may be present but is relatively less common compared with primary ovarian neoplasms.[25]

Acutely, patients may present with mass-related complications, such as ovarian torsion[26,27] or hemorrhage/rupture.[28] Such patients will have severe pain and clinical instability, requiring urgent surgical exploration.[28] A rare "pseudo-Meigs" syndrome has also been described in patients with colorectal or gastric metastases to the ovaries, characterized by large-volume benign ascites and pleural effusions, analogous to the classical syndrome described with benign ovarian fibromas. These patients also require timely surgical resection for symptom relief.[29]

Tumor cells may also promote overgrowth of normal ovarian stroma, leading to uncommon clinical manifestations. Patients may rarely develop "massive ovarian edema," with pronounced ovarian enlargement and abdominal pain despite small tumor deposits.[30] Over time, this process can induce excessive ovarian hormonal secretion, leading to endocrine symptoms, such as hirsutism or abnormal uterine bleeding.[19,22]

INITIAL WORKUP AND IMAGING OF OVARIAN METASTASES

Patients with nonspecific or acute symptoms will often undergo abdominal ultrasound (US), transvaginal pelvic US, and/or contrast-enhanced abdominopelvic computed tomography (CT) for initial evaluation.[31–34] Patients with a history of cancer often receive routine follow-up with contrast-enhanced CT, or potentially fluorodeoxyglucose (FDG) -PET/CT.[35]

Although abdominal US will often be unrevealing (in the absence of liver metastases or ascites), pelvic US and CT are frequently the first modalities to detect ovarian metastases.[36–38]

In the United States, pelvic US in average-risk patients is increasingly interpreted in the context of American College of Radiology (ACR), US Ovarian-Adnexal Reporting and Data System (O-RADS), a 2019 classification system that stratifies tumors based on overall likelihood of malignancy and recommended follow-up.[37,39] Because most metastatic ovarian tumors have large solid components, irregular multilocular cysts, and/or increased vascularity,[38] they are likely to be classified as US O-RADS category 4 (intermediate risk of malignancy, 10%–50%) or US O-RADS category 5 (high risk of malignancy, >50%). O-RADS 4 observations are often recommended to undergo pelvic MR imaging for definitive characterization, whereas O-RADS 5 masses prompt direct surgical referral to gynecologic oncology.[39]

CT may show obvious aggressive features in large ovarian masses (irregular solid components, cysts with thick, nodular septations), or acute complications, such as hemorrhage.[36,37] However, due to its limited soft tissue contrast, it may not enable complete characterization of equivocal adnexal findings, for which pelvic MR imaging may be required.[37,40] Despite its weaknesses in the pelvis, CT is particularly valuable for its large field-of-view, which may enable visualization of an unsuspected GI malignancy or a pattern of distant metastases atypical for ovarian cancer (eg, many liver metastases without peritoneal disease). If present, such findings suggest a secondary cause for an indeterminate ovarian mass, directing management toward endoscopy/tissue sampling rather than gynecologic surgery.[41] Nonetheless, certain GI tumors may remain occult on CT, such as small intraluminal tumors in decompressed bowel or infiltrative gastric malignancies.[42,43]

On FDG-PET/CT, patients with ovarian metastases may have nonspecific enlargement or variably increased, heterogeneous FDG uptake in the ovaries.[44] This may be challenging to differentiate from even physiologic processes in the adnexa due to the lack of IV contrast and obscuration of pelvic organs by excreted radiotracer in the bladder.[45] In the absence of widespread metastatic disease, US, contrast-enhanced CT, and/or MR imaging is often required for complete evaluation.

MR IMAGING PROTOCOL FOR ADNEXAL NEOPLASMS (PRIMARY OR METASTATIC)

MR imaging is considered the gold-standard imaging technique for pelvic masses, given its superior soft-tissue contrast and numerous available sequences for tissue characterization.[37] Its lack of ionizing radiation is also optimal for young or pregnant patients.[46] Female pelvic MR imaging protocols vary by institution but should include several key sequences for complete assessment of indeterminate adnexal masses,[47] detailed in later discussion. Our complete protocol is detailed in **Table 1**.

Multiplanar T2-weighted imaging (T2WI) is essential for anatomic localization and evaluation of both fluid and soft tissue components of pelvic masses. Sequences are typically obtained in the axial and sagittal planes, without fat-saturation

Table 1
MR imaging protocol for pelvic masses

Sequence	Sequence Type	Coverage	Slice-Thickness/Gap	Voxel	TR	TE	FOV
Coronal T2W	TSE	Center over pelvis	4/default	0.7 × 0.7	3000–5000	110	To cover
Sagittal T2W	TSE Multivane	Center over pelvis	3/1 mm	0.6 × 0.6	3000–5000	100	To cover
Axial DWI	EPI	Pelvic inlet/outlet	4mm/default	2.19 × 2.2	Shortest	Shortest	To cover
Axial T2w HR	TSE	Pelvic inlet/outlet	3mm/default	0.5 × 0.8	2500–6000	110	To cover
Axial T1w Dixon	TSE	Pelvic inlet/outlet	3mm/-	1.2 × 1.2	Shortest	Shortest	To cover
Pre 4D Thrive	FFE	Pelvic inlet/outlet	4mm/-	0.8 × 0.8	Shortest	Shortest	To cover
Axial 4D Thrive Dyn	TFE	Pelvic inlet/outlet	4mm/-	0.8 × 0.8	Shortest	Shortest	To cover
(+)Sagittal e-Thrive	TFE	Center over pelvis	3mm/-	0.5 × 0.5	Shortest	Shortest	To cover
(+)Axial e-Thrive	TFE	Whole pelvis	3mm/-	1.5 × 1.5	Shortest	Shortest	To cover

(FS). We obtain an additional coronal sequence with a large field-of-view for a general overview of the pelvis and lower abdomen, which is useful to identify hydronephrosis or other masses.[47]

Precontrast T1-weighted imaging (T1WI) with FS is essential to evaluate for intrinsically T1-hyperintense contents (hemorrhagic or proteinaceous debris). This sequence should be coupled with either T1WI without FS or in-phase/out-of-phase (OOP) sequences to assess for the presence of intralesional fat.[47]

Postcontrast T1WI with FS, using a gadolinium-based contrast agent, is necessary to assess for enhancing soft tissue components and mural nodularity within adnexal masses. In particular, dynamic contrast-enhanced sequences are useful to evaluate the rate and persistence of lesion enhancement. These can be used to create time-intensity curves, which are used by both adnexal lesions magnetic resonance imaging (ADNEX-MR) and ACR O-RADS MR imaging classification schema to help radiologists determine the risk of malignancy for indeterminate adnexal masses.[48,49] Subtraction images may be created to confirm true enhancement.[47] In a pregnant patient, postcontrast sequences may be deferred due to theoretic risks of gadolinium exposure to the fetus but may still be performed (following informed patient consent) if deemed essential for diagnosis.[46]

Finally, diffusion-weighted imaging (DWI) should be performed to increase the sensitivity for malignancy.[47] By identifying tissues with high cellularity,[47] DWI can draw attention to otherwise subtle metastases in the pelvis, including small peritoneal nodules.[37] It is also useful to definitively diagnose T2-hypointense solid ovarian masses as benign fibrous tumors.[49]

GENERAL MR IMAGING FEATURES OF OVARIAN METASTASES

Given substantial differences in tumor origin and behavior, no general diagnostic imaging criteria exist for metastatic ovarian masses. Although MR imaging can show general features of malignancy,[49,50] it may not allow for the definitive diagnosis of a primary or secondary tumor,[50,51] prompting tissue sampling and pathologic analysis. A radiologist's most valuable clue to a metastasis may only be history of a primary cancer, or a primary tumor seen elsewhere in the field-of-view.[37]

Nonetheless, several imaging characteristics are repeatedly used to describe metastatic carcinomas involving the ovaries[36,52–56]: bilateral, solid, hypervascular, and heterogeneous. Metastases also tend to be smaller than primary tumors (<13 cm).[56]

On MR imaging, metastatic masses may be heterogeneously T2-hyperintense[57] with variable areas of cystic change and mildly T2-hypointense solid components.[36,37,58,59] By ACR O-RADS MR imaging,[49] the frequent presence of solid, hyperenhancing components suggests most metastases would qualify as O-RADS MR imaging 4 (intermediate risk, 50% risk of malignancy) or O-RADS MR imaging 5 (high risk, >50% risk of malignancy).

Imaging features of ovarian metastases are summarized in **Table 2**.

MR IMAGING OF GASTRIC CANCER METASTASES AND KRUKENBERG TUMORS

Most gastric adenocarcinoma metastases to the ovaries are ultimately diagnosed as KTs,[11,50,54,60] although metastases from rare colorectal or breast cancers may share a similar histology. Imaging of this pathologic tumor subtype is the topic of numerous studies,[27,28,60–67] warranting dedicated review.

By imaging, KTs are often solid,[68] with a smooth, lobulated margin and oval shape.[50,54,69] More than 60% are bilateral.[19] KTs variably accompany other metastases or peritoneal disease.[50,68]

On MR imaging, KTs are usually T2-hyperintense (due to intracellular mucin in tumor cells), with central areas of patchy or linear T2-hypointensity (corresponding to fibrotic stroma).[50,54,59,67] KTs with a prominent stromal component have the potential to mimic fibroma-thecomas; however, in contrast with these benign, slowly enhancing, "T2-DWI dark" tumors,[49] KTs demonstrate more rapid growth,[50] more avid enhancement, and impeded diffusion.[60] Occasionally, KTs may also contain well-demarcated intratumoral cysts with hyperenhancing walls.[61,65]

KTs have a unique tendency to present during pregnancy,[20,36] with various case reports describing potential imaging findings in this setting.[62–64,66,70] An example of bilateral KTs diagnosed in a pregnant woman is included in **Fig. 1**.

KTs undergo "luteinization" in pregnant patients, with increased stromal proliferation and abnormal production of sex steroid hormones.[19] Luteinized KTs have more pronounced T2-hypointense stroma, and may even develop associated intratumoral microscopic fat, which can manifest on MR imaging as areas of T1-hyperintensity with dropout of signal on OOP imaging.[64] This differs from teratomas (mature or immature), which have T1-hyperintense macroscopic fat that shows signal dropout on FS-T1WI and "India-ink" artifact on OOP imaging.[37] KTs may also undergo rapid growth after delivery,[36] with increased risk for hemorrhage or rupture.[28] Hematoma may show heterogeneous T1 hyperintensity that persists on FS-T1WI and OOP sequences.

Table 2
Key MR imaging findings of ovarian metastases

Primary Cancer Type	Features of Ovarian Mass(es) Suggestive of Metastases
General ovarian metastases	Bilateral, heterogeneous, solid components, hypervascular; <13 cm; known history of primary cancer; primary cancer also seen in FOV
Krukenberg/gastric	Solid, oval, well-circumscribed; bilateral; T2-hyperintense with T2-hypointense stroma; rare microscopic fat or hemorrhage in pregnancy
Colorectal	Multilocular cystic or mixed cystic-solid; bilateral; mille-feuille sign; mucinous tumors may mimic primary mucinous ovarian neoplasms (stained-glass appearance on T2WI)
Appendix	Cystic ovarian mass(es) + pseudomyxoma peritonei; distended appendix containing T2-hyperintense mucin
Breast	Solid, small, bilateral, hyperenhancing; clinical history of advanced-stage cancer
Gynecologic	Solid or mixed cystic/solid; large primary endometrial or cervical mass ± pelvic nodal metastases
Lymphoma	Solid, bilateral; homogeneously T2-intermediate signal; hypoenhancement; lymphadenopathy/splenomegaly
Pancreaticobiliary	Cystic or mixed cystic/solid; can mimic primary mucinous neoplasms
Urothelial	Cystic; direct extension from locally invasive primary
Melanoma	Solid, mixed cystic/solid; possible intrinsic T1-hyperintensity from melanin

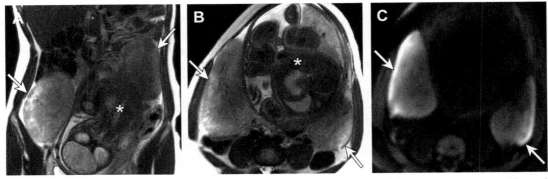

Fig. 1. Krukenberg tumors due to signet-ring adenocarcinoma in a 30-year-old pregnant woman at 33 weeks gestation. Pelvic MR imaging with coronal T2WI (*A*), axial T2WI (*B*), and DWI (*C*) shows large, solid bilateral ovarian masses (*white arrows*), which have mild peripheral T2 hyperintensity, profuse T2-hypointense central stroma, and impeded diffusion. Gravid uterus is noted (*asterisk*).

Of note, other pathologic subtypes of gastric cancer can also cause ovarian metastases. Intestinal-subtype gastric cancer much more rarely affects the ovaries, usually in older patients. The imaging appearance of these tumors differs significantly from KTs, more often mixed cystic and solid, with variable signal on T1WI and T2WI and areas of necrosis.[36,50,71]

MR IMAGING OF COLORECTAL CANCER METASTASES

Colorectal cancer metastases to the ovaries most often arise from primary rectosigmoid adenocarcinomas. These metastases are frequently larger than the primary tumor and are bilateral in 50% to 80% of patients (with unilateral tumors more likely to involve the right ovary).[36,50,72,73]

By imaging, ovarian metastases from colorectal cancers are usually multilocular cystic or mixed cystic/solid; this contrasts with KTs, which tend to be solid and smaller in size.[54,68,69] Margins are typically smooth,[69] although internal necrosis is common.[50,54] Peritoneal metastatic disease is present in 20% to 50% of cases,[50,73] whereas concurrent liver metastases are present in 25%.[73]

The "mille-feuille" sign (layered, stacked soft tissue along the margins of a cystic mass) is a recently identified morphology seen in colorectal cancer metastases on CT and MR imaging. This sign is reported to have a high specificity with high interrater agreement but is yet to undergo further validation.[74]

Colorectal cancer metastases with mucinous histology classically mimic primary ovarian neoplasms. On MR imaging, mucinous masses of any origin may contain multilocular cystic areas with a "stained glass" appearance on T2WI, as well as thickened septations and solid components.[36,50,54,71]

Although tumor morphology may be nearly identical in primary and secondary mucinous masses, bilaterality is particularly uncommon among primary tumors, and its presence should suggest metastases.[54] A surgical algorithm classifying all bilateral mucinous tumors and any unilateral mucinous tumor less than 10 cm as metastatic is reportedly 90% accurate in a small series.[75] However, only bilaterality is confirmed to be predictive of metastasis (95%) in a subsequent validation study.[76]

An example of metastatic rectal cancer involving the ovaries is shown in **Fig. 2.**

MR IMAGING OF APPENDICEAL CANCER METASTASES

Appendiceal tumors are rare GI malignancies, with more variable histology: potential subtypes include low-grade and high-grade mucinous neoplasia, mucinous adenocarcinoma, colonic-type adenocarcinoma, goblet cell carcinoma, and neuroendocrine neoplasms. Low-grade mucinous neoplasms are most likely to involve the ovaries.[36]

Any adnexal masses (typically cystic) in the setting of pseudomyxoma peritonei should raise concern for appendiceal ovarian metastases.[50] Pseudomyxoma peritonei is defined as disseminated intraperitoneal mucinous tumor due to rupture of an appendiceal mucinous neoplasm. On MR imaging, loculated mucinous deposits are found throughout the peritoneal cavity, which are markedly T2-hyperintense (only slightly less than simple ascites) and have minimal to no enhancement, based on the cellularity of the underlying tumor. Organ surfaces, classically the liver capsule

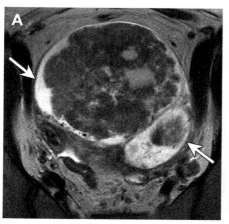
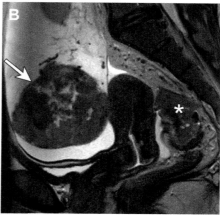

Fig. 2. Rectal adenocarcinoma metastatic to bilateral ovaries in a 37-year-old woman. Pelvic MR imaging with axial (A) and sagittal (B) T2WI shows bilateral mixed cystic/solid ovarian masses (*white arrows*), with heterogeneous solid components. There is an associated circumferential high rectal mass (*asterisk*).

may seem scalloped.[36,57] Pseudomyxoma is not typically seen in primary mucinous ovarian neoplasms, implying a secondary cause.[54] A dilated appendix containing T2-hyperintense mucin may also be seen in the pelvis, which confirms the diagnosis of primary appendiceal mucinous neoplasm.[36]

Appendiceal ovarian metastases are frequently bilateral; if unilateral, they also tend to involve the right ovary,[50] analogous to colorectal cancers. They are primarily multilocular cystic or mixed cystic/solid.[36,54]

An example of a metastatic appendiceal mucinous neoplasm involving the right ovary (with associated ovarian torsion) and pelvic pseudomyxoma peritonei is shown in **Fig. 3**.

MR IMAGING OF BREAST CANCER METASTASES

As the most common malignancy among women worldwide,[15] breast cancer is a relatively common cause for ovarian metastases. Primary cancer subtypes include invasive ductal and invasive lobular carcinoma.[77] Greatest risk of ovarian involvement among premenopausal patients is conferred by lobular histology or advanced stage disease.[78,79] Ovarian metastases usually present late after a known breast cancer diagnosis and are unlikely to be symptomatic.[11,80]

Given that many patients with breast cancer are diagnosed at early stages, and patients occasionally have breast cancer gene 1 (*BRCA1*) or *BRCA2* mutations (increasing their risk for both breast and primary ovarian cancers), accurate clinical history is particularly important for radiologists. In general, most adnexal masses among patients with a history of breast cancer are benign.[81] However, a new adnexal mass in a patient with stage 4 breast cancer is more likely to be a metastasis,[77] although a similar finding in a patient with stage 1 disease is more likely due to a benign ovarian process.[79] Similarly, a BRCA-positive patient is more likely to present with primary ovarian malignancy than a metastasis.[50,54]

By imaging, ovarian metastases from breast cancer are often bilateral, solid, small (≤5 cm), and hypervascular.[17,36,54,79] Solid components have heterogeneous T2 signal on MR imaging.[77] If mass(es) have a cystic component, thickened septations are uniformly present.[77] Necrosis and heterogeneous enhancement are also common.[82]

Examples of metastatic breast cancer to the ovaries are shown in **Fig. 4**.

MR IMAGING OF GYNECOLOGIC CANCER METASTASES

Both endometrial and cervical cancers may metastasize to the ovaries.[52] Adnexal metastases are particularly important to identify in premenopausal patients with early stage disease because they may not always undergo oophorectomy at the time of surgical treatment.[36,83,84]

Pelvic MR imaging is obtained for presurgical planning after initial diagnosis of cervical or uterine cancers, particularly when pathologic condition shows a high-risk disease.[50] Incidental ovarian masses may be detected on these scans, and both imaging and pathologic features of the primary tumor can aid in characterization.

Among patients with endometrial cancer, deep myometrial invasion (≥50%), lymph node metastases, and nonendometroid (serous/clear cell) histology are risk factors for adnexal involvement.[83] Among patients with cervical cancer, large tumor

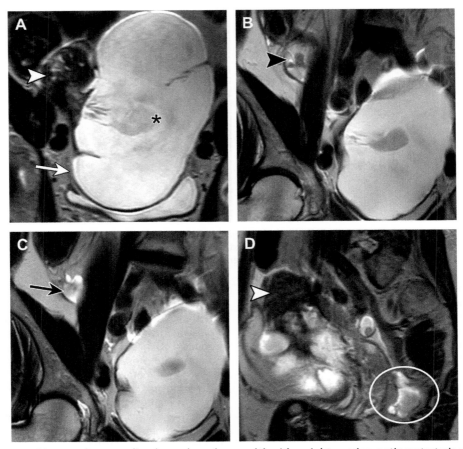

Fig. 3. Ruptured low-grade appendiceal neoplasm (mucocele) with a right ovarian cystic metastasis and consequent right ovarian torsion in a 63-year-old woman. Pelvic MR imaging with coronal (*A–C*), and sagittal (*D*) T2WI shows a large cystic right ovarian mass (*white arrow*) with thin septations and mucinous debris (*asterisk*). There is a twisted right ovarian pedicle with a "whirlpool sign" (*white arrowhead*). The appendix is mildly dilated, containing T2-hyperintense mucin (*black arrowhead*). There are associated loculated intraperitoneal mucinous deposits adjacent to the appendix (*black arrow*) and in the right cul-de-sac (*circle*).

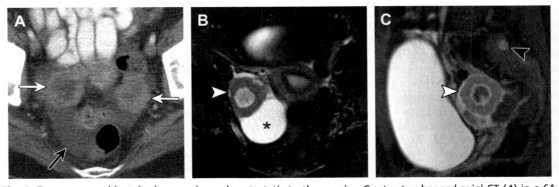

Fig. 4. Breast cancer (ductal adenocarcinoma) metastatic to the ovaries. Contrast-enhanced axial CT (*A*) in a 64-year-old woman with a history of breast cancer 17 years prior shows small bilateral solid ovarian masses with central necrosis (*white arrow*). There is associated pelvic ascites (*black arrow*). Pelvic MR imaging with axial fat sat-T2WI (*B*) and sagittal postcontrast fat sat-T1WI (*C*) in a 37-year-old woman with a history of breast cancer diagnosed 2 years prior shows a solid right ovarian mass (*white arrowhead*) with central necrosis, a physiologic right ovarian cyst (*asterisk*), and a sacral bone metastasis (*black arrowhead*).

size, deep cervical stromal invasion, uterine or vaginal invasion, lymph node metastases, and adenocarcinoma histology (rather than squamous) all increase the risk of ovarian metastases.[65,84] Thus, a large primary tumor and advanced-stage disease should prompt a radiologist to thoroughly investigate the adnexa; metastasis should be provided as a differential consideration for an aggressive-appearing ovarian mass.

By US or MR imaging, ovarian metastases from endometrial and squamous cervical cancers tend to be bilateral and solid.[85,86] However, they may also be mixed cystic or mixed cystic/solid, particularly when caused by cervical adenocarcinoma,[50,52,85] which can mimic a primary ovarian neoplasm. Primary tumor size may help with differentiation. For example, a large, unilateral, complex cystic ovarian mass in the setting of a small, noninvasive primary tumor is more suggestive of a synchronous primary ovarian neoplasm than a metastasis.[50]

An example of cervical adenocarcinoma with ovarian involvement is shown in **Fig. 5**.

MR IMAGING OF LYMPHOMA/LEUKEMIA METASTASES

Secondary ovarian involvement by lymphoma or leukemia occurs in the setting of disseminated, widespread disease, most frequently diffuse large B-cell lymphoma.[37]

By imaging, ovarian metastases are large, bilateral solid masses with extraovarian extension.[36] On MR imaging, masses consist of homogeneous, T2-intermediate soft tissue, with only mild enhancement on postcontrast sequences.[54,87]

In contrast to metastases from extraovarian carcinomas, lymphomatous metastases are often associated with extensive abdominopelvic lymphadenopathy and splenomegaly.[36,87] Other lymphomatous masses may be also seen in the pelvis, such as bulky masses that encase bowel without causing obstruction.[37]

An example of leukemic infiltration of the ovary is shown in **Fig. 6**.

IMAGING OF OTHER RARER METASTASES

Ovarian metastases from numerous other primary cancers are described, including pancreaticobiliary adenocarcinoma, renal cell carcinoma, urothelial carcinoma, small bowel and esophageal adenocarcinoma, lung cancer (adenocarcinoma or small cell), melanoma, neuroendocrine neoplasm, gastrointestinal stromal tumor, hepatocellular carcinoma, and sarcoma.[11] These tumors are primarily the subject of isolated case reports or small case series, and their rarity precludes a definitive review of their imaging features. However, several cancer types have notable features that can be helpful for radiologists to recognize.

Pancreaticobiliary metastases tend to be cystic, and can mimic primary mucinous neoplasms, similar to colorectal cancers. Bilaterality and history of cancer favors metastases.[53,54,88]

Urothelial cancer may spread to the ovaries, particularly in locally advanced, muscle-invasive disease with lymphovascular invasion.[37] Metastatic ovarian lesions often have a complex cystic appearance.[89–91]

Melanoma may have either solid or mixed cystic/solid morphology.[92] Although intrinsic T1

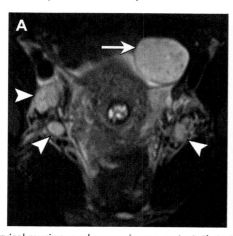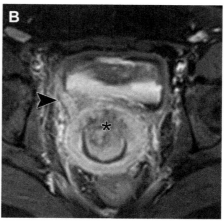

Fig. 5. Cervical mucinous adenocarcinoma metastatic to the left ovary in a 20 year-old woman. Pelvic MR imaging with axial fat sat-T2WI (*A*) and postcontrast fat sat-T1WI (*B*) shows a small left ovarian mass (*white arrow*), with loss of normal follicular architecture and central T2-hyperintense mucin. There is an associated infiltrative, hypoenhancing cervical mass (*asterisk*) with anterior vaginal, parametrial and posterior bladder involvement (*black arrowhead*). There are multiple enlarged T2-hyperintense pelvic sidewall lymph nodes (*white arrowheads*).

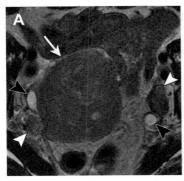
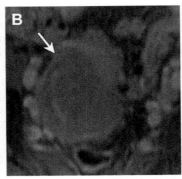
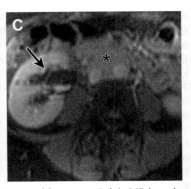

Fig. 6. Acute myeloid leukemia with involvement of the right ovary in a 53 year-old woman. Pelvic MR imaging with axial T2WI (*A*) and postcontrast fat sat-T1WI (*B, C*) shows a large, sold right ovarian mass (*white arrow*), which is mildly T2-hypointense, relatively homogeneous, and hypoenhancing. There are associated enlarged bilateral iliac lymph nodes (*white arrowhead*) and confluent para-aortic lymphadenopathy (*asterisk*). The mass also causes distal ureteral obstruction (*black arrowhead*) and right hydronephrosis (*black arrow*).

hyperintensity may indicate the presence of melanin on MR imaging,[93] this may be absent in amelanotic melanoma and can be mimicked by hemorrhage. An example of metastatic melanoma to the ovary is shown in **Fig. 7**.

CLINCHING THE DIAGNOSIS: ROLE OF BIOPSY, PATHOLOGY, AND TUMOR MARKERS

Ovarian masses considered indeterminate or suspicious for metastatic disease by imaging generally require a definitive pathologic diagnosis. Although surgery is the traditional mainstay for diagnosis and treatment, percutaneous sampling by interventional radiology is increasingly performed in patients who are poor surgical candidates or for whom the preferred surgeon (surgical oncology or gynecologic oncology) is uncertain.[37,94] Ovarian mass biopsies are now

known to be safe and effective: A 27-patient series showed 100% diagnostic yield, without any acute or long-term complications (including peritoneal seeding).[95]

Of note, ovarian masses that perplex radiologists are often also challenging for pathologists, who must use a combination of histologic features, complex immunohistochemistry, and novel molecular profiling to establish the precise diagnosis.[3,11,72] Referral to a tertiary care center with multidisciplinary tumor board discussion is indicated for such cases. If pathologic condition suggests a metastasis from a previously undiagnosed primary cancer, a patient must undergo further evaluation (such as endoscopy, CT, PET/CT, or breast imaging) to complete staging.

Serum tumor markers are also frequently obtained in patients with suspected ovarian

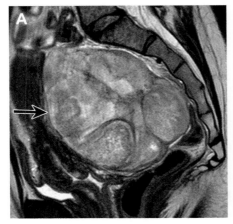
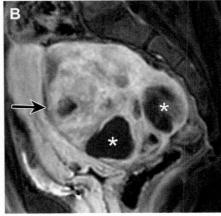

Fig. 7. Melanoma metastatic to the right ovary in a 41 year-old woman. Pelvic MR imaging with sagittal T2WI (*A*) and FS-T1WI (*B*), and postcontrast FS-T1WI shows a large, heterogenous right ovarian mass (*black arrow*), which is T2 hyperintense and hyperenhancing, with multifocal areas of necrosis (*asterisk*). There is associated mass effect on the uterus, rectosigmoid colon, and pelvic floor.

malignancy, which mainly play a supportive role in diagnosis, prognosis, and surveillance.[96] Cancer antigen (CA)-125 is classically elevated in 80% of primary epithelial ovarian cancers but may also be elevated due to ovarian metastases (in up to 70% of cases). This limits the specificity of this marker alone to discern tumor origin.[3] Elevation in CEA or CA 19-9 (with comparatively lower CA-125) is more likely in metastatic disease[96] but this is not reliable in practice.[97] More importantly, elevation of both CA-125 and CA 19-9 is associated with poor overall survival, which may help guide management and patient expectations.[24]

MANAGEMENT AND PROGNOSIS

Treatment of patients with ovarian metastases varies based on the type and extent of primary malignancy, as well as the severity of clinical symptoms. In general, patients with isolated or symptomatic ovarian metastatic disease undergo resection, and subsequently receive adjuvant chemotherapy for their primary cancer. However, patients who are poor surgical candidates or have widespread metastatic disease may only undergo chemotherapy.[3]

Surgical resection is a type of "metastasectomy" or cytoreductive surgery (CRS), consisting of salpingo-oophorectomy plus variable hysterectomy and debulking of peritoneal metastatic disease.[24] For patients with metastases of GI origin, hyperthermic intraperitoneal chemotherapy may also be performed during surgery.[3,98] Although surgery may not be curative, ovarian metastases may be more resistant to chemotherapy[99]; hence, surgery is often the only effective method to completely and rapidly resolve large, symptomatic tumors. Additionally, a successful CRS (to no residual visible disease, R0) is consistently shown to have survival benefits among patients with colorectal cancer,[3] as well as probable benefits in gastric and breast cancers.[3,79,98]

Despite advances in cancer treatment, prognosis for patients with ovarian metastases remains poor, particularly those with concurrent peritoneal carcinomatosis, nongynecologic primary malignancies, and diagnosis in pregnancy.[3,20,100] Survival varies based on specific tumor-related and patient-related factors but is largely worse than primary ovarian malignancy: overall 5-year survival rate is only 18.5%, compared with 40.0% in primary ovarian cancer.[3]

SUMMARY

Metastases to the ovaries are a challenging imaging diagnosis, and radiologists may struggle to differentiate between primary and secondary ovarian neoplasms in young women. Clinical context is key: a history of known primary extraovarian cancer, especially an aggressive subtype or advanced stage, should increase suspicion for metastases but is unfortunately lacking in many cases. Pelvic MR imaging provides the best opportunity to characterize indeterminate adnexal masses as malignant. Although no imaging features identify metastases with complete certainty, ovarian tumors that are bilateral, primarily solid, heterogeneous, and/or hyper-enhancing should potentially be considered suspicious for metastases. Conversely, a large, unilateral, cystic, or mixed cystic/solid mass, in the absence of peritoneal disease, is more suggestive of a primary ovarian neoplasm. Ultimately, most patients require a pathologic diagnosis and surgical resection. Nonetheless, radiologists play an essential role in suggesting the possibility of metastases when imaging appearances are atypical, as well as identifying unsuspected, incidental primary tumors, which can drastically affect the course of patient care.

CLINICS PEARLS

- The most common causes of ovarian metastases are colorectal, gastric, breast, and gynecologic carcinomas. Therefore, radiologists should carefully assess the adnexa in follow-up imaging of patients with known extraovarian malignancy, and should always scrutinize the GI tract on imaging of patients with indeterminate adnexal masses.

- MR imaging is the most accurate modality to evaluate indeterminate adnexal masses. ACR O-RADS MR imaging can be used to determine risk of malignancy (whether primary or metastatic).

- In a patient with an incidental, malignant-appearing adnexal mass, consider ovarian metastasis if known (advanced) malignancy, young age, bilateral tumors, and tumors with hypervascular, irregular, heterogeneous solid components. Note that stomach and breast malignancies tend to be solid, whereas colorectal metastases tend to be cystic.

- Metastatic mucinous ovarian tumors are notoriously challenging to differentiate from primary tumors but generally tend to be smaller (<13 cm), more often bilateral, and more frequently associated with peritoneal metastatic disease.

- Tissue sampling is often necessary to establish a definitive pathologic diagnosis. Percutaneous ovarian mass biopsy is safe and effective for this purpose.
- Radiologist recognition of adnexal metastases is important because patients may undergo targeted surgical resection, which has potential benefits for patient outcomes and symptom relief.

DISCLOSURE

A.P. Wasnik:None related to this article. Unrelated disclosures include book royalty, Elsevier Inc.; royalty, intellectual property, licensed by the University of Michigan to Applied Morphomics, Inc; research support, Sequana Medical, NV payable to University of Michigan; Research grant support, National Institute of Diabetes and Digestive and Kidney Diseases (R01-DK124779) payable to University of Michigan.

REFERENCES

1. Riihimaki M, Thomsen H, Sundquist K, et al. Clinical landscape of cancer metastases. Cancer Med 2018;7(11):5534–42.
2. Karpathiou G, Chauleur C, Hathroubi S, et al. Secondary Tumors of the Gynecologic Tract: A Clinicopathologic Analysis. Int J Gynecol Pathol 2019; 38(4):363–70.
3. Kubecek O, Laco J, Spacek J, et al. The pathogenesis, diagnosis, and management of metastatic tumors to the ovary: a comprehensive review. Clin Exp Metastasis 2017;34(5):295–307.
4. Ajani MA, Iyapo O, Salami A, et al. Secondary Ovarian Neoplasms in a Tertiary Hospital in Southwestern Nigeria. Ann Ib Postgrad Med 2019;17(1): 19–23.
5. Alvarado-Cabrero I, Rodriguez-Gomez A, Castelan-Pedraza J, et al. Metastatic ovarian tumors: a clinicopathologic study of 150 cases. Anal Quant Cytopathol Histpathol 2013;35(5):241–8.
6. Antila R, Jalkanen J, Heikinheimo O. Comparison of secondary and primary ovarian malignancies reveals differences in their pre- and perioperative characteristics. Gynecol Oncol 2006;101(1): 97–101.
7. de Waal YR, Thomas CM, Oei AL, et al. Secondary ovarian malignancies: frequency, origin, and characteristics. Int J Gynecol Cancer 2009;19(7): 1160–5.
8. Demopoulos RI, Touger L, Dubin N. Secondary ovarian carcinoma: a clinical and pathological evaluation. Int J Gynecol Pathol 1987;6(2):166–75.
9. Khunamornpong S, Suprasert P, Chiangmai WN, et al. Metastatic tumors to the ovaries: a study of 170 cases in northern Thailand. Int J Gynecol Cancer 2006;16(Suppl 1):132–8.
10. Yada-Hashimoto N, Yamamoto T, Kamiura S, et al. Metastatic ovarian tumors: a review of 64 cases. Gynecol Oncol 2003;89(2):314–7.
11. Lerwill MF, Young R H. Metastatic Tumors of the Ovary. In: Kurman R, Ellenson LH, Ronnett B, editors. Blaustein's Pathology of the Female Genital Tract. Cham: Springer; 2019. https://doi.org/10. 1007/978-3-319-46334-6_18.
12. Bruls J, Simons M, Overbeek LI, et al. A national population-based study provides insight in the origin of malignancies metastatic to the ovary. Virchows Arch 2015;467(1):79–86.
13. Moore RG, Chung M, Granai CO, et al. Incidence of metastasis to the ovaries from nongenital tract primary tumors. Gynecol Oncol 2004;93(1):87–91.
14. Zhang JJ, Cao DY, Yang JX, et al. Ovarian metastasis from nongynecologic primary sites: a retrospective analysis of 177 cases and 13-year experience. J Ovarian Res 2020;13(1):128.
15. Jemal A, Bray F, Center MM, et al. Global cancer statistics. CA Cancer J Clin 2011;61(2):69–90.
16. Center MM, Jemal A, Ward E. International trends in colorectal cancer incidence rates. Cancer Epidemiol Biomarkers Prev 2009;18(6):1688–94.
17. Guerriero S, Alcazar JL, Pascual MA, et al. Preoperative diagnosis of metastatic ovarian cancer is related to origin of primary tumor. Ultrasound Obstet Gynecol 2012;39(5):581–6.
18. Lee SJ, Bae JH, Lee AW, et al. Clinical characteristics of metastatic tumors to the ovaries. J Korean Med Sci 2009;24(1):114–9.
19. Kiyokawa T, Young RH, Scully RE. Krukenberg tumors of the ovary: a clinicopathologic analysis of 120 cases with emphasis on their variable pathologic manifestations. Am J Surg Pathol 2006; 30(3):277–99.
20. Kodama M, Moeini A, Machida H, et al. Fetomaternal outcomes of pregnancy complicated by Krukenberg tumor: a systematic review of literature. Arch Gynecol Obstet 2016;294(3):589–98.
21. Stewart CJ, Leung YC, Whitehouse A. Fallopian tube metastases of non-gynaecological origin: a series of 20 cases emphasizing patterns of involvement including intra-epithelial spread. Histopathology 2012;60(6B):E106–14.
22. Agnes A, Biondi A, Ricci R, et al. Krukenberg tumors: Seed, route and soil. Surg Oncol 2017; 26(4):438–45.
23. Duarte I, Llanos O. Patterns of metastases in intestinal and diffuse types of carcinoma of the stomach. Hum Pathol 1981;12(3):237–42.
24. Sal V, Demirkiran F, Topuz S, et al. Surgical Treatment of Metastatic Ovarian Tumors From

Extragenital Primary Sites. Int J Gynecol Cancer 2016;26(4):688–96.

25. Bruchim I, Ben-Harim Z, Piura E, et al. Preoperative clinical and radiological features of metastatic ovarian tumors. Arch Gynecol Obstet 2013; 288(3):615–9.

26. Jung YE, Lee JW, Kim BG, et al. Ovarian metastasis from pulmonary adenocarcinoma. Obstet Gynecol Sci 2013;56(5):341–4.

27. Sandhu S, Arafat O, Patel H, et al. Krukenberg tumor: a rare cause of ovarian torsion. J Clin Imaging Sci 2012;2:6.

28. La Fianza A, Cassani C, Ori Belometti G. Intralesional hemorrhage in Krukenberg tumor: a case report and review of the literature. J Ultrasound 2013;16(2):89–91.

29. Nagakura S, Shirai Y, Hatakeyama K. Pseudo-Meigs' syndrome caused by secondary ovarian tumors from gastrointestinal cancer. A case report and review of the literature. Dig Surg 2000;17(4): 418–9.

30. Tanaka YO, Takazawa Y, Matsuura M, et al. MR Imaging of Secondary Massive Ovarian Edema Caused by Ovarian Metastasis from Appendiceal Adenocarcinoma. Magn Reson Med Sci 2019; 18(2):111–2.

31. Bhosale PR, Javitt MC, Atri M, et al. ACR Appropriateness Criteria(R) Acute Pelvic Pain in the Reproductive Age Group. Ultrasound Q 2016;32(2): 108–15.

32. Expert Panel on Gastrointestinal I, Scheirey CD, Fowler KJ, et al. ACR Appropriateness Criteria((R)) Acute Nonlocalized Abdominal Pain. J Am Coll Radiol 2018;15(11S):S217–31.

33. Expert Panel on GYN, Imaging OB, Henrichsen TL, et al. ACR Appropriateness Criteria(R) Postmenopausal Acute Pelvic Pain. J Am Coll Radiol 2021; 18(5S):S119–25.

34. Expert Panel on Women's I, Maturen KE, Akin EA, et al. ACR Appropriateness Criteria((R)) Postmenopausal Subacute or Chronic Pelvic Pain. J Am Coll Radiol 2018;15(11S):S365–72.

35. Benson AB, Venook AP, Al-Hawary MM, et al. Colon Cancer, Version 2.2021, NCCN Clinical Practice Guidelines in Oncology. J Natl Compr Canc Netw 2021;19(3):329–59.

36. Karaosmanoglu AD, Onur MR, Salman MC, et al. Imaging in secondary tumors of the ovary. Abdom Radiol (NY) 2019;44(4):1493–505.

37. Taylor EC, Irshaid L, Mathur M. Multimodality Imaging Approach to Ovarian Neoplasms with Pathologic Correlation. Radiographics 2021;41(1): 289–315.

38. Testa AC, Ferrandina G, Timmerman D, et al. Imaging in gynecological disease (1): ultrasound features of metastases in the ovaries differ depending on the origin of the primary tumor. Ultrasound Obstet Gynecol 2007;29(5):505–11.

39. Andreotti RF, Timmerman D, Strachowski LM, et al. O-RADS US Risk Stratification and Management System: A Consensus Guideline from the ACR Ovarian-Adnexal Reporting and Data System Committee. Radiology 2020;294(1):168–85.

40. Expert Panel on Women's I, Atri M, Alabousi A, et al. ACR Appropriateness Criteria((R)) Clinically Suspected Adnexal Mass, No Acute Symptoms. J Am Coll Radiol 2019;16(5S):S77–93.

41. Heatley MK. Mucinous tumours of the ovary–primary and metastatic. J Clin Pathol 2012;65(7): 577–9.

42. Balthazar EJ, Siegel SE, Megibow AJ, et al. CT in patients with scirrhous carcinoma of the GI tract: imaging findings and value for tumor detection and staging. AJR Am J Roentgenol 1995;165(4): 839–45.

43. Gollub MJ, Schwartz LH, Akhurst T. Update on colorectal cancer imaging. Radiol Clin North Am 2007;45(1):85–118.

44. Park SH, Lee JJ, Kim HO, et al. 18F-Fluorodeoxyglucose (FDG)-positron emission tomography/computed tomography in mucosa-associated lymphoid tissue lymphoma: variation in 18F-FDG avidity according to site involvement. Leuk Lymphoma 2015;56(12):3288–94.

45. Bouchelouche K. PET/CT in Bladder Cancer: An Update. Semin Nucl Med 2022. https://doi.org/10.1053/j.semnuclmed.2021.12.004.

46. Tirada N, Dreizin D, Khati NJ, et al. Imaging Pregnant and Lactating Patients. Radiographics 2015; 35(6):1751–65.

47. Sakala MD, Shampain KL, Wasnik AP. Advances in MR Imaging of the Female Pelvis. Magn Reson Imaging Clin N Am 2020;28(3):415–31.

48. Sadowski EA, Robbins JB, Rockall AG, et al. A systematic approach to adnexal masses discovered on ultrasound: the ADNEx MR scoring system. Abdom Radiol (NY) 2018;43(3):679–95.

49. Sadowski EA, Thomassin-Naggara I, Rockall A, et al. O-RADS MRI Risk Stratification System: Guide for Assessing Adnexal Lesions from the ACR O-RADS Committee. Radiology 2022; 204371. https://doi.org/10.1148/radiol.204371.

50. Willmott F, Allouni KA, Rockall A. Radiological manifestations of metastasis to the ovary. J Clin Pathol 2012;65(7):585–90.

51. Brown DL, Zou KH, Tempany CM, et al. Primary versus secondary ovarian malignancy: imaging findings of adnexal masses in the Radiology Diagnostic Oncology Group Study. Radiology 2001; 219(1):213–8.

52. Ahmed SA, Taieb HA. Variations in radiological features between primary and secondary ovarian

malignancies. Egypt J Radiol Nucl Med 2018; 49(3):828–37.

53. Chang WC, Meux MD, Yeh BM, et al. CT and MRI of adnexal masses in patients with primary nonovarian malignancy. AJR Am J Roentgenol 2006; 186(4):1039–45.

54. Koyama T, Mikami Y, Saga T, et al. Secondary ovarian tumors: spectrum of CT and MR features with pathologic correlation. Abdom Imaging 2007; 32(6):784–95.

55. Shinagare AB, Gujrathi I, Cochon L, et al. Predictors of malignancy in incidental adnexal lesions identified on CT in patients with prior non-ovarian cancer. Abdom Radiol (NY) 2022;47(1):320–7.

56. Xu Y, Yang J, Zhang Z, et al. MRI for discriminating metastatic ovarian tumors from primary epithelial ovarian cancers. J Ovarian Res 2015;8:61.

57. Szklaruk J, Tamm EP, Choi H, et al. MR imaging of common and uncommon large pelvic masses. Radiographics 2003;23(2):403–24.

58. Imaoka I, Wada A, Kaji Y, et al. Developing an MR imaging strategy for diagnosis of ovarian masses. Radiographics 2006;26(5):1431–48.

59. Jung SE, Lee JM, Rha SE, et al. CT and MR imaging of ovarian tumors with emphasis on differential diagnosis. Radiographics 2002;22(6):1305–25.

60. Zulfiqar M, Koen J, Nougaret S, et al. Krukenberg Tumors: Update on Imaging and Clinical Features. AJR Am J Roentgenol 2020;215(4):1020–9.

61. Cho JY, Seong CK, Kim SH. Krukenberg tumor findings at color and power Doppler US; correlation with findings at CT, MR imaging, and pathology. Case reports. Acta Radiol 1998;39(3):327–9.

62. Chou MM, Ho ES, Lin NF, et al. Color Doppler sonographic appearance of a Krukenberg tumor in pregnancy. Ultrasound Obstet Gynecol 1998; 11(6):459–60.

63. Co PV, Gupta A, Attar BM, et al. Gastric cancer presenting as a krukenberg tumor at 22 weeks' gestation. J Gastric Cancer 2014;14(4):275–8.

64. Jeong YY, Kang HK, Seo JJ, et al. Luteinized fat in Krukenberg tumor: MR findings. Eur Radiol 2002; 12(Suppl 3):S130–2.

65. Kim SH, Kim WH, Park KJ, et al. CT and MR findings of Krukenberg tumors: comparison with primary ovarian tumors. J Comput Assist Tomogr 1996;20(3):393–8.

66. Mendoza-Rosado F, Nunez-Isaac O, Espinosa-Marron A, et al. Krukenberg tumor as an incidental finding in a full-term pregnancy: a case report. J Med Case Rep 2021;15(1):304.

67. Ha HK, Baek SY, Kim SH, et al. Krukenberg's tumor of the ovary: MR imaging features. AJR Am J Roentgenol 1995;164(6):1435–9.

68. Choi HJ, Lee JH, Kang S, et al. Contrast-enhanced CT for differentiation of ovarian metastasis from gastrointestinal tract cancer: stomach cancer versus colon cancer. AJR Am J Roentgenol 2006; 187(3):741–5.

69. Choi HJ, Lee JH, Seo SS, et al. Computed tomography findings of ovarian metastases from colon cancer: comparison with primary malignant ovarian tumors. J Comput Assist Tomogr 2005;29(1):69–73.

70. Goidescu IG, Nemeti G, Preda A, et al. Krukenberg tumor in pregnancy: a rare case and review of the literature. J Matern Fetal Neonatal Med 2021;1–6. https://doi.org/10.1080/14767058.2021.1946788.

71. Laurent PE, Thomassin-Piana J, Jalaguier-Coudray A. Mucin-producing tumors of the ovary: MR imaging appearance. Diagn Interv Imaging 2015;96(11):1125–32.

72. Kir G, Gurbuz A, Karateke A, et al. Clinicopathologic and immunohistochemical profile of ovarian metastases from colorectal carcinoma. World J Gastrointest Surg 2010;2(4):109–16.

73. Li X, Zhang W, Ding P, et al. Clinical characteristics and prognostic factors of colorectal cancer patients with ovarian metastasis: a multicenter retrospective study. Int J Colorectal Dis 2021;36(6): 1201–8.

74. Kurokawa R, Nakai Y, Gonoi W, et al. Differentiation between ovarian metastasis from colorectal carcinoma and primary ovarian carcinoma: Evaluation of tumour markers and "mille-feuille sign" on computed tomography/magnetic resonance imaging. Eur J Radiol 2020;124:108823.

75. Seidman JD, Kurman RJ, Ronnett BM. Primary and metastatic mucinous adenocarcinomas in the ovaries: incidence in routine practice with a new approach to improve intraoperative diagnosis. Am J Surg Pathol 2003;27(7):985–93.

76. Khunamornpong S, Suprasert P, Pojchamarnwiputh S et al. Primary and metastatic mucinous adenocarcinomas of the ovary: Evaluation of the diagnostic approach using tumor size and laterality. Gynecol Oncol 2006;101(1):152–7.

77. Abd El hafez A, Monir A. Diagnostic spectrum of ovarian masses in women with breast cancer; magnetic resonance imaging: histopathology correlation. Ann Diagn Pathol 2013;17(5):441–7.

78. Moore EK, Roylance R, Rosenthal AN. Breast cancer metastasising to the pelvis and abdomen: what the gynaecologist needs to know. BJOG 2012; 119(7):788–94.

79. Tian W, Zhou Y, Wu M, et al. Ovarian metastasis from breast cancer: a comprehensive review. Clin Transl Oncol 2019;21(7):819–27.

80. Peters IT, van Zwet EW, Smit VT, et al. Prevalence and Risk Factors of Ovarian Metastases in Breast Cancer Patients < 41 Years of Age in the Netherlands: A Nationwide Retrospective Cohort Study. PLoS One 2017;12(1):e0168277.

81. Simpkins F, Zahurak M, Armstrong D, et al. Ovarian malignancy in breast cancer patients with an

adnexal mass. Obstet Gynecol 2005;105(3): 507–13.

82. Reinert T, Nogueira-Rodrigues A, Kestelman FP, et al. The Challenge of Evaluating Adnexal Masses in Patients With Breast Cancer. Clin Breast Cancer 2018;18(4):e587–94.

83. Baiocchi G, Clemente AG, Mantoan H, et al. Adnexal Involvement in Endometrial Cancer: Prognostic Factors and Implications for Ovarian Preservation. Ann Surg Oncol 2020;27(8):2822–6.

84. Cheng H, Huo L, Zong L, et al. Oncological Outcomes and Safety of Ovarian Preservation for Early Stage Adenocarcinoma of Cervix: A Systematic Review and Meta-Analysis. Front Oncol 2019;9: 777.

85. Kuria M, Gitau S, Warfa K. Cervical cancer with bilateral ovarian metastases: case report and review of literature. BJR Case Rep 2018;4(4): 20180047.

86. Moro F, Leombroni M, Pasciuto T, et al. Synchronous primary cancers of endometrium and ovary vs endometrial cancer with ovarian metastasis: an observational study. Ultrasound Obstet Gynecol 2019;53(6):827–35.

87. Slonimsky E, Korach J, Perri T, et al. Gynecological Lymphoma: A Case Series and Review of the Literature. J Comput Assist Tomogr 2018;42(3):435–40.

88. Meriden Z, Yemelyanova AV, Vang R, et al. Ovarian metastases of pancreaticobiliary tract adenocarcinomas: analysis of 35 cases, with emphasis on the ability of metastases to simulate primary ovarian mucinous tumors. Am J Surg Pathol 2011; 35(2):276–88.

89. Badin J, Abello A, Gupta M, et al. Urothelial Carcinoma of the Bladder With a Rare Solitary Metastasis to the Ovary. Urology 2020;135:24–7.

90. Bus MT, Cordeiro ER, Anastasiadis A, et al. Urothelial carcinoma in both adnexa following perforation during transurethral resection of a non-muscle-invasive bladder tumor: a case report and literature review. Expert Rev Anticancer Ther 2012;12(12): 1529–36.

91. Taylor BL, Matrai CE, Smith AL, et al. Gynecologic Organ Involvement During Radical Cystectomy for Bladder Cancer: Is It Time to Routinely Spare the Ovaries? Clin Genitourin Cancer 2019;17(1): e209–15.

92. Abe Y, Takeuchi M, Matsuzaki K, et al. A case of metastatic malignant melanoma of the ovary with a multilocular cystic appearance on MR imaging. Jpn J Radiol 2009;27(10):458–61.

93. Moselhi M, Spencer J, Lane G. Malignant melanoma metastatic to the ovary: presentation and radiological characteristics. Gynecol Oncol 1998; 69(2):165–8.

94. Spencer JA, Anderson K, Weston M, et al. Image guided biopsy in the management of cancer of the ovary. Cancer Imaging 2006;6:144–7.

95. Thabet A, Somarouthu B, Oliva E, et al. Image-guided ovarian mass biopsy: efficacy and safety. J Vasc Interv Radiol 2014;25(12):1922–1927 e1.

96. Rao S, Smith DA, Guler E, et al. Past, Present, and Future of Serum Tumor Markers in Management of Ovarian Cancer: A Guide for the Radiologist. Radiographics 2021;41(6):1839–56.

97. Moro F, Pasciuto T, Djokovic D, et al. Role of CA125/CEA ratio and ultrasound parameters in identifying metastases to the ovaries in patients with multilocular and multilocular-solid ovarian masses. Ultrasound Obstet Gynecol 2019;53(1): 116–23.

98. Lionetti R, De Luca M, Travaglino A, et al. Treatments and overall survival in patients with Krukenberg tumor. Arch Gynecol Obstet 2019;300(1): 15–23.

99. Sugarbaker PH, Liang J. Ovarian metastases from right colon cancer treated with systemic cancer chemotherapy, a case report. Int J Surg Case Rep 2018;47:25–9.

100. Lionetti R, De Luca M, Travaglino A, et al. Prognostic factors in Krukenberg tumor. Arch Gynecol Obstet 2019;300(5):1155–65.

Magnetic Resonance Imaging of Acute Adnexal Pathology

Erica B. Stein, MD*, Kimberly L. Shampain, MD

KEYWORDS

• Adnexa • Ovary • Torsion • Pelvic pain

KEY POINTS

- Acute pelvic pain is a common presenting symptom in women.
- Pelvic ultrasound (US) is considered first-line imaging for the evaluation of pelvic pain.
- Pelvic magnetic resonance imaging (MRI) can be useful in the imaging evaluation of sonographically indeterminate adnexal masses and/or acute pathology.

Abbreviations	
MRI	imagnetic resonance imaging
US	ultrasound
PID	pelvic inflammatory disease
TOA	tubo-ovarian abscess

INTRODUCTION

Acute pelvic pain is a common presenting symptom in women both in the emergency department and in the outpatient setting. By definition, acute pelvic pain is new, noncyclical pain, that lasts less than three months in duration. Acute pelvic pain can present with nonspecific symptoms and determining the etiology can be challenging for the treating clinician. The first step in working up pelvic pain in a reproductive-aged woman is to exclude pregnancy, as acute pelvic pain in pregnant women includes additional considerations. In addition, one must consider pre versus postmenopausal status when evaluating a woman with acute pelvic pain. Given the overlap in presenting signs and symptoms, the differential for acute pelvic pain is often quite broad, encompassing many organ systems (eg, gynecologic,

urologic, musculoskeletal). Many of the common etiologies for acute pelvic pain are self-limited, such as ruptured hemorrhagic cyst in menstruating women. Imaging plays a pivotal role in narrowing the differential diagnosis and elucidating more critical time-sensitive pathologies such as ovarian torsion, tubo-ovarian abscess (TOA), or ectopic pregnancy.

IMAGING OF ACUTE PELVIC PAIN

According to the American College of Radiology (ACR) Appropriateness Criteria, the first-line imaging modality for acute pelvic pain when gynecologic or obstetric pathologies are suspected is pelvic ultrasound (US).[1,2] Ideally, this would include both transabdominal and transvaginal sonography. Pelvic US is widely available, portable, and without ionizing radiation. Unfortunately, there

University of Michigan, Department of Radiology, 1500 East Medical Center Drive B1 D502, Ann Arbor, MI 48109, USA
* Corresponding author.
E-mail address: erst@med.umich.edu

Magn Reson Imaging Clin N Am 31 (2023) 109–120
https://doi.org/10.1016/j.mric.2022.04.001

are some limitations with US. Sonographic evaluation of the pelvis can be challenging secondary to limitations with body habitus, decreased visualization due to adjacent shadowing bowel gas or calcified uterine leiomyomas, and range of technologist expertise resulting in operator dependence.

Computed tomography (CT) may be ordered in the emergency setting when nongynecologic pathology is suspected (eg, appendicitis or diverticulitis). While not commonly used as the initial imaging modality, CT can assist in the diagnosis of acute gynecologic pathologies such as ruptured hemorrhagic cyst, pyosalpinx, or TOA.

Magnetic resonance imaging (MRI) has limited availability in the emergent setting due to lengthy examination time and high associated cost. As a result, pelvic MRI is not considered first-line imaging per the ACR Appropriateness Criteria, but *may be appropriate* in certain clinical scenarios for problem-solving and lesion characterization.[1,2] The purpose of this review is to familiarize the audience with both common and less frequently encountered gynecologic and obstetric pathologies that can be diagnosed with MRI.

NONOBSTETRIC ACUTE ADNEXAL PATHOLOGY
Hemorrhagic cyst

At imaging, functional follicles in premenopausal women are routinely identified as cysts containing simple fluid. Occasionally, bleeding can occur within a follicle. Hemorrhagic cysts are often detected incidentally, but other times the patient may present with acute onset of pelvic pain. Most hemorrhagic cysts are less than 5 cm, but can enlarge to greater than 10 cm.[3] There are 3 factors that are thought to contribute to the pain: stretching of the ovarian capsule by the intracystic hemorrhage, mass effect, or leaking of fluid or blood related to cyst rupture.[4]

At MRI, hemorrhagic cysts may demonstrate variable signal on T1 and T2-weighted imaging based on the age of the intralesional blood products. If the blood products are subacute, there is usually an intermediate signal on T1WI and low signal on T2WI due to the presence of deoxyhemoglobin.[4] Typically, increased signal intensity is seen on T1WI as the blood products age secondary to the presence of methemoglobin. Occasionally, hemorrhagic cysts demonstrate layering blood-fluid or hematocrit levels (**Fig. 1**). Sometimes the cyst has already ruptured at the time of imaging evaluation and there is no dominant follicle or corpus luteum. This can be a diagnostic challenge as the hemorrhagic cyst has deflated, but the presence of hemoperitoneum in the pelvis can be a clue to the diagnosis.[5] Even a small amount of hemoperitoneum in the cul-de-sac can cause irritation of the peritoneal lining. MRI diagnostic clues include T1-weighted hyperintense fluid in the dependent pelvis and a crenulated ovarian cyst, suggestive of recent rupture/deflation.

Adnexal torsion
Ovarian torsion Ovarian torsion is a gynecologic surgical emergency for which the ovary twists along its vascular pedicle. If not diagnosed in a timely fashion, torsion will result in vascular compromise, ultimately leading to ischemia or infarction of the ovary. Risk factors for ovarian torsion include prior pelvic surgery, ovulation induction medication, and intraovarian lesions acting as a lead point.[3,6,7] Lead point intraovarian lesions are present in approximately 50% to 80% of reported cases of torsion and are often large (>4-5 cm) but usually benign.[3,6,7] The most common benign lead point etiologies for torsion include corpus luteum or physiologic follicle and dermoid cyst/teratoma, accounting for approximately 17% of all ovarian torsion cases.[8,9] Interestingly,

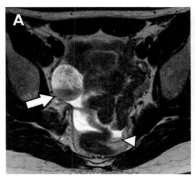
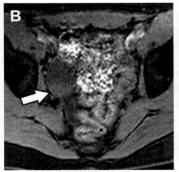
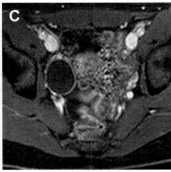

Fig. 1. Hemorrhagic right ovarian cyst. Pelvic MRI with axial T2WI (*A*) axial precontrast T1WI (*B*) and axial postcontrast T1WI (*C*) shows a circumscribed unilocular right adnexal cyst with nonsimple fluid and layering blood products (*arrows*) and trace hemoperitoneum (*arrowhead*).

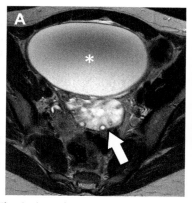 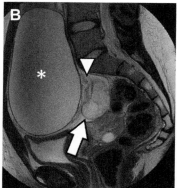 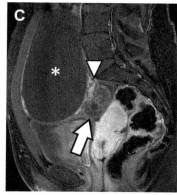

Fig. 2. Torsed right ovary secondary to large cystic mass acting as a lead point. Pelvic MRI with axial T2WI (*A*) sagittal T2WI (*B*) and sagittal postcontrast T1WI (*C*) shows an enlarged and medialized right ovary with peripheralized follicles and hypoenhancement (*arrows*); a thickened vascular pedicle (*arrowheads*); and an adjacent 13.4 cm unilocular cyst (*asterisks*). Ovarian torsion was surgically confirmed, secondary to a benign serous cystadenofibroma.

intraovarian lesions related to malignancy, endometriosis, or infection often make the ovary more adherent and less likely to torse.[3,10]

Symptoms of ovarian torsion classically include sudden onset of unilateral pelvic/lower abdominal pain, potentially accompanied by nausea, vomiting, and fever.[9,10] This may be a challenging diagnosis to make clinically due to nonspecific or vague symptoms and overlap with nongynecologic etiologies. If US is nondiagnostic or equivocal for ovarian torsion, MRI can be helpful in the acute setting.[1,9]

The features of ovarian torsion at MRI are similar to those at US, including ovarian enlargement, peripherally located follicles, and twisting of the vascular pedicle. If an intraovarian lead point is present, MRI is particularly helpful with lesion characterization (**Fig. 2**).

The appearance of the ovary may vary depending on the stage of presentation. In early torsion, the enlarged and edematous ovary exhibits hyperintense stroma on T2WI with peripheralized follicles[11–13] (see **Fig. 2**; **Fig. 3**). In later stages of torsion, the ovary becomes more heterogeneous on T2WI secondary to hemorrhage and necrosis. If left untreated, the ovary eventually becomes hypointense on both T1 and T2-weighted imaging and is nonenhancing on the T1-weighted postcontrast sequences due to infarction[6,11] (**Fig. 4**).

The twisted vascular pedicle is pathognomonic for ovarian torsion and the most specific finding on MRI, but unfortunately is seen in less than one-third of patients[8,9] (see **Fig. 3**). The twisted vascular pedicle may appear as a thickened and edematous adnexal structure with a swirled configuration.

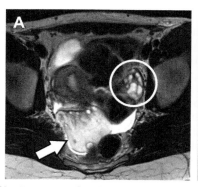 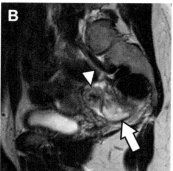 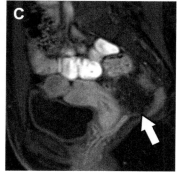

Fig. 3. Hypoperfused right ovary from torsion. Pelvic MRI with axial T2WI (*A*) sagittal T2WI (*B*) and sagittal postcontrast T1WI (*C*) shows an enlarged and hypoenhancing right ovary with T2W hyperintense signal of the ovarian stroma, peripheralized follicles, and swirled appearance of the vascular pedicle (*arrowhead*). A normal left ovary is seen (circle). A markedly edematous right ovary secondary to torsion was confirmed at surgery.

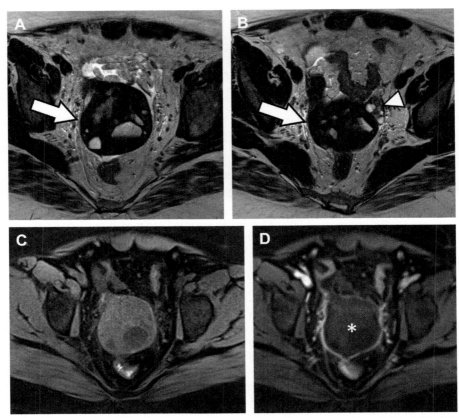

Fig. 4. Devascularized right ovary from torsion in a patient with prior hysterectomy. Pelvic MRI with axial T2WI (*A, B*) axial precontrast T1WI (*C*) and axial postcontrast T1WI (*D*) shows an enlarged and medialized right ovary (*arrows*) with pronounced hypointense T2W signal of the ovarian stroma with lack of internal enhancement (*asterisk*). A normal left ovary is seen (*arrowhead*). A hemorrhagic and torsed right ovary was confirmed at surgery.

Isolated fallopian tube torsion Isolated fallopian tube torsion is rare and occurs when the fallopian tube twists about its vascular pedicle. It is more common in adolescents and premenopausal women, and the prevalence is approximately one in 1.5 million women.[14-16] Clinical presentation may mimic that of ovarian torsion and often, the diagnosis is only made after surgical exploration. Interestingly, tubal torsion more commonly occurs on the right side. This may be due to nearby sigmoid mesentery partially immobilizing the left fallopian tube or higher rates of surgical exploration of right, rather than left, lower quadrant pain due to concern for acute appendicitis.[15,17]

Isolated fallopian tube torsion can be a diagnostic challenge for radiologists, occasionally presenting as a midline cystic mass (either in the posterior cul-de-sac or cranial to the uterus) with a normal ipsilateral ovary.[18] At MRI, the tube may appear swirled or twisted, while the ovary maintains a normal appearance (**Fig. 5**).

Infected endometrioma
Endometriosis is a fairly common, benign condition affecting approximately 10% of reproductive age women in which normal endometrial tissue is present in an abnormal location, outside of the uterine cavity.[19] Endometriomas are cystic endometriotic lesions in the ovaries, commonly referred to as chocolate cysts due to the thick dark brown liquid contained within them.[20] Secondary TOA formation can occur in the setting of ovarian endometrioma, a potentially life-threatening condition which can result in infertility, ectopic pregnancy, and chronic pelvic pain.[21]

Patients with ovarian endometriomas demonstrate a higher predisposition to TOA when compared with the general population with the incidence of endometrioma-associated TOA reported to be 2.15% - 2.3%.[22] Risk factors associated with this condition include lower genital tract infection by organisms including *Neisseria gonorrhea, Chlamydia trachomatis, Escherichia coli, Mycoplasma genitalium,* and *Gardnerella vaginalis,* as

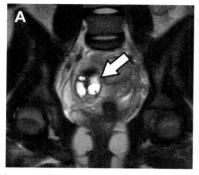 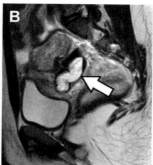 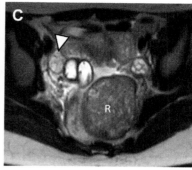

Fig. 5. Isolated right fallopian tube torsion. Noncontrast pelvic MRI with coronal T2WI (*A*) sagittal T2WI (*B*) and axial T2WI (*C*) shows a dilated fallopian tube (*arrows*) with layering hemorrhage in a twisted "u" shaped configuration with a normal right ovary (*arrowhead*). Pathology confirmed hematosalpinx with extensive stromal hemorrhage and necrosis related to tubal torsion. R = rectum.

well as spontaneous rupture of endometriotic cysts. Rupture results in release of intracystic hemorrhagic content, which can act as a nutrient-rich milieu for bacteria, increasing risk for superimposed infection.[23]

Endometriomas demonstrate the pathognomonic feature of "shading" on T2-weighted imaging in which there is low signal throughout the entire lesion or in variable parts of the lesion, typically dependently, due to the layering of protein and iron content. This is in contradistinction to ovarian hemorrhagic cysts which usually do not demonstrate T2-weighted "shading." This is helpful in differentiating these two entities because both endometriomas and hemorrhagic cysts often demonstrate high signal intensity on T1-weighed images.[24] The characteristic MRI appearance of superinfection resulting in TOA will be discussed further in the TOA subsection of pelvic inflammatory disease below.

Pelvic inflammatory disease

Pelvic inflammatory disease (PID) is an infection of the female genital tract which occurs in an ascending manner, extending from the vagina to the cervix, uterus, fallopian tubes, ovaries, and potentially peritoneal cavity, and may present with cervicitis, endometritis, salpingitis, hydrosalpinx, oophoritis, and peritonitis.[25] Sexually transmitted diseases, most commonly *Chlamydia trachomatis* and *Neisseria gonorrhoeae*, account for more than 85% of acute PID cases.[26] Below is a discussion of three entities which fall under the umbrella of PID and can present acutely with characteristic MRI findings.

Pyosalpinx Pyosalpinx, for which the fallopian tube is filled with pus, presents on MRI as a distended fallopian tube, dilated with fluid of varying signal intensities on T1 and T2-weighted imaging

due to its complex nature. Diffusion-weighted imaging (DWI) is particularly helpful in the setting of infection, as purulent fluid will impede diffusion. With pyosalpinx, the fluid restricts diffusion, and the tube wall may be thickened and hyperenhancing[27] (**Fig. 6**). This is in contrast to hydrosalpinx, which is often incidental and asymptomatic, and refers to tube dilation from simple fluid.

Tubo-ovarian abscess TOA occurs with continued ascending infection with resultant formation of a complex mass involving the ovary and fallopian tube and subsequent distortion and destruction of the normal adnexal anatomy.[28] The treatment of TOA may require intravenous antibiotics and percutaneous drainage, with imaging suggestive of TOA often necessitating inpatient rather than outpatient management.[29] In older women, TOA may also be seen secondary to complicated diverticulitis and may not accompany a typical picture of PID.

On MRI, TOA typically presents as a complex adnexal mass containing a fluid component with thickened, hyperenhancing walls and septations as well as perilesional edema[27] (**Fig. 7**). Due to its complex appearance, TOA may prove challenging to differentiate from ovarian malignancy on MRI. The presence of a complex fluid-filled tubular structure (eg, pyosalpinx), in close proximity to the lesion in question may aid in TOA diagnosis as this would not be an expected finding with ovarian malignancy.[30]

Fitz-Hugh–Curtis syndrome Fitz-Hugh–Curtis syndrome (FHCS) is a manifestation of the most extreme aspect of ascending infection, that of peritonitis in the perihepatic space, seen on imaging as hepatic capsular/subcapsular hyperemia and associated edema. In the acute/subacute stage, the typical MRI appearance of FHCS is

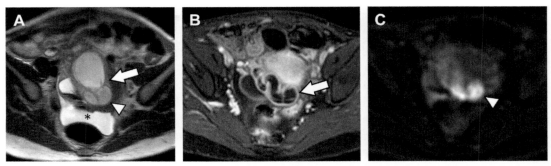

Fig. 6. Right pyosalpinx. Pelvic MRI with axial T2WI (A) axial postcontrast T1WI (B) and axial DWI (C) shows a dilated right fallopian tube (*arrows*) with thickened and enhancing walls containing nonsimple fluid that impedes diffusion (*arrowheads*), and small volume of ascites (*asterisk*). Patient was treated for pelvic inflammatory disease and pyosalpinx with intravenous antibiotics with resolution of pelvic pain and fever.

hepatic capsular and subcapsular enhancement on arterial phase postcontrast images[27] (**Fig. 8**). As FHCS becomes chronic, typical MRI findings include enhancement in the peripheral liver on delayed portal venous phase postcontrast images due to the development of subcapsular fibrosis, focal perihepatic ascites, and fibrous adhesive bands in the perihepatic space.[31]

FHCS may present differently than less widespread PID, with patients reporting upper

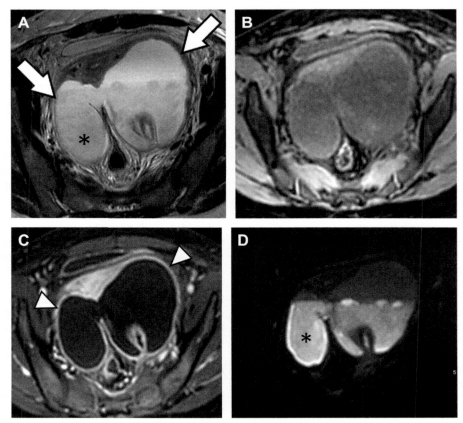

Fig. 7. Bilateral tubo-ovarian abscesses that communicate in the midline. Pelvic MRI with axial T2WI (A) axial precontrast T1WI (B) axial postcontrast T1WI (C) and axial DWI (D) shows bilateral thick-walled cystic adnexal masses (*arrows*) with nonsimple fluid that impedes diffusion (*asterisks*), and thickened enhancing walls (*arrowheads*). Given the size and complexity of the abscesses that did not respond to intravenous antibiotics and percutaneous drainage, surgical management was pursued, and pathology confirmed bilateral ovarian abscesses.

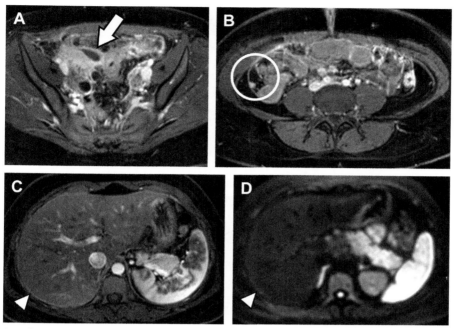

Fig. 8. Pelvic inflammatory disease with perihepatitis (Fitz-Hugh–Curtis syndrome). Abdominopelvic MRI with axial postcontrast PV phase T1WI (*A, B*) axial postcontrast arterial phase T1WI (*C*) and axial DWI (*D*) shows extensive inflammation throughout the pelvis with a small rim-enhancing abscess abutting the uterine fundus (*arrow*). There is smooth thickening and enhancement of the peritoneum in the right paracolic gutter (circle), adjacent to a nonenlarged appendix, and subtle early hepatic capsular enhancement with associated impeded diffusion (*arrowheads*). Patient was treated conservatively with antibiotics and symptoms improved. PV = portal venous.

abdominal pain in addition to pelvic pain. Chronic FHCS can result in longstanding intractable upper abdominal pain. If FHCS is suspected, extended field of view imaging must be performed to include the entire abdomen and pelvis rather than pelvis only.[27]

OVARIAN HYPERSTIMULATION SYNDROME

Ovarian hyperstimulation syndrome (OHSS) is an iatrogenic condition related to assisted reproductive technology (ART) and administration of human chorionic gonadotropin (hCG). In this clinical syndrome, bilateral ovarian enlargement occurs secondary to numerous follicles with acute onset of ascites. Acute pelvic pain may occur from a variety of etiologies, including rapid enlargement of a follicle, rupture of a follicle, hemorrhage into a follicle, stretching of the ovarian capsule, or ovarian torsion.[32] The marked enlargement of the ovaries increases the risk for torsion, with an incidence of approximately 7.5% in patients with OHSS.[33] Fluid shifts from the intravascular to the third space occur in the setting of increased capillary permeability, resulting in ascites and pleural effusions.[34]

At MRI, symmetrically enlarged ovaries are the hallmark of this diagnosis. The ovaries are often

greater than 12 cm, containing numerous follicles of variable size that are T1-weighted hypointense and T2-weighted hyperintense (**Fig. 9**).[35] There may be occasional T1-weighted hyperintensity in the follicles due to hemorrhage. It is important to differentiate OHSS from a cystic ovarian neoplasm. In OHSS, there should be no abnormal enhancing soft tissue associated with the cystic follicles, and some normal ovarian stroma should be present centrally.[35,36] The ascites is often simple appearing on MRI, but may occasionally contain some T1-weighted hyperintensity due to a ruptured hemorrhagic follicle. Acute hemoperitoneum is not typical for OHSS and, if present, another etiology should be explored.

RUPTURED TERATOMA

Ovarian teratomas are fairly common, representing 20% of adult and 50% of pediatric ovarian tumors, with potential complications including ovarian torsion, malignant transformation, and rupture.[37,38] Rupture, which occurs in 1% to 4% of cases, can lead to acute or chronic peritonitis secondary to spread of liquid sebum into the peritoneal cavity.[37,39] Acute teratoma rupture can result in chemical peritonitis, often the result of

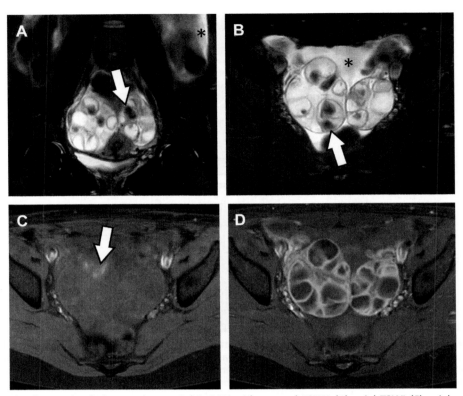

Fig. 9. Ovarian hyperstimulation syndrome. Pelvic MRI with coronal T2W1 (A) axial T2WI (B) axial precontrast T1WI (C) and axial postcontrast T1WI (D) shows enlarged ovaries with multiple follicles (some of which contain hemorrhage (arrows)), moderate volume of ascites in the pelvis and lower quadrants (asterisks), and follicular wall enhancement.

trauma, infection, labor, or torsion, and necessitates urgent surgical exploration. Chronic rupture resulting in recurrent leakage with chronic peritonitis is more common than sudden rupture and can result in gliosis (chronic granulomatous peritonitis) leading to peritoneal adhesions.[39]

Teratoma diagnosis can be made on MRI when intralesional fat is present in an adnexal mass. At MRI, fat is seen as high signal intensity on T1-weighted imaging with signal drop out on chemical-selective fat-saturated T1-weighted imaging.[38,40] Teratoma rupture can be diagnosed when wall discontinuity is visualized or fat-fluid levels are present in the peritoneum (Fig. 10). If a site of discontinuity cannot be identified, the combination of imaging findings of ascites and distorted, compressed lesion shape can be used to suggest the diagnosis of rupture, typically treated

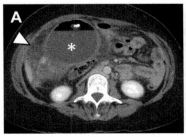
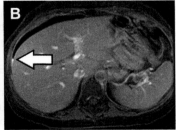
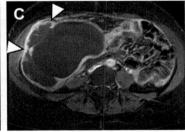

Fig. 10. Ruptured right ovarian teratoma that had undergone malignant degeneration. Axial contrast-enhanced abdominopelvic CT (A) shows a right ovarian teratoma (asterisk) with fat-fluid levels and extensive infiltration of the surrounding fat (arrowhead). Abdominopelvic MRI with axial T2WI (B) and axial postcontrast T1WI (C) shows fat-fluid level in the right upper quadrant related to intraperitoneal fat (arrow) and irregular wall and septal enhancement of the teratoma (arrowheads). Following exploratory laparotomy, ruptured teratoma was confirmed with invasive poorly differentiated squamous cell carcinoma arising in a mature cystic teratoma.

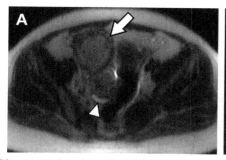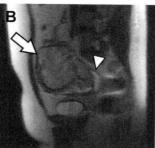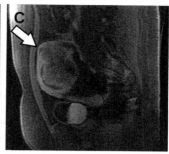

Fig. 11. Right adnexal ectopic pregnancy. Pelvic MRI obtained after indeterminate pelvic ultrasound with axial T2WI (*A*) sagittal T2WI (*B*) and sagittal postcontrast T1WI (*C*) shows a cystic and solid structure in the right adnexa (*arrows*) with an adjacent tubular fluid-filled structure (*arrowheads*), likely a fallopian tube in this patient with a rising B-HCG and no IUP identified on ultrasound. There is patchy enhancement of the ectopic pregnancy and nonenhancement of the adjacent fallopian tube. Due to the large size of the ectopic pregnancy, patient underwent embolization of the arterial supply to the extrauterine pregnancy.

surgically.[39] Both acute and chronic rupture recurrent leakage) can present with omental infiltration (diffuse or localized), ascites, and omental and bowel inflammatory masses, resulting in an imaging appearance which can be confused for tuberculous peritonitis and peritoneal carcinomatosis.[41] Thus, when these findings are seen in a patient with ovarian teratoma, lesion rupture should

be considered, and the wall should be inspected thoroughly for discontinuity.[39]

Obstetric Acute Adnexal Pathology

Tubal ectopic pregnancy
An ectopic pregnancy occurs when a fertilized oocyte implants outside of the endometrial cavity, most commonly within the ampullary portion of

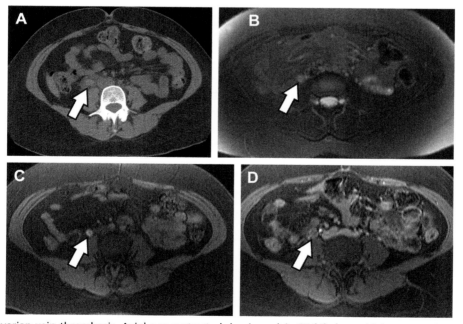

Fig. 12. Ovarian vein thrombosis. Axial noncontrast abdominopelvic CT (*A*) shows high attenuation within the expanded right gonadal vein (*arrow*) with inflammatory infiltration of the adjacent fat, suggestive of acute gonadal vein thrombus. Confirmatory pelvic MRI with axial T2WI (*B*) axial precontrast T1WI (*C*) and axial postcontrast T1WI (*D*) shows asymmetric expansion and hyperintensity of the right gonadal vein with a nonenhancing filling defect (*arrows*).

the fallopian tube. Ectopic pregnancies occur in approximately 2% of all pregnancies with risk factors including ART, prior pelvic or tubal surgery, and history of PID.[42] Ectopic pregnancy should be considered a possible diagnosis in any premenopausal woman presenting with acute pelvic pain and a positive B-hCG level. Pelvic US is the first-line imaging modality to assess for an intrauterine pregnancy (IUP). Occasionally, the sonographic results may be unclear and MRI may be performed. MRI can help determine the location of a suspected ectopic pregnancy, especially if management and treatment decisions depend on the exact location (eg, tubal, abdominal, or within a rudimentary horn) (**Fig. 11**).[43]

OVARIAN VEIN THROMBOSIS

Ovarian vein thrombosis (OVT) is associated with pregnancy, malignancy, pelvic surgery, and PID as these conditions result in increased incidence of venous stasis, hypercoagulability, and inflammation.[44] OVT affects the right ovarian vein in 80% to 90% of cases due to its length, valve incompetency, and absence of retrograde flow.[45,46] OVT often presents with fever, leukocytosis, and lower abdominal pain.[47] If OVT is not recognized, and left untreated, the thrombus can expand into the renal vein and inferior vena cava (IVC), with potential for pulmonary embolism.[48]

MRI is particularly well suited to assess the superior most aspect of OVT as the appearance of the IVC on contrast-enhanced CT can be confusing secondary to mixing artifacts from the draining renal veins at this level. Furthermore, given the often young age and pregnant status of these patients, MRI is ideal given the lack of ionizing radiation.[48] OVT demonstrates variable signal on T1-weighted imaging, determined by age of the methemoglobin within the thrombus. It appears on T2-weighted images as intermediate to high signal intensity and may contain a dark peripheral rim secondary to hemosiderin. On postcontrast images, there may be a filling defect within the vessel with surrounding perivascular hyperenhancement due to associated inflammation[48–50] (**Fig. 12**).

SUMMARY

Acute pelvic pain is a common presenting symptom in both pre and postmenopausal women. The clinical history, physical examination findings, and laboratory markers may paint a confusing picture and radiologic imaging plays a crucial role in diagnosis. While pelvic US is considered first-line imaging, MRI may be helpful in the acute setting

to problem-solve in certain clinical scenarios. MRI can assist in diagnosis due to superior soft-tissue contrast resolution, even when noncontrast technique is used in pregnant patients. In addition, MRI images a larger field-of-view compared with pelvic US and can assist in fully assessing large lesions and identifying the site of origin.[9] When contrast is administered, adnexal mass enhancement kinetics, or absence of enhancement as seen in ovarian torsion, can further aid in lesion characterization. Thus, radiologists must have baseline familiarity with the MRI appearance of acute pelvic pathology, specifically for cases in which sonographic studies are nondiagnostic or indeterminate and MRI is needed for urgent diagnosis.

CLINICS CARE POINTS

- Per the ACR Appropriateness Criteria (ACR-AC), pelvic US is first-line imaging for acute pelvic pain in pregnant and nonpregnant women.
- Pelvic MRI *may be* appropriate if US is inconclusive or nondiagnostic, according to the ACR-AC.
- The most common etiologies for benign lead point in the setting of ovarian torsion are corpus luteum or physiologic follicle and dermoid cyst/teratoma.
- If TOA presents in a postmenopausal patient, consider both gynecologic and nongynecologic etiologies.

DISCLOSURE

The authors have no relevant disclosures.

REFERENCES

1. Bhosale PR, Javitt MC, Atri M, et al. ACR Appropriateness Criteria(R) Acute Pelvic Pain in the Reproductive Age Group. Ultrasound Q 2016;32(2) 108–15.
2. Expert Panel on GYN, Imaging OB, Henrichsen TL et al. ACR Appropriateness Criteria(R) Postmenopausal Acute Pelvic Pain. J Am Coll Radiol 2021 18(5S):S119–25.
3. Olpin JD, Strachowski L. Imaging of Acute Pelvic Pain: Nonpregnant. Radiol Clin North Am 2020 58(2):329–45.

4. Knoepp US, Mazza MB, Chong ST, et al. MR Imaging of Pelvic Emergencies in Women. Magn Reson Imaging Clin N Am 2017;25(3):503–19.

5. Patel MD, Young SW, Dahiya N. Ultrasound of Pelvic Pain in the Nonpregnant Woman. Radiol Clin North Am 2019;57(3):601–16.

6. Rha SE, Byun JY, Jung SE, et al. CT and MR imaging features of adnexal torsion. Radiographics 2002; 22(2):283–94.

7. Stark JE, Siegel MJ. Ovarian torsion in prepubertal and pubertal girls: sonographic findings. AJR Am J Roentgenol 1994;163(6):1479–82.

8. Duigenan S, Oliva E, Lee SI. Ovarian torsion: diagnostic features on CT and MRI with pathologic correlation. AJR Am J Roentgenol 2012;198(2):W122–31.

9. Somberg Gunther M, Kanmaniraja D, Kobi M, et al. MRI of Acute Gynecologic Conditions. J Magn Reson Imaging 2020;51(5):1291–309.

10. Chang HC, Bhatt S, Dogra VS. Pearls and pitfalls in diagnosis of ovarian torsion. Radiographics 2008; 28(5):1355–68.

11. Nepal P, VanBuren W, Khandelwal K, et al. Problem-solving with MRI in acute abdominopelvic conditions, part 2: gynecological, obstetric, vascular, and renal diseases. Emerg Radiol 2021;28(6): 1173–83.

12. Singh A, Danrad R, Hahn PF, et al. MR imaging of the acute abdomen and pelvis: acute appendicitis and beyond. Radiographics 2007;27(5):1419–31.

13. Uyeda JW. Utility of MR Imaging in Abdominopelvic Emergencies. Radiol Clin North Am 2019;57(4): 705–15.

14. Ferrera PC, Kass LE, Verdile VP. Torsion of the fallopian tube. Am J Emerg Med 1995;13(3):312–4.

15. Gross M, Blumstein SL, Chow LC. Isolated fallopian tube torsion: a rare twist on a common theme. AJR Am J Roentgenol 2005;185(6):1590–2.

16. Raziel A, Mordechai E, Friedler S, et al. Isolated recurrent torsion of the Fallopian tube: case report. Hum Reprod 1999;14(12):3000–1.

17. Bondioni MP, McHugh K, Grazioli L. Isolated fallopian tube torsion in an adolescent: CT features. Pediatr Radiol 2002;32(8):612–3.

18. Harmon JC, Binkovitz LA, Binkovitz LE. Isolated fallopian tube torsion: sonographic and CT features. Pediatr Radiol 2008;38(2):175–9.

19. Vercellini P, Viganò P, Somigliana E, et al. Endometriosis: pathogenesis and treatment. Nat Rev Endocrinol 2014;10(5):261–75.

20. Exacoustos C, De Felice G, Pizzo A, et al. Isolated Ovarian Endometrioma: A History Between Myth and Reality. J Minim Invasive Gynecol 2018;25(5): 884–91.

21. Cacciatore B, Leminen A, Ingman-Friberg S, et al. Transvaginal sonographic findings in ambulatory patients with suspected pelvic inflammatory disease. Obstet Gynecol 1992;80(6):912–6.

22. Kubota T, Ishi K, Takeuchi H. A study of tubo-ovarian and ovarian abscesses, with a focus on cases with endometrioma. J Obstet Gynaecol Res 1997;23(5): 421–6.

23. Gao Y, Qu P, Zhou Y, et al. Risk factors for the development of tubo-ovarian abscesses in women with ovarian endometriosis: a retrospective matched case-control study. BMC Womens Health 2021;21(1):43.

24. Foti PV, Farina R, Palmucci S, et al. Endometriosis: clinical features, MR imaging findings and pathologic correlation. Insights Imaging 2018;9(2):149–72.

25. Soper DE. Pelvic inflammatory disease. Obstet Gynecol 2010;116(2 Pt 1):419–28.

26. Brunham RC, Gottlieb SL, Paavonen J. Pelvic inflammatory disease. N Engl J Med 2015;372(21):2039–48.

27. Czeyda-Pommersheim F, Kalb B, Costello J, et al. MRI in pelvic inflammatory disease: a pictorial review. Abdom Radiol (N Y) 2017;42(3):935–50.

28. Revzin MV, Mathur M, Dave HB, et al. Pelvic Inflammatory Disease: Multimodality Imaging Approach with Clinical-Pathologic Correlation. Radiographics 2016;36(5):1579–96.

29. Demirtas O, Akman L, Demirtas GS, et al. The role of the serum inflammatory markers for predicting the tubo-ovarian abscess in acute pelvic inflammatory disease: a single-center 5-year experience. Arch Gynecol Obstet 2013;287(3):519–23.

30. Kim SH, Kim SH, Yang DM, et al. Unusual causes of tubo-ovarian abscess: CT and MR imaging findings. Radiographics 2004;24(6):1575–89.

31. Nishie A, Yoshimitsu K, Irie H, et al. Fitz-Hugh-Curtis syndrome. Radiologic manifestation. J Comput Assist Tomogr 2003;27(5):786–91.

32. Cicchiello LA, Hamper UM, Scoutt LM. Ultrasound evaluation of gynecologic causes of pelvic pain. Obstet Gynecol Clin North Am 2011;38(1):85–114, viii.

33. Mashiach S, Bider D, Moran O, et al. Adnexal torsion of hyperstimulated ovaries in pregnancies after gonadotropin therapy. Fertil Steril 1990;53(1):76–80.

34. Kumar P, Sait SF, Sharma A, et al. Ovarian hyperstimulation syndrome. J Hum Reprod Sci 2011; 4(2):70–5.

35. Jung BG, Kim H. Severe spontaneous ovarian hyperstimulation syndrome with MR findings. J Comput Assist Tomogr 2001;25(2):215–7.

36. Baron KT, Babagbemi KT, Arleo EK, et al. Emergent complications of assisted reproduction: expecting the unexpected. Radiographics 2013;33(1):229–44.

37. Comerci JT Jr, Licciardi F, Bergh PA, et al. Mature cystic teratoma: a clinicopathologic evaluation of 517 cases and review of the literature. Obstet Gynecol 1994;84(1):22–8.

38. Outwater EK, Siegelman ES, Hunt JL. Ovarian teratomas: tumor types and imaging characteristics. Radiographics 2001;21(2):475–90.

39. Park SB, Kim JK, Kim KR, et al. Imaging findings of complications and unusual manifestations of ovarian teratomas. Radiographics 2008;28(4):969–83.

40. Guinet C, Ghossain MA, Buy JN, et al. Mature cystic teratomas of the ovary: CT and MR findings. Eur J Radiol 1995;20(2):137–43.

41. Fibus TF. Intraperitoneal rupture of a benign cystic ovarian teratoma: findings at CT and MR imaging. AJR Am J Roentgenol 2000;174(1):261–2.

42. Centers for Disease C, Prevention. Ectopic pregnancy–United States, 1990-1992. MMWR Morb Mortal Wkly Rep 1995;44(3):46–8.

43. Gopireddy DR, Le R, Virarkar MK, et al. Magnetic Resonance Imaging Evaluation of Ectopic Pregnancy: A Value-Added Review. J Comput Assist Tomogr 2021;45(3):374–82.

44. Jacoby WT, Cohan RH, Baker ME, et al. Ovarian vein thrombosis in oncology patients: CT detection and clinical significance. AJR Am J Roentgenol 1990; 155(2):291–4.

45. Sinha D, Yasmin H, Samra JS. Postpartum inferior vena cava and ovarian vein thrombosis–a case report and literature review. J Obstet Gynaecol 2005;25(3):312–3.

46. Kominiarek MA, Hibbard JU. Postpartum ovarian vein thrombosis: an update. Obstet Gynecol Surv 2006;61(5):337–42.

47. Dunnihoo DR, Gallaspy JW, Wise RB, et al. Postpartum ovarian vein thrombophlebitis: a review. Obstet Gynecol Surv 1991;46(7):415–27.

48. Sharma P, Abdi S. Ovarian vein thrombosis. Clin Radiol 2012;67(9):893–8.

49. Martin B, Mulopulos GP, Bryan PJ. MRI of puerperal ovarian-vein thrombosis (case report). AJR Am J Roentgenol 1986;147(2):291–2.

50. Carpenter JP, Holland GA, Baum RA, et al. Magnetic resonance venography for the detection of deep venous thrombosis: comparison with contrast venography and duplex Doppler ultrasonography. J Vasc Surg 1993;18(5):734–41.

MR Imaging of Endometriosis of the Adnexa

Michelle D. Sakala, MD[a],*, Priyanka Jha, MBBS[b], Angela Tong, MD[c], Myles T. Taffel, MD[c], Myra K. Feldman, MD[d]

KEYWORDS

- Endometriosis • Endometrioma • Kissing ovaries • Hematosalpinx
- Endometriosis-associated ovarian cancer • Decidualized endometrioma
- Spontaneous hemorrhage in pregnancy

KEY POINTS

- Protocols should include pre-contrast T1-weighted imaging with fat saturation, T2-weighted imaging without fat saturation, opposed- and in-phase or Dixon imaging, administration of contrast media, and subtraction imaging to assist in the evaluation of endometriomas versus other masses, deep infiltrating endometriosis, and endometriosis-associated ovarian cancer.
- MR imaging is useful to characterize endometriomas based on multiplicity and bilaterality, associated deep infiltrating endometriosis, homogenous T1-weighted hyperintensity, T2 shading, T2 dark spot sign, and lack of fat or enhancing solid tissue. Hematosalpinges present as dilated thin-walled T1-weighted hyperintense fallopian tubes, although may not contain shading.
- Endometriosis-associated ovarian cancer is associated with larger lesions, loss of T2 shading, enhancing solid components, and diffusion restriction of solid components.
- Decidualized endometriosis can mimic malignant transformation of endometriosis due to solid projections within endometriomas; however, the projections have a characteristic rounded morphology, follow signal characteristics of decidualized placenta, and follow-up will show stabilization of growth. Spontaneous hemorrhage of endometriomas and other forms of endometriosis can occur during pregnancy.

INTRODUCTION

Endometriosis is the presence of ectopic endometrial glands outside of the uterus. It is estimated to occur in 10% of women and can cause lifelong chronic pain, disability, and infertility.[1] Routine transvaginal ultrasound is the first-line imaging modality to detect endometriomas and hematosalpinges, both of which are markers for deep infiltrating endometriosis (DIE).[2] MR imaging can provide a more comprehensive assessment by characterizing adnexal findings, detecting the presence and extent of DIE and evaluating malignancy risk. Endometriosis of the adnexa is often multifocal and can involve all adnexal structures including the ovaries, fallopian tubes, and broad ligaments. MR is also valuable in

Author Disclosure Statement:
[a] Department of Radiology, Division of Abdominal Imaging, University of Michigan-Michigan Medicine, 1500 East Medical Center Drive, Ann Arbor, MI 48109, USA; [b] Department of Radiology and Biomedical Imaging, University of California San Francisco, 505 Parnassus Avenue, Box 0628, San Francisco, CA 94143, USA; [c] Department of Radiology, New York University Langone Health, 660 1st Avenue, 3rd Floor, New York, NY 10016, USA; [d] Imaging Institute, Section of Abdominal Imaging, Cleveland Clinic, 9500 Euclid Avenue Mail Code A21, Cleveland, OH 44195, USA
* Corresponding author.
E-mail address: misakala@med.umich.edu

Magn Reson Imaging Clin N Am 31 (2023) 121–135
https://doi.org/10.1016/j.mric.2022.06.006
1064-9689/23/© 2022 Elsevier Inc. All rights reserved.

assessing adnexal manifestations of endometriosis in the setting of pregnancy, when the gravid uterus may limit ultrasound evaluation.

MR IMAGING PROTOCOL

An optimized MR imaging protocol is important to promote visualization and diagnosis of endometriosis and to characterize benign and malignant lesions. In this review, the authors focus on MR imaging protocol components crucial for characterization and assessment of the adnexa (**Table 1**).

The MR imaging protocol for endometriosis is designed to maximize the visualization of hemorrhagic products in endometriomas and the adjacent desmoplastic reaction elicited by repetitive, cyclical hemorrhage of this ectopic glandular tissue. Patient preparation can optionally include allowing the urinary bladder to be full, application of vaginal and/or rectal contrast, bowel preparation, and administration of a bowel antiperistaltic agent.[3–5] The most important sequence for both anatomic and endometriosis visualization is a T2 fast spin echo without fat suppression (FS). The background of T2 hyperintense fat contrasts the anatomic structures and the low signal of endometriomas and endometriotic implants. Two imaging planes should be used at minimum, most commonly the sagittal and axial planes.[5,6] An additional coronal plane may also be included for better localization. Conventional axial and coronal planes are sufficient; however, axial and coronal planes obliqued to the cervical canal or uterine ligaments may provide better visualization of disease in those regions.[3,7]

T1-weighted imaging (T1WI) with FS is important to include as blood products in endometriosis are typically T1 hyperintense and stand out against the suppressed fat signal. Again, at least two planes are recommended, typically sagittal small field-of-view and axial large field-of-view acquisitions.[3] A single axial plane of T1WI with opposed- and in-phase or Dixon imaging is imperative to distinguish blood products from bulk fat.[8]

Post-contrast T1WI is also important to include in the MR imaging protocol, especially when adnexal lesions are present. Although post-contrast imaging does not improve the detection of endometriomas or other deposits, it is helpful in distinguishing endometriomas from infectious ovarian lesions and for evaluating enhancing components associated with malignant transformation.[3,6,9] Subtraction images, where pre-contrast T1WI is subtracted from post-contrast T1WI, are an especially important tool as the hyperintense T1 signal in blood products may obscure enhancing components. Sagittal and axial imaging planes are recommended with optional coronal plane.[3]

Similar to post-contrast T1WI, diffusion-weighted image (DWI) helps to evaluate for malignancy and infection. DWI has the additional benefit of identifying abnormal lymph nodes or pelvic malignant implants in the setting of neoplasm.[9] Given the many fluid-filled structures in the pelvis such as the urinary bladder, bowel, and ovarian cysts, both a low b-value and a high b-value of at least 800 to 1000 s/mm^2 are recommended to suppress normal fluid signal.[9,10] Apparent diffusion coefficient (ADC) maps are also recommended to confirm true diffusion restriction.

Susceptibility-weighted imaging (SWI) may be helpful in identifying endometriosis through the visualization of hemosiderin from chronic blood products. SWI uses high-resolution gradient-recalled echo sequences with phase and magnitude

Table 1
Basics of a recommended MR imaging protocol for endometriosis

Sequence	Fat Suppression	Acquisition Planes	Notes
T2 FSE	No	Sagittal, axial	Optional planes: coronal, oblique coronal, oblique axial
T1WI	Yes	Sagittal, axial	Optional planes: coronal, oblique coronal, oblique axial
T1WI in and out of phase/Dixon	No	Axial	
T1WI post-contrast with fat suppression	Yes	Sagittal, axial	Optional planes: Coronal
Diffusion-weighted image	Yes	Axial	• Include high b-value of 800–1000 s/mm^2 • Include ADC map

Abbreviations: T1WI, T1-weighted image; T2 FSE, T2 fast spin echo.

information. It is more sensitive to susceptibility arti-fact than conventional T2*-weighted imaging, particularly with a 3-T field strength.[11] However, differentiating blood and calcification in vascular structures, calcification in the ovary, and foreign bodies such as tubal ligation clips may be difficult, and intended findings may be obscured by suscep-tibility from bowel gas. The utility of SWI in practice is, therefore, variable and uncommonly used.

ENDOMETRIOMAS

Endometriomas are a common manifestation of endometriosis. These ovarian or para-ovarian cysts contain ectopic endometrial elements and blood products of varying age due to repeated cyclic hemorrhage. They are often multiple and can be bilateral.[12–14] Endometriomas are frequently easily diagnosed with ultrasound and

MR imaging. In unclear cases, concomitant DIE on imaging, clinical history suggesting endometriosis, and chronicity can be used to differentiate endometriomas from other adnexal masses.

Endometriomas have markedly hyperintense and homogenous T1-weighted (T1W) signal inten-sity (SI) owing to frequent and short-interval cyclic accumulation of methemoglobin, high protein con-centration, and viscosity (**Fig. 1**). This appearance is most conspicuous on T1WI when fat saturation is applied. Heterogeneous signal may develop when acute on chronic hemorrhage is present, however, most of the T1W SI will remain markedly hyperintense and otherwise overall homogenous. Other lesions with T1W hyperintensity that can be mistaken for endometriomas include hemor-rhagic cysts, teratomas, mucin-containing tumors, and tubo-ovarian complex (**Table 2**).

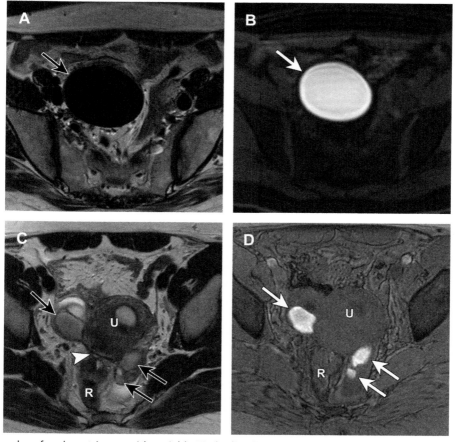

Fig. 1. Examples of endometriomas with variable T2 shading in two patients (*A* and *B* vs *C* and *D*). T2-weighted axial MR images (*A, C*) show endometriomas with T2-weighted hypointensity consistent with T2 shading (*black arrows*). T1-weighted axial MR images with fat saturation (*B, D*) showing corresponding marked homogenous hyperintense signal (*white arrows*). (*C*) and (*D*) Multiple endometriomas in both ovaries. The axial T2-weighted image (*C*) also shows a hypointense fibrotic deposit of deep infiltrating endometriosis between the ovaries overlying the posterior uterus (*white arrowhead*). U, uterus; R, rectum.

Table 2
Differentiating T1-weighted hyperintense lesions

T1-Weighted Hyperintense Lesions	Distinguishing Characteristics
Endometrioma	Often multiple and bilateral, homogenous marked T1W SI, T2 shading, T2 dark spot, does not resolve on short-term follow-up, can restrict diffusion, no internal enhancement
Hemorrhagic cyst	Singular and unilateral, heterogeneous or peripheral T1W SI, retractile clot is not as hypointense as T2 dark spot, T2 shading possible
Mature teratoma	T1W SI suppresses with fat suppression, India ink artifact with opposed-phase imaging indicates macroscopic fat, T1W SI can be heterogeneous due to other germ cell layers
Mucin-containing masses (eg, mucinous cystadenoma)	Variable T1W SI depending on mucin concentration, multilocular with variable SI between locules, hemorrhage can occur and sequela chronically persist resulting in T2 dark spot, calcifications can mimic T2 dark spot
Tubo-ovarian complex	Variable T1W SI, can be heterogeneous, enhancing thickened walls, restricts diffusion, other inflammatory changes including peritonitis

Abbreviations: SI, signal intensity; T1W, T1-weighted.

T2W imaging features of endometriomas include T2 shading and the T2 dark spot sign. T2 shading is signal intensity that is less than simple fluid and/or adjacent follicles on T2W imaging[12] (see **Fig. 1**). T2 shading results from the accumulation of deoxyhemoglobin, methemoglobin, and hemosiderin. T2 shading can have a variety of appearances ranging from marked to mild hypointensity, homogeneous to heterogeneous, and appear as a gradient of layering hypointensity within an otherwise hyperintense structure.[2] T2 shading alone is highly sensitive (83%) but less specific (45%) for endometriomas due to overlap with hemorrhage in cysts and malignant lesions.[14] A thickened T2W hypointense rim also reflects hemosiderin-laden macrophages and fibrous tissue in the wall of the endometrioma. Fluid–fluid levels may also reflect acute on chronic hemorrhage.

The T2 dark spot is a discrete and well-defined markedly T2W hypointense structure within or along the wall of an endometrioma, with an average size of 6.3 mm, thought to reflect chronic retracted blood clot.[14] There is often associated hyperintense T1W SI. The T2 dark spot does not enhance, an important feature that is assessed well on post-contrast subtraction imaging. The presence of an enhancing mural nodule is concerning for malignant transformation.

Endometriomas also restrict diffusion due to T2W hypointensity and "T2 blackout effect." ADC values are based on the slope of SI loss between acquisitions obtained with lower and higher b-values. Because the T2W SI is already low, there is less SI loss with higher b-values and the resultant ADC value is low[12](**Fig. 2**).

Differentiating Endometriomas from Other Adnexal Masses

Hemorrhagic cysts

Functional hemorrhagic cysts are frequently hyperintense on T1WI with shading on T2WI. Compared with endometriomas, the T1W hyperintense signal within hemorrhagic cysts is typically less pronounced, more heterogeneous, and often occupies only a portion of the cyst due to the quantity and age of the blood resulting in absence of or low concentration of methemoglobin. This yields a more heterogenous T1WI appearance or there may be a T1W hyperintense rim peripherally in the lesion[15](**Fig. 3**). Although heterogeneity is the more likely appearance, hemorrhagic cysts can still be homogenous on T1WI and have T2 shading,[15] making differentiation with endometriomas difficult. In such cases, follow-up imaging or comparison with recent prior imaging is helpful.

Hemorrhagic cysts tend to appear with menstrual cycles and decrease in size over time. Endometriomas, however, do not tend to regress unless treated hormonally. Hemorrhagic lesions less than 3 cm, such as follicles and corpus luteum cysts, can be difficult to differentiate from endometriomas, and chronicity may also be the only feature favoring endometrioma.[15] Given hemorrhagic cysts are physiologic, they are often unilateral and singular, rather than multiple and bilateral.

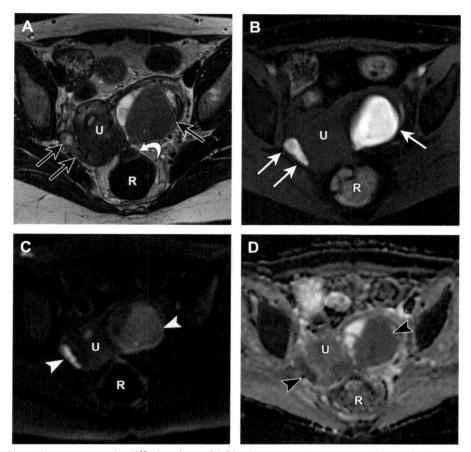

Fig. 2. Endometriomas can restrict diffusion due to highly viscous proteinaceous and hemorrhagic contents. Axial T2-weighted image (A) shows T2 shading in endometriomas bilaterally (black arrows). A hypointense fibrotic deep infiltrating endometriosis nodule tethers the uterus and anterior rectal wall (white curved arrow). Axial T1-weighted MR image with fat saturation (B) shows marked hyperintense homogenous signal within multiple endometriomas bilaterally (white arrows). Axial diffusion-weighted MR image (b-value = 800) (C) with intermediate to high signal within the endometriomas (white arrowheads). (D) Axial apparent diffusion coefficient map shows low signal within the endometriomas, confirming diffusion restriction (black arrowheads). U, uterus; R, rectum.

The T2 dark spot sign is also a useful imaging feature to distinguish endometriomas from hemorrhagic cysts (Fig. 4). This is a highly specific (93%) sign of chronic hemorrhage, usually indicative of an endometrioma. Unfortunately, the sensitivity is low (36%) and the absence of the sign does not mean a lesion is not an endometrioma.[14] In contrast to retracting blood clot in a hemorrhagic cyst (see Fig. 3), the T2 dark spot is markedly hypointense and smaller.

Teratomas

A mature cystic teratoma can be T1W hyperintense or have T1W hyperintense components (Fig. 5) due to its fat content. Tissue components from other germ cell layers are often present. The T1W hyperintense signal will become hypointense with frequency-selective fat saturation. Use of opposed- and in-phase gradient-echo imaging is also helpful where macroscopic lipid will be indicated by India ink artifact at the lipid–water interfaces or intracellular lipid will become hypointense on opposed-phase images.[16] However, if short tau inversion recovery imaging is used in the protocol, the loss of T1W SI is not frequency-specific and can occur with both fat and hemorrhage.[12] The T2W SI for fatty components in mature cystic teratomas is also high.[8]

Other masses containing hemorrhagic and proteinaceous contents

Mucin-containing masses can also be T1W hyperintense, but the intensity of mucin is variable

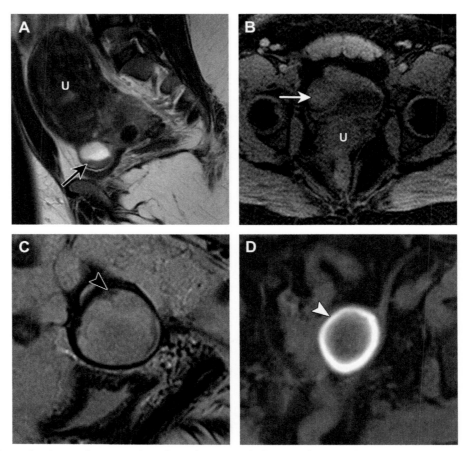

Fig. 3. Hemorrhagic cysts in two patients (*A* and *B* vs *C* and *D*). Sagittal T2-weighted MR image (*A*) shows a cyst with layering hypointense signal compatible with blood clot (*black arrow*). Incidental fibroids present in the uterus (U). Axial T1-weighted MR image with fat saturation (*B*) shows mild heterogeneous hyperintense signal within the hemorrhagic cyst at the level of the blood clot (*white arrow*). Sagittal T2-weighted MR from a different patient with a hemorrhagic cyst (*C*) shows mild internal T2-weighted hypointensity (*black arrowhead*). Axial T1-weighted image with fat saturation from the same patient (*D*) shows peripheral T1-weighted hyperintense signal (*white arrowhead*). Note the T2-weighted hypointensity in both cases is not as hypointense as for the T2 dark spot sign (see **Fig. 4**).

depending on viscosity. Mucinous cystadenomas are often multilocular, whereas endometriomas are often unilocular. The SI often differs between locules due to variable mucin content causing a stained-glass appearance[17,18] (**Fig. 6**). However, some mucinous neoplasms are unilocular, and the absence of heterogeneous T2 shading is helpful to distinguish from endometriomas.

Hemorrhage can also occur in other preexisting benign or malignant adnexal neoplasms. The T1W hyperintensity may not be as striking but the T2W sequelae of chronic hemorrhage, including a T2 dark spot, may exist due to the chronicity of the lesion. Peripheral calcification can also mimic the T2 dark spot, thus evaluation of both T1W and T2W sequences and comparison modalities is advised. Other mucin-containing tumors, such as

metastases and mucinous cystadenocarcinoma will often be heterogeneous with solid components and may be very large in size.[18]

Tubo-ovarian abscesses can also be T1W hyperintense and T2W hypointense and restrict diffusion due to protein-rich content and potential associated hemorrhage[19] (**Fig. 7**). The T1W hyperintensity can be homogenous or variable. Clinical context in addition to wall thickening and enhancement, inflammatory change, and pyosalpinx may assist in the diagnosis.

SUSCEPTIBILITY-WEIGHTED IMAGING OF ENDOMETRIOMAS

Some endometriomas do not show the typical features of T2 shading and T1W hyperintensity. These

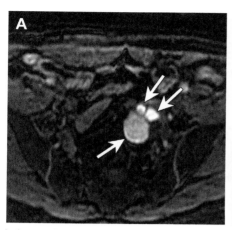
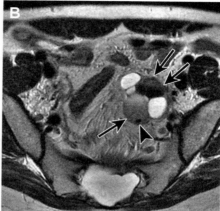

Fig. 4. T2 dark spot sign in an endometrioma. Axial T1-weighted MR image (*A*) shows homogenous hyperintense signal in multiple left endometriomas (*white arrows*). Axial oblique T2-weighted MR image (*B*) shows the corresponding variable appearance of T2 shading (*black arrow*) and a T2 dark spot (*black arrowhead*) in a posterior endometrioma. Incidental follicles present.

can be mistaken for non-endometriotic cysts due to higher fluid content or solid-appearing fibrotic masses due to markedly low T2W SI. In these atypical endometriomas, SWI may be helpful for diagnosing these lesions as endometriomas.

SWI depicts local magnetic field inhomogeneity as signal voids and may be used to detect the sequela of hemorrhage. Endometriomas may contain punctate or curved signal voids along the wall resulting from hemosiderin-laden macrophages or throughout the cyst due to deoxyhemoglobin and hemosiderin from repeat hemorrhage. A study of 42 pathology-proven endometriomas showed that adding SWI increased the MRI diagnosis in 76.2% to 97.6% of the endometriomas.[11]

Hemorrhagic cysts did not show signal voids, although there were only two in the study.[11] Of note, the amount of signal void and appearance may vary with the menstrual cycle and the phase of evolving blood products.[20]

OVARIAN POSITIONING

Endometriomas are associated with DIE, and the configuration of the ovaries and/or endometriomas may be a predictor of more severe disease.[21,22] When endometriotic implants occur in the posterior pelvis, they can elicit significant inflammation and fibrosis. The subsequent adhesion formation frequently extends between the

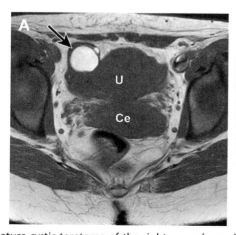
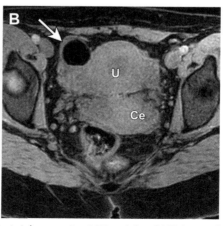

Fig. 5. Mature cystic teratoma of the right ovary (arrow). Axial precontrast T1-weighted MR image (*A*) shows a unilocular lesion with homogenous hyperintense signal (*black arrow*). Axial T1-weighted image with fat saturation (*B*) shows loss of signal within the lesion indicating macroscopic fat, characteristic of a mature cystic teratoma (*white arrow*). No internal enhancement. U, uterus; Ce, cervix.

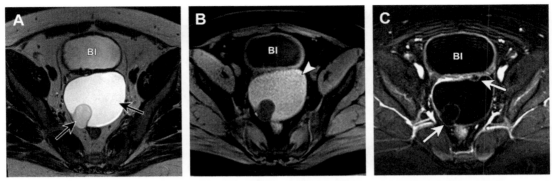

Fig. 6. Mucinous cystadenoma of the right ovary which is located posterior to the bladder. Axial T2-weighted MR image (*A*) shows a multilocular cystic mass with differing signal intensity within different locules (*black arrows*). Axial T1-weighted MR image with fat saturation (*B*) shows homogenous hyperintense signal in one of the locules due to variation in mucin content (*white arrowhead*). Axial post-contrast T1-weighted image with fat saturation (*C*) shows thin enhancing septations (*white arrows*) and no enhancing solid components. Bl, bladder.

ovaries and the surrounding pelvic structures (posterior uterine wall, uterosacral ligaments, and anterior rectum). When the ovaries are retracted posteriorly and medially and/or when situated next to each other, this is known as a "kissing ovary" configuration (**Fig. 8**). This appearance has been associated with higher severity of endometriosis on intraoperative staging.[22,23]

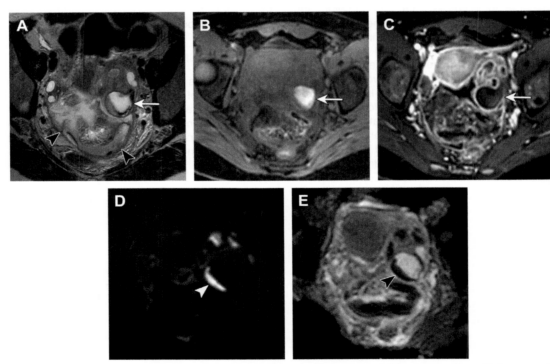

Fig. 7. Left tubo-ovarian abscess. Short axis oblique T2-weighted MR image (*A*) shows an enlarged left ovary with diffuse, mild increased signal intensity of the ovarian stroma and a cystic component (*white arrow*). Inflammatory peritoneal thickening (*black arrowheads*) and heterogeneous ascites are also present. Axial T1-weighted image with fat saturation (*B*) shows hyperintense signal within the left ovarian cystic structure (*white arrow*). Axial subtraction post-contrast T1-weighted image with fat saturation (*C*) shows rim enhancement of multiple locules, including the cystic structure (*white arrow*). Axial diffusion weighted image (b-value = 1600) (*D*) shows markedly hyperintense signal within the cystic component (*white arrowhead*). Axial apparent diffusion coefficient map (*E*) shows corresponding hypointensity of the cystic component which restricts diffusion (*black arrowhead*).

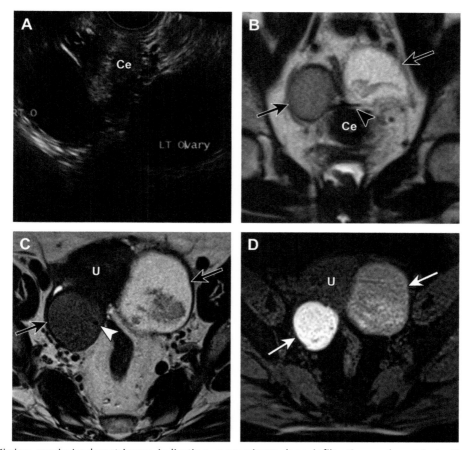

Fig. 8. Kissing ovaries/endometriomas indicating concomitant deep infiltrating endometriosis. Transvaginal pelvic ultrasound (*A*) shows bilateral cystic lesions oriented adjacent and posterior to the cervix (Ce). Coronal T2-weighted MR image (*B*) and axial T2-weighted MR image (*C*) show bilateral kissing ovaries (*black arrows*) posterior to the cervix (Ce) and uterus (U) with abutment of bilateral cystic lesions. There is a thin fibrotic band of adhesion between the ovaries and cervix (*black arrowhead*) and further adhesion along the uterus. There is T2 shading in both lesions and a T2 dark spot on the right (*white arrowhead*). Axial T1-weighted MR image (*D*) without contrast and with fat saturation shows typical T1-weighted hyperintensity of an endometrioma on the right and heterogeneity of the lesion on the left (*white arrows*). Given the pattern of disease, the left sided lesion is likely also an endometrioma, although a hemorrhagic cyst could also have this appearance.

FALLOPIAN TUBE INVOLVEMENT/ HEMATOSALPINX

Endometriosis is a frequent cause of fallopian tube dilation with approximately 30% of women having tubal involvement on laparoscopy.[24,25] Endometriotic implants most commonly involve the serosa and subserosa of the fallopian tubes and are not typically visible on imaging. These superficial implants elicit repetitive bouts of hemorrhage and fibrosis, which lead to peritubal adhesions and fallopian tube dilation.[26] Transmural or mucosal involvement is less commonly encountered.[27]

Hematosalpinx is highly suggestive of endometriosis, even in the absence of endometriosis elsewhere in the pelvis.[25,28] In fact, it may be the only finding indicative of underlying endometriosis.[24,27] The intraluminal appearance on T2WI is variable and frequently does not demonstrate T2 shading classically associated with endometriomas (**Fig. 9**). The absence of intraluminal T2W hypointensity may be related to the extraluminal location of the implants, which restricts the chronic, cyclical nature of hemorrhage deposition classically encountered within the ovary. Unlike pyosalpinx, the fallopian tube walls are typically thinner in the setting of endometriosis.[25]

BROAD LIGAMENT ENDOMETRIOSIS

Endometriosis can involve the broad ligament, which is the adnexal suspensory ligament and

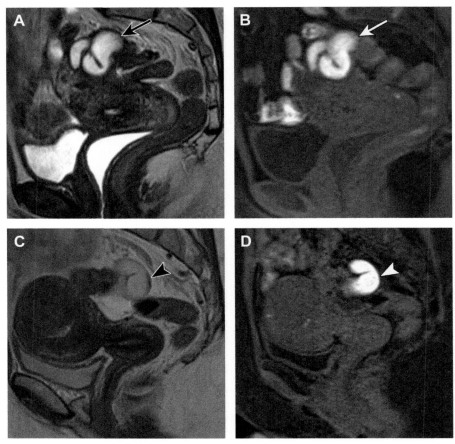

Fig. 9. Hematosalpinx in two patients (*A* and *B* vs *C* and *D*). Sagittal T2-weighted MR image (*A*) shows a dilated tubular structure posterior and superior to the uterus (*black arrow*) with hyperintensity and no shading. Corresponding sagittal T1-weighted MR image with fat saturation (*B*) shows diffuse hyperintense signal compatible with hematosalpinx (*white arrow*). Sagittal T2-weighted MR image (*C*) in a different patient shows a dilated tubular structure posterior to the uterine-cervical junction which is predominantly hyperintense but with layering hypointensity posteriorly consistent with T2 shading (*black arrowhead*). Corresponding sagittal T1-weighted MR image with fat saturation (*D*) shows hyperintensity consistent with hematosalpinx (*white arrowhead*).

serves as the mesentery to the ovary and fallopian tube. The broad ligament is the lateral extension of the anterior and posterior peritoneal surfaces of the uterus, which come together laterally and extend to the pelvic side wall and pelvic floor inferiorly. The presence of the broad ligament results in anterior and posterior peritoneal recesses. Endometriomas and DIE can therefore also involve the broad ligament, the recesses, and the adjacent but separate structures such as the ureters and uterosacral ligaments. The proximal round ligament courses through the broad ligament and can be involved by DIE. Endometriosis of the broad ligament can manifest as an adnexal extra-ovarian mass or endometrioma, isolated as unifocal disease, or be contiguous with adjacent DIE deposits[2,29] (**Fig. 10**).

ENDOMETRIOSIS-ASSOCIATED OVARIAN CANCER

Endometriosis-associated ovarian cancer (EAOC) is a subset of ovarian cancers defined as an ovarian cancer in association with ipsilateral or contralateral ovarian endometriosis, pelvic endometriosis, or histopathology showing endometriosis. The mechanism for transition from benign disease to malignancy is the subject of ongoing research but likely multifactorial including molecular genomic alterations, biologic modulators, and hormonal factors.[30]

This unique group of cancers tends to occur at an earlier age and is associated with better prognosis and outcomes as compared with ovarian cancers in the general population. The most common

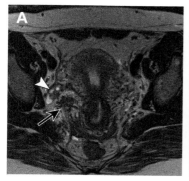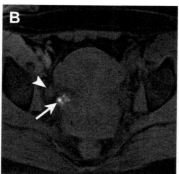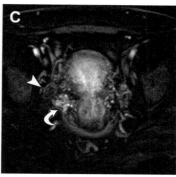

Fig. 10. Deep infiltrating endometriosis of the right broad ligament. This presented as a right adnexal mass separate from the right ovary (*white arrowhead*) in a patient with cyclic flank pain and hematuria. The mass was encasing the right ureter and caused cyclic hydronephrosis (not present at the time of MR imaging and not shown here). Axial T2-weighted MR image (*A*) shows an irregular T2-weighted hypointense mass (*black arrow*) between the uterus and cervix and right ovary. Axial T1-weighted MR image with fat saturation (*B*) shows intrinsic hyperintensity (*white arrow*) within the mass due to active glandular components of deep infiltrating endometriosis (DIE). Axial T1-weighted post-contrast MR image with fat saturation and subtraction (*C*) shows enhancement due to a chronic fibrotic component (also represented by T2-weighted hypointensity) of DIE (*curved white arrow*). The right ureter coursed into the posterior aspect of the mass.

histology for EAOC includes endometrioid adenocarcinoma and clear cell carcinoma followed by mucinous borderline tumors, endometrial stromal sarcoma, and Mullerian adenosarcomas.[31]

Clinical symptoms of EAOC are nonspecific and may overlap with endometriosis. Tumor markers such as CA-125 are not reliable to establish a diagnosis as they can be elevated in women with benign endometriosis and normal in women with ovarian cancers. Given that imaging studies are frequently performed for women with endometriosis, it is crucial that radiologists evaluate endometriomas for evidence of malignant transformation.[31]

MR imaging is more sensitive than ultrasound for distinguishing benign from malignant ovarian lesions and is an important tool in ovarian lesion assessment. Studies evaluating MR imaging features of EAOC have shown a larger lesion size among malignant lesions (11.2 cm) as compared with benign (7.8 cm).[32] The characteristic T2 shading of cyst fluid in benign endometriomas is often lost or absent in malignant lesions. This has been attributed to dilution of endometriotic cyst contents by serous or mucin-producing tumors. Benign endometriomas can contain internal septa due to hemorrhagic contents. Septa in benign lesions tend to be smooth and avascular, whereas septa in malignant lesions may be nodular and show post-contrast enhancement or restricted diffusion.[31] Enhancing mural nodules and papillary projections are imaging features of malignant ovarian lesions. These solid elements can show variable pre-contrast SI and may exhibit a restricted diffusion pattern on DWI. Post-contrast subtraction imaging is helpful to recognize enhancement of solid elements as lesions may have cyst fluid with intrinsic hyperintense signal on T1WI (**Fig. 11**).

DECIDUALIZED ENDOMETRIOSIS

Pregnancy is a progesterone-predominant state, where there is a relative decline in estrogen and increase in progesterone hormone levels.[33] Decidualization is a physiologic response of the eutopic normal endometrial lining to these hormonal changes in pregnancy, where the endometrium hypertrophies and becomes more vascular to support the growing fetus. Ectopic endometrium present in endometriomas and DIE can also respond to these hormonal changes and undergo decidualization.[33] Overall, as endometriosis is an estrogen driven disorder, the progesterone-predominant state of pregnancy favors an improvement in endometriosis.[33]

With decidualization, endometriomas can demonstrate a rapid growth, particularly early in pregnancy after which they may stabilize or continue to increase in size.[34–36] Decidualized endometriomas usually appear as unilocular or multilocular cystic masses with a solid component on ultrasound (**Fig. 12**). Rounded, smooth, highly vascularized, solid papillary projections in the internal wall of endometriomas seem to be the most consistently reported characteristic of decidualization.[37] In a study by Mascilini and colleagues, the smooth, rounded appearance of the papillary projections signaled benignity with a large majority of patients with decidualized endometriomas (82%) demonstrating this feature.[36]

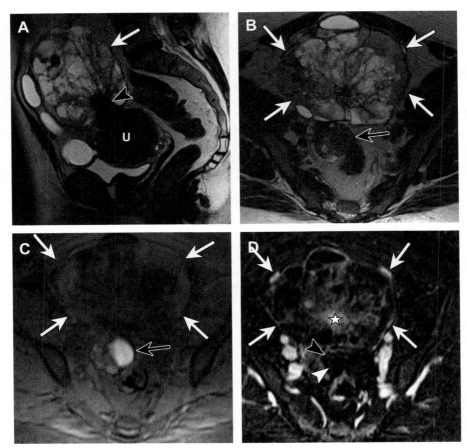

Fig. 11. Endometriosis-associated ovarian cancer. Premenopausal woman with chronic pelvic pain and irregular menses. Sagittal T2-weighted MR image (*A*) shows a large hypointense deep infiltrative endometriosis (DIE) lesion (*black arrowhead*) that extends from the posterior uterus (U) to the large left ovarian mass (*white arrow*). Axial T2-weighted MR image (*B*) shows a unilocular right ovarian lesion with T2 shading, characteristic of an endometrioma (*black arrow*) and the large, multiloculated left ovarian mass with numerous irregular septations and heterogeneous signal (*white arrows*). Axial pre-contrast T1-weighted image (*C*) with fat suppression shows homogeneous hyperintense signal within the unilocular right ovarian lesion characteristic of an endometrioma (*black arrow*). The large left ovarian lesion is heterogeneous (*white arrows*). Axial post-contrast T1-weighted MR image (*D*) with fat suppression and subtraction shows enhancement of solid elements (*star*) and irregular septations throughout the left ovarian mass (*white arrows*). Enhancing septa (*white arrowhead*) and nodule (*black arrowhead*) was also noted within the right ovarian lesion. Histopathology showed well-differentiated mixed epithelial carcinomas (seromucinous and endometrioid) arising in a background of endometriosis in both ovaries.

Differentiation with malignancy can be particularly challenging, especially in the absence of previous imaging documentation of endometriomas. On MR imaging, the mural nodules seen in malignancy are T1 hypointense and T2 hyperintense.[38] The decidualized solid components of endometriomas demonstrate SI similar to the decidualized endometrium or placenta and can be T2 hypointense.[11,35,39] Note that gadolinium-based contrast is not given during pregnancy to evaluate for enhancement due to potential safety concerns for the fetus. Solid components of both decidualized endometriomas and malignancy can restrict diffusion on DWI. Higher b-value DWI and ADC maps can be helpful for differentiation. Decidualized endometriomas show decreased signal at higher b-values (b-value = 1500), whereas cancers maintain their restricted diffusion, especially on higher b-values.[39] Takeuchi and colleagues also showed that decidualized endometriomas exhibit high SI on DWI (b-values = 800) due to T2 shine-through effect.[39] Despite this, given the current sparse literature on this topic, patient-centered decision-making is advised with close monitoring during pregnancy (**Fig. 13**). Conservative management can be pursued, if decidualized endometriosis is highly suspected, such as in scenarios wherein the growth of the mass stabilizes on follow-up.

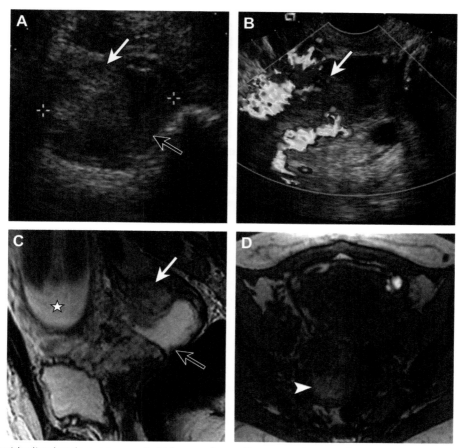

Fig. 12. Decidualized endometrioma mimicking ovarian malignancy. A 34-year-old woman found to have an incidental adnexal mass during routine obstetric ultrasound, proven to be a decidualized endometrioma after surgical resection at the time of cesarean section. Gray scale ultrasound (US) image (*A*) demonstrates a unilocular mass (calipers) with solid components (*black* and *white arrows*). As shown here, decidualization can be nonuniform presenting as solid nodules (*white arrow*) or solid tissue (*black arrow*) along the wall of the endometrioma. Color Doppler US (*B*) shows the mass to be markedly hypervascular. Note the smooth and rounded appearance of the solid component that has been described to be typical of decidualized endometriomas (*white arrow*). Sagittal T2-weighted MR image (*C*) shows the same cystic mass with nonuniform solid components (*white* and *black arrows*). Note the gestation in the uterus (*star*). Axial T1-weighted image (*D*) shows intrinsic T1 hyperintensity of the fluid contents (*white arrowhead*), which is suggestive of hemorrhagic contents, that can be seen in endometriomas. However, imaging distinction from malignancy remains challenging.

Spontaneous hemoperitoneum in pregnancy (SHiP) is unprovoked (nontraumatic) intraperitoneal bleeding during pregnancy and up to 42 days postpartum arising from endometriomas or DIE, particularly in patients status post fertility assistance with ovarian stimulation and in vitro fertilization.[40] In patients who underwent surgical interventions, active hemorrhage was noted from endometriotic implants, ruptured utero-ovarian vessels, hemorrhagic nodules of decidualized cells, and/or pseudoaneurysms. Imaging usually demonstrates unexplained intraperitoneal free fluid and hemorrhage. Presumed decidual reaction in DIE can result in pseudoaneurysms likely secondary to decidualization and neovascularity,

which can lead to catastrophic hemorrhage.[41] There are no current tools to identify patients at risk of SHiP; therefore, when unexplained hemoperitoneum is seen, hemorrhage related to endometriosis should be considered in the differential.

SUMMARY

Endometriomas are a common manifestation of endometriosis and can occur in isolation or associated with hematosalpinx or DIE. Utilization of a proper MR protocol can assist in differentiation with other adnexal masses and increase detection of EAOC. The hormonal changes of pregnancy can

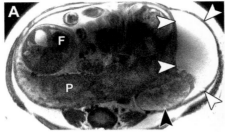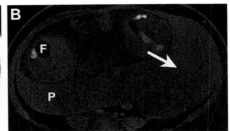

Fig. 13. 34-year-old woman with history of endometriosis presents with a large left adnexal mass in pregnancy. The mass was resected at the time of cesarean section delivery and found to represent a clear cell cancer. Axial T2-weighted image (*A*) shows a large cystic mass (*white arrowheads*) with a large solid component (*black arrowhead*). Axial T1-weighted image (*B*) does not demonstrate hyperintensity in the cyst fluid (*white arrow*), in contrast to **Fig. 11.** The mass and the solid component demonstrated exponential growth in pregnancy, which was suspicious for malignancy. F, fetus; P, placenta.

cause decidualization of endometriosis. A potential complication of endometriosis is spontaneous hemorrhage in pregnancy.

CLINICS CARE POINTS

- Endometriomas have marked homogenous T1-weighted hyperintensity, T2 shading, and some will have the T2 dark spot sign. They are often multiple and bilateral.

- Hematosalpinges appear as dilated tubular structures that are also hyperintense on T1-weighted imaging. However, T2 shading may or may not be present.

- Post contrast subtraction imaging is vital to evaluate for endometriosis associated ovarian cancer as lesions may have cyst fluid with intrinsic T1-weighted hyperintensity.

- Endometriomas can decidualize in pregnancy and mimic ovarian cancer due to solid components and rapid growth. Solid components will have smooth round projections and match signal of the endometrium and placenta. Growth tends to stabilize; however, if growth continues, suspect malignancy.

- If a pregnant or post-partum patient presents with nontraumatic abdominal pain and hemoperitoneum, evaluate for signs of endometriosis as a source because spontaneous hemorrhage in pregnancy can occur.

DISCLOSURE

Sakala - No disclosures. Jha- No disclosures. Tong- Research support from Siemens Heatlhcare in the form of hardware and software. Taffel- No disclosures. Feldman- No disclosures.

REFERENCES

1. Shafrir AL, Farland LV, Shah DK, et al. Risk for and consequences of endometriosis: A critical epidemiologic review. Best Pract Res Clin Obstet Gynaecol 2018;51:1–15.
2. Jha P, Sakala M, Chamie LP, et al. Endometriosis MRI lexicon: consensus statement from the society of abdominal radiology endometriosis disease-focused panel. Abdom Radiol (NY) 2020;45(6):1552–68.
3. Tong A, VanBuren WM, Chamié L, et al. Recommendations for MRI technique in the evaluation of pelvic endometriosis: consensus statement from the Society of Abdominal Radiology endometriosis disease-focused panel. Abdom Radiol 2020;45(6): 1569–86.
4. Brown MA, Mattrey RF, Stamato S, et al. MRI of the female pelvis using vaginal gel. AJR Am J Roentgenol 2005;185(5):1221–7.
5. Chassang M, Novellas S, Bloch-Marcotte C, et al. Utility of vaginal and rectal contrast medium in MRI for the detection of deep pelvic endometriosis. Eur Radiol 2010;20(4):1003–10.
6. Bazot M, Bharwani N, Huchon C, et al. European society of urogenital radiology (ESUR) guidelines: MR imaging of pelvic endometriosis. Eur Radiol 2017; 27(7):2765–75.
7. Bazot M, Gasner A, Ballester M, et al. Value of thin-section oblique axial T2-weighted magnetic resonance images to assess uterosacral ligament endometriosis. Hum Reprod 2011;26(2):346–53.
8. Taylor EC, Irshaid L, Mathur M. Multimodality Imaging Approach to Ovarian Neoplasms with Pathologic Correlation. RadioGraphics 2021;41(1):289–315.
9. Sakala MD, Shampain KL, Wasnik AP. Advances in MR Imaging of the Female Pelvis. Magn Reson Imaging Clin N Am 2020;28(3):415–31.
10. Kim HJ, Lee SY, Shin YR, et al. The Value of Diffusion-Weighted Imaging in the Differential Diagnosis of Ovarian Lesions: A Meta-Analysis. PLoS One 2016;11(2):e0149465.

11. Takeuchi M, Matsuzaki K, Nishitani H. Susceptibility-Weighted MRI of Endometrioma: Preliminary Results. AJR Am J Roentgenol 2008;191(5):1366–70.

12. Siegelman ES, Oliver ER. MR Imaging of Endometriosis: Ten Imaging Pearls. RadioGraphics 2012;32(6):1675–91.

13. Exacoustos C, De Felice G, Pizzo A, et al. Isolated Ovarian Endometrioma: A History Between Myth and Reality. J Minim Invasive Gynecol 2018;25(5):884–91.

14. Corwin MT, Gerscovich EO, Lamba R, et al. Differentiation of Ovarian Endometriomas from Hemorrhagic Cysts at MR Imaging: Utility of the T2 Dark Spot Sign. Radiology 2014;271(1):126–32.

15. Kanso HN, Hachem K, Aoun NJ, et al. Variable MR findings in ovarian functional hemorrhagic cysts. J Magn Reson Imaging 2006;24(2):356–61.

16. Allen BC, Hosseinzadeh K, Qasem SA, et al. Practical Approach to MRI of Female Pelvic Masses. AJR Am J Roentgenol 2014;202(6):1366–75.

17. Zhao SH, Qiang JW, Zhang GF, et al. MRI in differentiating ovarian borderline from benign mucinous cystadenoma: Pathological correlation. J Magn Reson Imaging 2014;39(1):162–6.

18. Laurent PE, Thomassin-Piana J, Jalaguier-Coudray A. Mucin-producing tumors of the ovary: MR imaging appearance. Diagn Interv Imaging 2015;96(11):1125–32.

19. Peyrot H, Montoriol PF, Canis M. Spontaneous T1-Hyperintensity Within an Ovarian Lesion: Spectrum of Diagnoses. Can Assoc Radiol J 2015;66(2):115–20.

20. Solak A, Sahin N, Genç B, et al. Diagnostic value of susceptibility-weighted imaging of abdominal wall endometriomas during the cyclic menstrual changes: a preliminary study. Eur J Radiol 2013;82(9):e411–416.

21. Redwine DB. Ovarian endometriosis: a marker for more extensive pelvic and intestinal disease. Fertil Steril 1999;72(2):310–5.

22. Williams JC, Burnett TL, Jones T, et al. Association between kissing and retropositioned ovaries and severity of endometriosis: MR imaging evaluation. Abdom Radiol (NY) 2020;45(6):1637–44.

23. Ghezzi F, Raio L, Cromi A, et al. Kissing ovaries": a sonographic sign of moderate to severe endometriosis. Fertil Steril 2005;83(1):143–7.

24. Gougoutas CA, Siegelman ES, Hunt J, et al. Pelvic endometriosis: various manifestations and MR imaging findings. AJR Am J Roentgenol 2000;175(2):353–8.

25. Revzin MV, Moshiri M, Katz DS, et al. Imaging Evaluation of Fallopian Tubes and Related Disease: A Primer for Radiologists. Radiographics 2020;40(5):1473–501.

26. Kim MY, Rha SE, Oh SN, et al. MR Imaging findings of hydrosalpinx: a comprehensive review. Radiographics 2009;29(2):495–507.

27. Outwater EK, Siegelman ES, Chiowanich P, et al. Dilated fallopian tubes: MR imaging characteristics. Radiology 1998;208(2):463–9.

28. Foti PV, Ognibene N, Spadola S, et al. Non-neoplastic diseases of the fallopian tube: MR imaging with emphasis on diffusion-weighted imaging. Insights Imaging 2016;7(3):311–27.

29. Trehan A, Trehan AK. Endometrioma contained within the broad ligament. BMJ Case Rep 2014;2014. bcr2013203441.

30. Nezhat F, Datta MS, Hanson V, et al. The relationship of endometriosis and ovarian malignancy: a review. Fertil Steril 2008;90(5):1559–70.

31. Robinson KA, Menias CO, Chen L, et al. Understanding malignant transformation of endometriosis: imaging features with pathologic correlation. Abdom Radiol 2019. https://doi.org/10.1007/s00261-019-01914-7.

32. Tanaka YO, Yoshizako T, Nishida M, et al. Ovarian carcinoma in patients with endometriosis: MR imaging findings. AJR Am J Roentgenol 2000;175(5):1423–30.

33. Navarro R, Poder L, Sun D, et al. Endometriosis in pregnancy. Abdom Radiol (NY) 2020;45(6):1741–53.

34. Guerriero S, Ajossa S, Piras S, et al. Serial ultrasonographic evaluation of a decidualized endometrioma in pregnancy. Ultrasound Obstet Gynecol 2005;26(3):304–6.

35. Takeuchi M, Matsuzaki K, Nishitani H. Magnetic resonance manifestations of decidualized endometriomas during pregnancy. J Comput Assist Tomogr 2008;32(3):353–5.

36. Mascilini F, Moruzzi C, Giansiracusa C, et al. Imaging in gynecological disease. 10: Clinical and ultrasound characteristics of decidualized endometriomas surgically removed during pregnancy. Ultrasound Obstet Gynecol 2014;44(3):354–60.

37. Frühauf F, Fanta M, Burgetová A, et al. Endometriosis in pregnancy - diagnostics and management. Ceska Gynekol 2019;84(1):61–7.

38. Miyakoshi K, Tanaka M, Gabionza D, et al. Decidualized ovarian endometriosis mimicking malignancy. AJR Am J Roentgenol 1998;171(6):1625–6.

39. Takeuchi M, Matsuzaki K, Harada M. Computed diffusion-weighted imaging for differentiating decidualized endometrioma from ovarian cancer. Eur J Radiol 2016;85(5):1016–9.

40. Lier MCI, Malik RF, Ket JCF, et al. Spontaneous hemoperitoneum in pregnancy (SHiP) and endometriosis - A systematic review of the recent literature. Eur J Obstet Gynecol Reprod Biol 2017;219:57–65.

41. Feld Z, Rowen T, Callen A, et al. Uterine artery pseudoaneurysm in the setting of deep endometriosis: an uncommon cause of hemoperitoneum in pregnancy. Emerg Radiol 2018;25(1):107–10.

MR Imaging of Mimics of Adnexal Pathology

Tugce Agirlar Trabzonlu, MD[a], Mallika Modak, PhD[a], Jeanne M. Horowitz, MD[a,*]

KEYWORDS

• MR imaging • Adnexal mass • Ovary • Ultrasound • Computed tomography • Neoplasm • Mimics

KEY POINTS

- Radiologists should be aware that many benign and malignant diseases can mimic adnexal pathologies on imaging, including uterine leiomyomas, abscesses, peritoneal inclusion cysts, gastrointestinal masses such as mucocele of the appendix, colorectal cancer, gastrointestinal stromal tumor, and retroperitoneal cystic and solid masses of developmental, lymphatic, neoplastic, neurogenic, and mesenchymal origin.
- A step-wise approach when identifying the origin of a pelvic mass on imaging is to first determine if the mass is intraperitoneal or extraperitoneal, then ovarian or non-ovarian in origin. Subsequent differentiation of whether the mass is cystic or solid can assist in narrowing the differential diagnosis.
- On MR imaging, the ovaries are best seen on T2-weighted imaging. Visualization of discrete normal ovaries can exclude an ovarian etiology of a pelvic mass.
- Clues on MR imaging and other modalities that suggest an ovarian etiology of a pelvic mass include embedding of part of an ovary in the tumor ("embedded organ sign"); asymmetrically enlarged ovarian veins extending to the pelvic mass ("ovarian vascular pedicle sign"); and if the mass deforms the surface of an adjacent ovary into a "beak" shape forming a sharp angle ("beak sign").
- Gynecologic masses mimicking ovarian masses are most often leiomyomas. Two radiologic signs that confirm these are uterine in origin include the "claw sign" and the "bridging vessel sign."

INTRODUCTION

Radiologists frequently encounter adnexal pathology in their daily practice.[1] Although most of these abnormalities are ovarian in origin, 5.1% of the patients who underwent surgery for a suspected ovarian mass were found to have lesions of extra-ovarian origin.[2] Determining the source of a pelvic mass is crucial in directing patient management. Mimics of ovarian pathology typically require a different treatment approach from ovarian cancers.[3,4] Identifying the etiology of a mass may be challenging due to complex pelvic anatomy and overlapping imaging appearances. Knowledge of pelvic anatomic spaces and the expected imaging characteristics of pelvic masses can narrow the differential and assist in making a

definitive diagnosis.[5] In this article, the authors review pelvic imaging modalities, pelvic anatomy, and how to determine if a mass is of ovarian origin. Then, the authors review and illustrate imaging findings of non-adnexal abnormalities which can masquerade as ovarian in nature, including uterine leiomyomas, intraperitoneal cystic and solid masses of mesenteric or gastrointestinal (GI) origin, and extraperitoneal cystic and solid masses.

IMAGING

Pelvic ultrasound (US) is often the appropriate first-line imaging tool when a gynecologic abnormality is suspected; pelvic masses are usually detected with US or, alternatively, computed

[a] Department of Radiology, Northwestern University Feinberg School of Medicine, 676 North Saint Clair Street, Suite 800, Chicago, IL 60611 USA
* Corresponding author. Department of Radiology, Northwestern Memorial Hospital, 676 North Saint Clair Street Suite 800, Chicago, IL 60611.
E-mail address: jeanne.horowitz@nm.org

Magn Reson Imaging Clin N Am 31 (2023) 137–148
https://doi.org/10.1016/j.mric.2022.06.007
1064-9689/23/© 2022 Elsevier Inc. All rights reserved.

tomography (CT) if non-gynecologic pathology is of concern.[6] MR imaging is often used for problem-solving after initial US or CT to further characterize pelvic masses.[4,6,7]

ANATOMY

To determine the anatomic origin of a pelvic mass, the radiologist should first look for the important anatomic landmarks in the pelvis and their displacement relative to the mass to determine if the mass is intraperitoneal or extraperitoneal. Then, the radiologist should search for organ-specific clues to determine if is the lesion is of ovarian or extra-ovarian origin.[8]

Determining the Compartment of the Pelvic Mass

The peritoneum is the biggest serous membrane in the body with two layers: visceral and parietal peritoneum. The outer parietal peritoneum lines the abdominal wall, and the inner visceral peritoneum envelopes most of the organs in the abdominal cavity.[9] The organs that are surrounded by the peritoneum are referred to as intraperitoneal, and organs that are located inferior and/or posterior to the peritoneum are referred to as extraperitoneal.[5] In the female pelvis, there is caudal reflection of the peritoneum over the dome of the bladder, the anterior and posterior surface of the uterus, and rectouterine pouch.[9] Posteriorly, the rectum is divided into intraperitoneal and extraperitoneal portions by the anterior peritoneal reflection.[10] The intraperitoneal organs in the pelvis include the ovaries, small bowel, transverse and sigmoid colon, and upper third of the rectum. The extraperitoneal space contains the bladder, uterus, vagina, ureters, ascending and descending colon, lower two-thirds of the rectum, iliac vasculature, and lymphatics.[5]

The layers of the peritoneum covering the uterus extend laterally to the pelvic sidewalls as broad ligaments,[9] which surround the fallopian tubes and ovaries.[3] The suspensory ligament of the ovary is derived from the superolateral part of the broad ligament that anchors the ovary to the pelvic sidewalls. It contains vessels, lymphatics, and nerves extending to the ovary.[11]

Intraperitoneal masses tend to displace the iliac vessels and uterus laterally. There can be posterior and lateral displacement of the ureter. Masses in the rectouterine pouch may displace the uterus anteriorly and the rectum posteriorly.

In contrast, extraperitoneal masses typically displace the adjacent extraperitoneal structures anteriorly and medially. Extraperitoneal masses can encase the iliac vessels or efface the adjacent pelvic wall musculature.[3,8] However, a large pelvic mass can involve both the intraperitoneal and extraperitoneal spaces.[3,8]

Determining Whether the Intraperitoneal Mass Is Ovarian or Non-Ovarian in Origin

Identifying normal ovaries and the phantom organ sign

If a large mass originates from a small organ, the organ can become nonvisible, known as the "phantom organ" sign.[8] Seeing discrete normal ovaries can exclude an ovarian etiology. The ovaries are ovoid or almond-shaped structures, typically present within the ovarian fossa on either side of the uterus, anterior or anteromedial to the ureter.[11]

In premenopausal women, most of the ovaries are easily identified. On CT, the characteristic imaging appearance is well circumscribed ovoid structures with low or fluid-attenuation corresponding to small follicles. In postmenopausal patients, visualization of the ovaries can be difficult related to their small size and paucity of follicles. On CT imaging, they are typically uniform soft tissue attenuation.[11] Tracking the ovarian veins leads to the suspensory ligaments of the ovaries and is helpful in identification of the normal ovaries, especially in postmenopausal patients.[11] The ovarian veins course anteriorly to the psoas muscle and drain to the inferior vena cava on the right and the left renal vein on the left.[12]

On MR imaging, the ovaries can be most easily seen on T2-weighted imaging. Premenopausal ovaries contain central stroma demonstrating a relatively low T2 signal and surrounding peripheral follicles with high T2 signal.[6] Postmenopausal ovaries are identified as predominantly solid structures with increased stromal tissue, demonstrating a relatively decreased homogenous T2 signal. They can contain small senescent follicles. Some ovaries appear as nodular tissue at the proximal ends of the round ligaments.[3,6]

The suspensory ligaments can be used as an anatomic landmark to identify ovaries or masses arising from the ovaries. On MR imaging, they can be identified as narrow fan-shaped soft tissue bands extending from the ovaries to the lateral pelvic wall, best seen on axial and sagittal T2-weighted images.[8,13] Although demonstrating the suspensory ligament in association with a pelvic mass can be helpful in identifying the ovarian origin, the depiction of this ligament with MR imaging is often difficult.[13]

Embedded organ sign

If at least a part of the ovary is embedded in the tumor, the tumor is likely ovarian in origin, the "embedded organ sign." When an extra-ovarian tumor extrinsically compresses the adjacent ovary, it causes deformation of the adjacent ovarian surface, the "negative embedded organ" sign.[14]

Ovarian vascular pedicle sign

Asymmetrically enlarged ovarian veins extending to a pelvic mass suggest that the mass is ovarian, known as the "ovarian vascular pedicle sign." Lee and colleagues[15] reported that sensitivity and positive predictive values of the ovarian vascular pedicle sign on CT to confirm ovarian origin were 92% and 97%, respectively. However, it should be noted that a large pelvic mass not arising from the ovary can compress the ipsilateral ovarian vein and mimic ovarian pathology.[8]

Beak sign

If a mass deforms the surface of an adjacent ovary into a "beak" forming a sharp angle, ovarian origin is favored, referred to as the "beak sign."[8,14]

MIMICS OF ADNEXAL PATHOLOGIES
Gynecologic Masses Mimicking Adnexal Pathologies

Pedunculated or parasitic uterine fibroids

Leiomyomas are the most common gynecologic neoplasms with a prevalence of approximately 70% to 80% by age 50 years.[16] US is the preferred initial imaging modality to detect leiomyomas. On US, fibroids are well circumscribed solid masses, sometimes with a whorled appearance. They can be of varying echogenicity.[17] However, a very enlarged fibroid uterus can prevent optimal assessment on US due to a limited field of view. MR imaging, with its excellent soft tissue contrast, is often the preferred modality for fibroid mapping for surgical or uterine artery embolization planning, determination of leiomyoma degeneration, and distinguishing between leiomyomas and adnexal masses.[16]

On MRI, a nondegenerated uterine leiomyoma is a well-defined mass demonstrating homogenous decreased signal intensity on T2-weighted images relative to the myometrium. Degenerated uterine fibroids have variable appearance on T2-weighted and pre-contrast and post-contrast T1-weighted images. A pedunculated subserosal leiomyoma, a parasitic leiomyoma, or a para-ovarian leiomyoma can mimic an ovarian fibroma, fibrothecoma, or Brenner tumor, as these ovarian tumors contain a large fibrous component that has similar imaging characteristics on MR imaging to that of a leiomyoma.[16] If there is cystic degeneration, the fibroid can mimic a cystic ovarian tumor as both demonstrate high signal intensity on T2-weighted images and low signal intensity on T1-weighted images.[5]

There are two radiologic signs that confirm that a fibroid is uterine in origin. The "claw sign" shows sharp angles at the edges of the leiomyoma where myometrium extends around it. The "bridging vessel sign" indicates vessels anchoring the leiomyoma to the uterus (**Fig. 1**). Differentiation of a pedunculated uterine fibroid from an adnexal mass is especially important in pregnant patients to avoid surgery and continue conservative management before delivery.[16] An example of a fibroid mimicking an adnexal mass is shown in **Fig. 2**.

Non-Gynecologic Intraperitoneal Diseases Mimicking Adnexal Pathologies

Bowel abscess mimicking an adnexal mass

A common complication of perforated appendicitis and diverticulitis is abscess formation. Because of the close proximity of the appendix to the right ovary and the sigmoid colon to the left ovary, an abscess from complicated appendicitis or diverticulitis can be mistaken for an adnexal mass. Usually, an abscess in this setting is not a diagnostic dilemma and is easily distinguished from an adnexal mass on CT with associated inflammatory changes of the appendix or involved colon.[18,19] If the patient's presentation for medical care is delayed, a large thick-walled fluid collection can sometimes be seen in the pelvis, and it can be difficult to exclude an adnexal etiology.[19] The demonstration of an ipsilateral normal ovary in this scenario can exclude adnexal origin. In some cases, there can be secondary reactive involvement of the ipsilateral ovary or a fistula extending to the ovary which can cloud the clinical picture.[18,20] Follow-up imaging after the symptoms have resolved can also exclude an adnexal mass if a normal ipsilateral ovary is seen after treatment.

Peritoneal inclusion cysts mimicking an adnexal mass

Peritoneal inclusion cysts are a nonneoplastic process secondary to reactive mesothelial proliferation and can be seen in the setting of prior pelvic surgery, endometriosis, pelvic inflammatory disease, or trauma.[3,5] The mesothelial cells in the peritoneum normally reabsorb fluid in the peritoneal cavity. Impaired reabsorption of the fluid in the presence of adhesions results in accumulation of fluid and formation of cysts that conform to the shape of adjacent structures.[3,21] These cysts are generally incidentally detected in premenopausal patients with active ovaries. However, sometimes they can cause pelvic pain or swelling.[5] These lesions can mimic cystic ovarian neoplasms, such

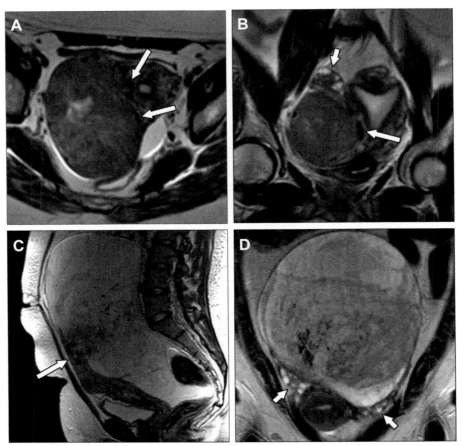

Fig. 1. Two patients demonstrating the "bridging vessel" sign. (*A, B*) On axial and coronal T2-weighted MR images, bridging vessels (*long arrows*) are seen between the uterus and a subserosal fibroid, indicating its uterine origin. The coronal MR image shows a separate, normal ovary with small follicles (*short arrow*). (*C, D*) In a 29-year old woman with a large central pelvic mass (pathologically proven degenerated fibroid), bridging vessels are seen on sagittal T2-weighted MR imaging (*C, long arrow*), and normal ovaries are seen separately on coronal T2 MR images (*D, short arrows*).

as benign or borderline tumors (**Fig. 3**). On US, they appear as a unilocular or a multilocular cyst in close proximity to the adjacent ovary. Low-resistance vascularity can be seen on color Doppler imaging within thin septations where small vessels course through mesothelial tissue.[5] Peritoneal inclusion cysts and their relationship with the adjacent structures are better demonstrated with MR imaging. On MR imaging, they appear as unilocular or multilocular cysts. The septations of the cysts should be thin and can demonstrate smooth enhancement without nodularity.[3] Peritoneal inclusion cysts can envelop the ovary and form an "entrapped" or "spider in a web" appearance.[3] Hemorrhage can occur within peritoneal inclusion cysts, demonstrated as high signal intensity on T1-weighted MR imaging and relative low intensity on T2-weighted MR imaging.[5]

Intraperitoneal Mass of Gastrointestinal Origin Mimicking an Adnexal Mass

Intraperitoneal masses of gastrointestinal (GI) origin can mimic ovarian cancer, including mucocele of the appendix, primary colon cancer, and GI stromal tumor (GIST).

Mucocele of the appendix

Mucocele of the appendix refers to a dilated appendix containing intraluminal mucin secondary to mucosal hyperplasia, appendiceal cystadenoma or cystadenocarcinoma, or chronic obstruction.[22] An appendiceal mucocele appears on CT as a well circumscribed tubular or spherical low-attenuation mass.[23] They are typically found adjacent to the base of the cecum, in the expected location of the appendix. After detection of a mucocele, radiologists should thoroughly assess

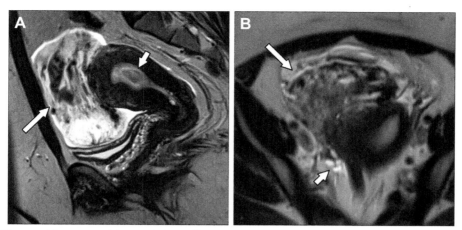

Fig. 2. A 33-year-old woman with a pathologically proven uterine fibroid mimicking an ovarian sclerosing stromal tumor or granulosa cell tumor. On sagittal (*A*) and axial (*B*) T2-weighted MR imaging, a right-sided pelvic mass (*long arrows*) shows heterogeneous high T2 signal with low signal intensity internal nodules, which can be seen in sclerosing stromal tumors of the ovary, granulosa cell tumors, and leiomyomas. An endometrial polyp in this case (*A, short arrow*) also raises suspicion for an ovarian sex cord stromal tumor. However, a normal right ovary is identified (*B, short arrow*), indicating that this is of uterine origin.

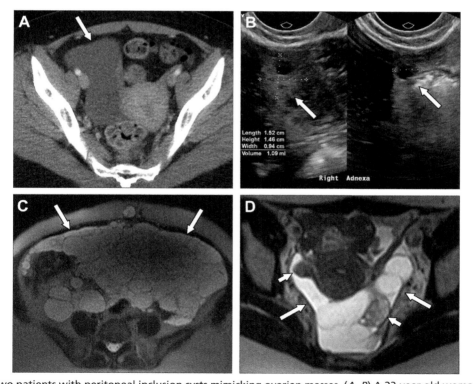

Fig. 3. Two patients with peritoneal inclusion cysts mimicking ovarian masses. (*A, B*) A 22-year old woman with a 10-cm right pelvic cystic mass on axial contrast-enhanced CT (*A, long arrow*) thought to be of ovarian origin. Pelvic US (*B*) demonstrates a normal right ovary (*arrows*). This was demonstrated to be a peritoneal inclusion cyst on surgical pathology. (*C, D*) In a different patient, large septated pelvic cystic lesions on axial T2-weighted MR imaging conform to the peritoneal cavity (*C, D, long arrows*), surrounding normal ovaries (*short arrows*), consistent with peritoneal inclusion cysts.

for extraluminal mucin. Extraluminal mucin appears as low-attenuating deposits in the periappendiceal space, peritoneal cavity, or on abdominal visceral surfaces, such as on the ovaries and the bowel.[22] Calcifications may often be present within the wall of the appendiceal mucocele, best identified via CT. On US, mucoceles can be identified by the very specific "onion skin sign," marked by echogenic concentric layers.[18] The close proximity of the mucocele to the cecum can help distinguish this pathology from adnexal masses and is best appreciated on MR imaging. Identification of a normal right ovary can also exclude an adnexal mass (**Fig. 4**).

Primary colorectal cancer

Primary colorectal cancer can sometimes be mistaken for an adnexal mass.[24] On CT and MR imaging, primary colorectal cancers typically appear as a soft tissue mass narrowing the lumen of the colon due to nodular wall thickening.[25] MR imaging plays a key role in primary staging of rectal cancer.[24] However, local extension of tumors derived from the sigmoid colon and cecum to nearby structures such as the adnexa may make it difficult to determine the tumor's origin. Anatomically, the relationship of the mass and its contiguity with the inferior mesenteric vein as opposed to the gonadal vein is useful in distinguishing sigmoid colon cancers.[26]

Gastrointestinal stromal tumors

GISTs are another type of GI neoplasm that can mimic ovarian cancers (**Fig. 5**). GISTs are mesenchymal neoplasms that originate from GI pacemaker cells. Although they primarily arise from the stomach, they can occur at any point along the GI tract and may mimic adnexal pathologies.[27] On CT, GISTs demonstrate soft tissue attenuation, with central necrosis resulting in internal areas of lower attenuation.[27] GISTs are often exophytic and grow into surrounding structures, which can make it challenging to identify their origin and distinguish them from adnexal pathology on CT. Thus, MR imaging may provide an alternative method of better discrimination of GISTs from neighboring abdominal and pelvic structures due to superior soft tissue contrast.[28] Overall, the appearance of GISTs on MR imaging is variable due to potential necrotic or cystic areas within the masses. The ultimate diagnosis of GISTs relies on histopathology.

Diffuse Peritoneal Processes: A Mimicker of Advanced Ovarian Cancer

Peritoneal involvement of tumor is frequently seen in patients with ovarian cancer. The differential diagnosis for diffuse intraperitoneal processes which can mimic advanced ovarian cancer includes pseudomyxoma peritonei, peritoneal metastases/carcinomatosis from GI primary tumor, lymphoma (**Fig. 6**), and less common entities such as primary malignant mesothelioma, primary peritoneal serous papillary carcinoma, disseminated peritoneal leiomyomatosis, peritoneal tuberculosis, splenosis, and primary lymphangiomatosis.[3,29,30]

Other than ovarian cancer, GI carcinomas such as gastric, pancreatic, and colorectal carcinomas are the most common tumors that spread to the peritoneum. On CT, the imaging findings vary from discrete nodules to infiltrative masses with or without ascites.[3,29] On MR imaging, peritoneal carcinomatosis shows gradual enhancement after intravenous contrast administration and is best shown on images acquired 5 to 10 minutes following contrast injection.[29] CT is commonly used to assess for peritoneal carcinomatosis as it is widely available with fast acquisition time.[29] CT has been shown to have sensitivity of 68% and specificity of 88% in the detection of the peritoneal metastases. MR imaging has been demonstrated to have the highest sensitivity for the detection of peritoneal metastases in ovarian and patients with GI cancer with a sensitivity rate of 92% and specificity rate of 85%.[31] It has been shown that MR imaging is superior in detection of tumor smaller than 1 cm. Diffusion-weighted imaging can enhance detection of the peritoneal and omental implants secondary to better contrast resolution.[29,32] In the presence of diffuse peritoneal disease, the stomach, pancreas, and colon should be carefully examined in addition to the ovaries to determine the origin of the primary tumor.

Extraperitoneal Non-Gynecological Diseases Mimicking Adnexal Pathologies

Owing to their location and large size, many extraperitoneal entities in the pelvis may appear intraperitoneal in location and can mimic adnexal diseases.[30] The most common entities that affect the pelvic retroperitoneum are the direct involvement of gynecologic, bladder or GI tumors. However, primary neoplastic and nonneoplastic entities of these regions can occur.[3] Extraperitoneal masses can be developmental, neurogenic lymphatic, or mesenchymal in etiology.[33,34] Assessment with pelvic MR imaging is important in these cases to evaluate the complex anatomy of the pelvis and the relationship of the mass to the adjacent pelvic structures.[30] Identification of normal ovaries and differentiation of whether the mass is cystic or solid assist in narrowing the differential diagnosis.[35]

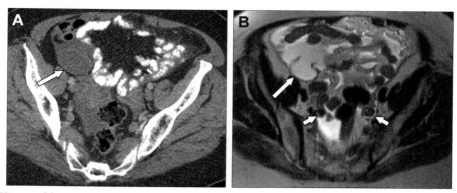

Fig. 4. A 69-year-old woman with a ruptured low grade appendiceal mucinous neoplasm (LAMN), mimicking an ovarian cystic mass on CT (*A, long arrow*). On axial T2-weighted MRI (*B*), the right pelvic cystic mass (LAMN) had ruptured (*long arrow*), and the LAMN was located adjacent to the cecum (not shown). Small right and left ovaries were identified by tracing the gonadal vessels (*short arrows*).

Cystic Extraperitoneal Lesions Mimicking Adnexal Pathologies

Extraperitoneal cystic lesions can be congenital, developmental, or lymphatic in origin.[5] Spinal meningeal cysts are diverticula/herniations of the dural sac from a congenital sacral defect into the presacral space. On MR imaging, these are unilocular cysts that have a connection with the spinal canal and demonstrate signal intensity similar to that of cerebrospinal fluid.[35,36]

Developmental cystic lesions
Developmental cysts located in the presacral and retrorectal space include dermoid, epidermoid, and enteric cysts such as tailgut and duplication

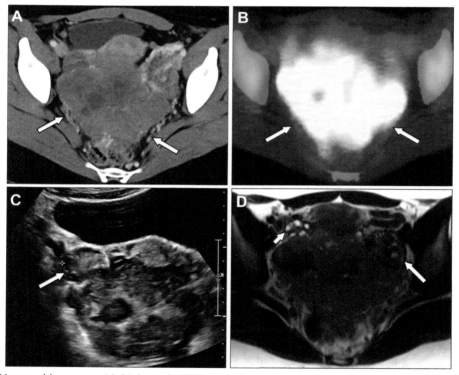

Fig. 5. A 31-year-old woman with high-grade GIST mimicking an ovarian mass, diagnosed on biopsy of a metastasis. Axial contrast-enhanced CT (*A*) shows a large solid enhancing mass in the central pelvis of uncertain origin (*arrows*), and normal ovaries are not well seen. PET/CT (*B*) shows this is a malignant, hypermetabolic mass (*arrows*). Pelvic US (*C*) and axial T2-weighted MR imaging (*D*) demonstrate a normal size right ovary adjacent to the mass (*short arrows*). The GIST has also spread to involve the left ovary (*D, long arrow*).

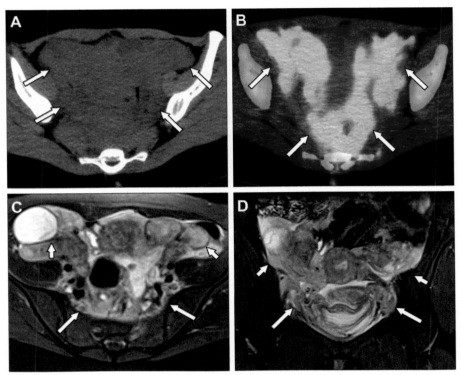

Fig. 6. A 28-year-old with B cell lymphoma mimicking diffuse peritoneal metastatic disease from ovarian cancer. Extensive tumor in the pelvis is seen on noncontrast CT (*A, arrows*), difficult to assess the origin without contrast. Axial-fused PET/CT shows extensive hypermetabolic peritoneal metastatic disease (*B, arrows*). Axial and coronal T2 fat saturated MR imaging shows intermediate T2 signal tumor to be both intraperitoneal and extraperitoneal (*C, D, long arrows*), with ovarian enlargement, also indicating lymphomatous involvement of the ovaries (*short arrows*).

cysts.[30,37] Rarely, a severe congenital ureteropelvic junction obstruction can mimic an ovarian mass (**Fig. 7**).

An epidermoid cyst is a unilocular cyst in the presacral space demonstrating high signal intensity on T2-weighted imaging with heterogeneous T1-signal intensity.[36] Demonstration of diffusion restriction secondary to protein-rich content can be helpful in distinguishing an epidermoid cyst from other cystic lesions.[35]

A dermoid cyst consists of well-differentiated elements from two or more germ cell layers and contains intralesional fat. On MR imaging, it is a T2 hyperintense cystic lesion with T1 hyperintense areas that show signal drop on fat-saturated sequences consistent with intralesional macroscopic fat. These lesions can contain calcifications.[21,35,36]

A rectal duplication cyst can be separate from or communicate with the adjacent rectum. A rectal duplication cyst has discrete mucosal and submucosal layers from the adjacent rectum, but a common muscularis propria.[3,36]

A tailgut cyst or embryonic hindgut hamartoma is a rare developmental cyst that originates from the remnant of the hindgut. On MR imaging, these appear as a multilocular cystic lesion with variable T1 and T2 signal intensity secondary to mucin and protein components. Septations can show mild enhancement.[3]

Retrorectal lesions are surgically removed secondary to the risk of malignancy and malignant transformation.[35] In one meta-analysis of retrorectal lesions, 30% were malignant. Of congenital lesions in this series, 60 tailgut cysts out of 1033 congenital lesions were malignant (6%).[38]

Cystic lesions lymphatic in origin

A lymphocele is a nonneoplastic entity which is usually seen as a complication of lymphadenectomy beginning approximately 3 weeks after surgery. On MR imaging, these appear as T2 hyperintense uniloculated or multiloculated fluid-filled lesions at the surgical site that extend along and conform to the morphology of the adjacent structures. Lymphoceles can become complicated secondary to hemorrhage or infection.[5,35]

Lymphangioleiomyomatosis is a rare entity seen in premenopausal women and is characterized by

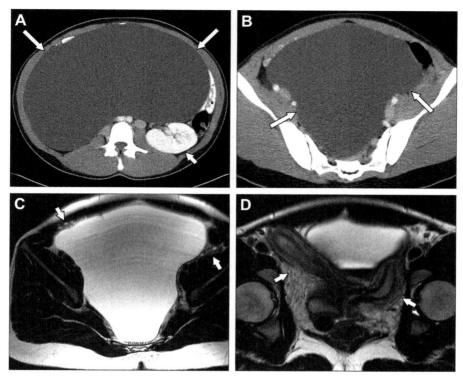

Fig. 7. A 18-year-old woman with very large congenital ureteropelvic junction (UPJ) obstruction mimicking a cystic ovarian mass. A large cystic, non-enhancing mass fills the abdomen and pelvis on contrast-enhanced CT (A, B, *long arrows*). A single left kidney is present (A, *short arrow*), and normal ovaries are difficult to identify in the pelvis on CT (B). Axial T2-weighted MR imaging allows more confident identification of normal ovaries with small follicles (C, *arrows*). Uterus demonstrates didelphys configuration (D, *arrows*). No normal right kidney parenchyma was seen on imaging, but renal histology was identified on surgical pathology.

cystic retroperitoneal masses. Associated cystic lung disease can aid in differential diagnosis.[5]

A cystic lymphangioma is a lymphatic malformation. Rarely, these lesions can be seen in the retroperitoneal region.[5]

Cystic degeneration of metastatic lymph nodes from genitourinary malignancies can also mimic adnexal lesions. The determination of the retroperitoneal location of the lymph node stations helps in differentiating lymphadenopathy from adnexal masses.[5]

Solid or Predominantly Solid Extraperitoneal Lesions Mimicking Adnexal Pathologies

Solid or predominantly solid extraperitoneal diseases that can mimic adnexal pathologies include neurogenic tumors, mesenchymal neoplasms, lymphoma, or vascular entities such as an aneurysm or a pseudoaneurysm.[33,34,39]

Neurogenic tumors

Neurogenic tumors in the pelvis include schwannomas, neurofibromas, gangliogliomas, paragangliomas, and malignant nerve sheath tumors. These masses have similar imaging characteristics as well-circumscribed, predominantly solid masses. They can contain calcifications.[39,40]

Schwannomas arise from the nerve sheath. On US, they are well circumscribed hypoechoic masses demonstrating internal vascularity. When large in size, they can contain areas of cystic/myxoid degeneration, hemorrhage, or calcifications. On MR imaging, they can be homogenous or heterogeneous depending on cystic or hemorrhagic components. The solid components of these masses demonstrate enhancement. Some schwannomas can demonstrate a target sign, with myxomatous peripheral high T2 signal and a fibrous central low T2 signal. Some schwannomas demonstrate a thin margin of high T1 signal fat surrounding the lesion. Some schwannomas demonstrate bands of relatively T2 low signal corresponding to fascicular bands within the tumor.[3,33,40]

Neurofibromas also arise from nerve sheaths and can be solitary or multiple in the setting of neurofibromatosis. They can undergo malignant transformation. Similar to schwannomas, these

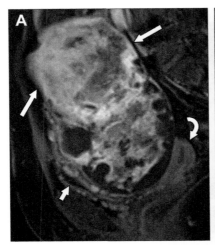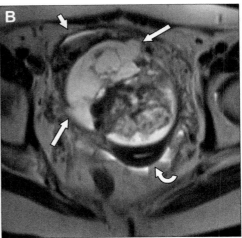

Fig. 8. A 64-year-old woman with large solitary fibrous tumor of the bladder mimicking ovarian cancer. A large central pelvic mass shows the areas of solid enhancement on sagittal T1 fat-saturated MR imaging (*A, long arrows*) and heterogeneous T2 signal with cystic components on axial T2-weighted MR imaging (*B, long arrows*). This mass compresses the bladder (*A, B, short arrows*) and uterus (*A, B, curved arrows*). Normal ovaries were not identified.

can demonstrate cystic or myxoid degeneration or demonstrate the target sign.[40]

Gangliogliomas are rare benign tumors arising from sympathetic ganglia. These masses often manifest in young adults. On imaging, these lesions are solid masses that show gradual contrast enhancement.[40]

Paragangliomas arise from chromaffin cells within the paraganglia. Patients with paragangliomas usually present with symptoms of catecholamine release such as hypertension, headache, or palpitations.[40]

Mesenchymal tumors

Mesenchymal tumors of the pelvis include many benign and malignant entities and can mimic adnexal lesions if large at presentation. These tumors include benign neoplastic processes such as leiomyomas, myxomas, chordomas, solitary fibrous tumors (**Fig. 8**), and malignant entities such as sarcomas.[33,39]

SUMMARY

Radiologists must be able to use pelvic anatomy and expected imaging characteristics to determine whether a mass is ovarian in origin or is a "mimic" of an adnexal pathology. MR imaging is often used as a problem-solving tool when characterizing pelvic masses. Knowledge of pelvic anatomy, intraperitoneal and extraperitoneal spaces, and the differential for cystic and solid pelvic masses is key to avoid misclassifying a mass "mimic" as an ovarian neoplasm. Common adnexal mass mimics that are important to

recognize include uterine leiomyomas, abscesses, peritoneal inclusion cysts, GI masses such as mucocele of the appendix, colorectal cancer, GIST, and extraperitoneal cystic and solid masses of developmental, lymphatic, neoplastic, neurogenic, and mesenchymal origin.

CLINICS CARE POINTS

- Radiologists should be aware that many benign and malignant diseases can mimic adnexal pathologies, and determination of the origin of the mass is crucial in directing patient management to prevent unnecessary interventions.

- Distinguishing a mimicker from adnexal pathology can be a diagnostic challenge due to complex pelvic anatomy and overlapping imaging features; however, MR imaging can be used as a problem-solving tool to narrow the differential diagnosis and assist in making a more definitive diagnosis.

- Mimics of adnexal masses include uterine leiomyomas, abscesses, peritoneal inclusion cysts, gastrointestinal masses, and extraperitoneal cystic and solid masses.

DISCLOSURE

The authors have nothing to disclose.

REFERENCES

1. Szklaruk J, Tamm EP, Choi H, et al. MR imaging of common and uncommon large pelvic masses. Radiographics 2003;23(2):403–24.
2. Ozat M, Altinkaya SO, Gungor T, et al. Extraovarian conditions mimicking ovarian cancer: a single center experience of 15 years. Arch Gynecol Obstet 2011;284(3):713–9.
3. Nougaret S, Nikolovski I, Paroder V, et al. MRI of Tumors and Tumor Mimics in the Female Pelvis: Anatomic Pelvic Space-based Approach. Radiographics 2019;39(4):1205–29.
4. Spencer JA, Forstner R, Cunha TM, et al. ESUR Female Imaging Sub-Committee. ESUR guidelines for MR imaging of the sonographically indeterminate adnexal mass: an algorithmic approach. Eur Radiol 2010;20(1):25–35.
5. Moyle PL, Kataoka MY, Nakai A, et al. Nonovarian cystic lesions of the pelvis. Radiographics 2010;30(4):921–38.
6. Spencer JA, Ghattamaneni S. MR imaging of the sonographically indeterminate adnexal mass. Radiology 2010;256(3):677–94.
7. Forstner R, Thomassin-Naggara I, Cunha TM, et al. ESUR recommendations for MR imaging of the sonographically indeterminate adnexal mass: an update. Eur Radiol 2017;27(6):2248–57.
8. Horta M, Cunha TM. Pitfalls in imaging of female pelvic masses. Curr Radiol Rep 2017;(5):53.
9. Pannu HK, Oliphant M. The subperitoneal space and peritoneal cavity: basic concepts. Abdom Imaging 2015;40(7):2710–22.
10. Gollub MJ, Maas M, Weiser M, et al. Recognition of the anterior peritoneal reflection at rectal MRI. AJR Am J Roentgenol 2013;200(1):97–101.
11. Saksouk FA, Johnson SC. Recognition of the ovaries and ovarian origin of pelvic masses with CT. Radiographics 2004;24(Suppl 1):S133–46.
12. Karaosmanoglu D, Karcaaltincaba M, Karcaaltincaba D, et al. MDCT of the ovarian vein: normal anatomy and pathology. AJR Am J Roentgenol 2009;192(1):295–9.
13. Kaniewska M, Gołofit P, Heubner M, et al. Suspensory ligaments of the female genital organs: MRI evaluation with intraoperative correlation. Radiographics 2018;38(7):2195–211.
14. Nishino M, Hayakawa K, Minami M, et al. Primary retroperitoneal neoplasms: CT and MR imaging findings with anatomic and pathologic diagnostic clues. Radiographics 2003;23(1):45–57.
15. Lee JH, Jeong YK, Park JK, et al. Ovarian vascular pedicle" sign revealing organ of origin of a pelvic mass lesion on helical CT. AJR Am J Roentgenol 2003;181(1):131–7.
16. Deshmukh SP, Gonsalves CF, Guglielmo FF, et al. Role of MR imaging of uterine leiomyomas before and after embolization. Radiographics 2012;32(6):E251–81.
17. Wilde S, Scott-Barrett S. Radiological appearances of uterine fibroids. Indian J Radiol Imaging 2009;19(3):222–31.
18. Moris D, Paulson EK, Pappas TN. Diagnosis and management of acute appendicitis in adults: a review. JAMA 2021;326(22):2299–311.
19. Montgomery RS, Wilson SE. Intraabdominal abscesses: image-guided diagnosis and therapy. Clin Infect Dis 1996;23(1):28–36.
20. Panghaal VS, Chernyak V, Patlas M, et al. CT features of adnexal involvement in patients with diverticulitis. AJR Am J Roentgenol 2009;192(4):963–6.
21. Elsherif SB, Agely A, Gopireddy DR, et al. Mimics and pitfalls of primary ovarian malignancy imaging. Tomography 2022;8(1):100–19.
22. Leonards LM, Pahwa A, Patel MK, et al. Neoplasms of the Appendix: Pictorial Review with Clinical and Pathologic Correlation. Radiographics 2017;37(4):1059–83.
23. Bennett GL, Tanpitukpongse TP, Macari M, et al. CT diagnosis of mucocele of the appendix in patients with acute appendicitis. AJR Am J Roentgenol 2009;192(3):W103–10.
24. Van Cutsem E, Verheul HMW, Flamen P, et al. Imaging in Colorectal Cancer: Progress and Challenges for the Clinicians. Cancers 2016;8(9). https://doi.org/10.3390/cancers8090081.
25. Horton KM, Abrams RA, Fishman EK. Spiral CT of colon cancer: imaging features and role in management. Radiographics 2000;20(2):419–30.
26. Okamoto D, Asayama Y, Yoshimitsu K, et al. Exophytic colon cancer mimicking an ovarian tumor: the value of evaluation of the venous anatomy on MDCT. CMIG Extra: Cases 2005;29(4):1–4.
27. Levy AD, Remotti HE, Thompson WM, et al. Gastrointestinal stromal tumors: radiologic features with pathologic correlation. Radiographics 2003;23(2):283–304, 456; [quiz: 532].
28. Dimitrakopoulou-Strauss A, Ronellenfitsch U, Cheng C, et al. Imaging therapy response of gastrointestinal stromal tumors (GIST) with FDG PET, CT and MRI: a systematic review. Clin Transl Imaging 2017;5(3):183–97.
29. Levy AD, Shaw JC, Sobin LH. Secondary tumors and tumorlike lesions of the peritoneal cavity: imaging features with pathologic correlation. Radiographics 2009;29(2):347–73.
30. Masch WR, Kamaya A, Wasnik AP, et al. Ovarian cancer mimics: how to avoid being fooled by extraovarian pelvic masses. Abdom Radiol (Ny) 2016;41(4):783–93.
31. van 't Sant I, Engbersen MP, Bhairosing PA, et al. Diagnostic performance of imaging for the detection of peritoneal metastases: a meta-analysis. Eur Radiol 2020;30(6):3101–12.

32. Nougaret S, Addley HC, Colombo PE, et al. Ovarian carcinomatosis: how the radiologist can help plan the surgical approach. Radiographics 2012;32(6):1775–800 [discussion: 1800-1803].

33. Rajiah P, Sinha R, Cuevas C, et al. Imaging of uncommon retroperitoneal masses. Radiographics 2011;31(4):949–76.

34. Reiter MJ, Schwope RB, Lisanti CJ. Algorithmic approach to solid adnexal masses and their mimics: utilization of anatomic relationships and imaging features to facilitate diagnosis. Abdom Imaging 2014;39(6):1284–96.

35. Chandramohan A, Bhat TA, John R, et al. Multimodality imaging review of complex pelvic lesions in female pelvis. Br J Radiol 2020;93(1116):20200489.

36. Janvier A, Rousset P, Cazejust J, et al. MR imaging of pelvic extraperitoneal masses: a diagnostic approach. Diagn Interv Imaging 2016;97(2):159–70.

37. Dahan H, Arrivé L, Wendum D, et al. Retrorectal developmental cysts in adults: clinical and radiologic-histopathologic review, differential diagnosis, and treatment. Radiographics 2001;21(3):575–84.

38. Baek SK, Hwang GS, Vinci A, et al. Retrorectal tumors: a comprehensive literature review. World J Surg 2016;40(8):2001–15.

39. Shanbhogue AK, Fasih N, Macdonald DB, et al. Uncommon primary pelvic retroperitoneal masses in adults: a pattern-based imaging approach. Radiographics 2012;32(3):795–817.

40. Rha SE, Byun JY, Jung SE, et al. Neurogenic tumors in the abdomen: tumor types and imaging characteristics. Radiographics 2003;23(1):29–43.

MR imaging of the Adnexa
Technique and Imaging Acquisition

Andrea G. Rockall, MRCP, FRCR[a,b,*], Aurélie Jalaguier-Coudray, MD[c], Isabelle Thomassin-Naggara, MD, PhD[d,e]

KEYWORDS

- MR imaging • Dynamic contrast-enhanced T1-weighted sequence • Time–intensity curves
- O-RADS MRI • Ovarian cancer • Adnexal mass

KEY POINTS

- To ensure accurate use of the O-RADS MRI score, excellent MR imaging technique is essential and includes the following:
- Good patient preparation.
- Clear radiographic instructions and excellent MR imaging technique.
- Standard anatomical imaging for mass morphology.
- Diffusion and perfusion sequences for functional information.
- Recognizing some potential pitfalls that can prepare the imaging team to mitigate challenges.

INTRODUCTION

MR imaging has a high diagnostic accuracy and reproducibility to classify adnexal masses as benign or malignant, using a risk stratification scoring system, the Ovarian-Adnexal Reporting and Data System MR imaging (O-RADS MRI) score.[1] The information gained at MR imaging may be used for treatment planning for masses that remain indeterminate or suspicious for cancer following ultrasound.[2] The use of the published lexicon ensures that radiologists are using the same terminology for each finding, which also aids with reproducibility between radiologists.[3] In order to achieve this high diagnostic accuracy and reproducibility, it is important to ensure high technical quality of the MR scan.[4] In this article, we describe the important technical aspects to achieve the best possible MR images for interpretation. In addition, we cover some frequently asked questions, with tips to overcome certain challenges.

Patient Preparation

The first step to achieve excellent image quality is to provide the patient with important information about the scheduled examination. An informative patient information pamphlet should be provided to let the patient know what to expect at the time of their appointment and a point of contact in the department of radiology. This will ensure that the patient can ask any questions in advance of their appointment, avoiding any unnecessary stress or unexpected difficulties on the day, in addition to checking for any potential contraindications to MR imaging. Good communication via patient information packets before scheduled MR imaging is likely to improve patient compliance at the time of image acquisition.

The scheduling of the MR appointment can be at any time during the menstrual cycle. Ideally the patient should fast (apart from drinking water) for at least 3 hours and be scanned with the bladder partially filled. One technique to ensure the

a Division of Cancer and Surgery, Imperial College London, Hammersmith Campus, ICTEM Building, London W12 0NN, United Kingdom; b Department of Radiology, Imperial College Healthcare NHS Trust, London, United Kingdom; c Service de Radiologie, Institut Paoli Calmettes, Marseille, France; d Service de Radiologie, Hôpital Tenon, Sorbonne Université, Paris, France; e Institute for Computing and Data Sciences, Sorbonne Université, Paris, France
* Corresponding author.
E-mail address: a.rockall@imperial.ac.uk

Magn Reson Imaging Clin N Am 31 (2023) 149–161
https://doi.org/10.1016/j.mric.2022.09.002
1064-9689/23/© 2022 Elsevier Inc. All rights reserved.

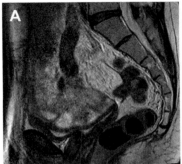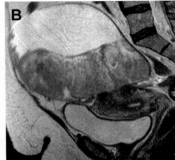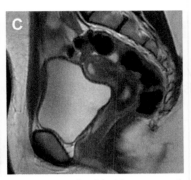

Fig. 1. Sagittal T2WI of the pelvis. (*A*) Empty bladder and no antiperistaltic agent. The bladder cannot be adequately evaluated due to underdistension, and bowel movement obscures the pelvic anatomy of this patient who is status posthysterectomy. (*B*) The bladder is appropriately full allowing assessment of the bladder and vesico-uterine reflection. (*C*) The bladder is overly distended, resulting in the displacement of the uterus and compression of pelvic structures.

appropriate level of bladder filling is to ask the patient to void their bladder approximately 30 minutes to 1 hour before the appointment (**Fig. 1**). The bladder will then be partially distended but not too full to be uncomfortable during the study. A partially full bladder allows good visualization of the bladder and the vesico-uterine pouch, which can be difficult to assess when the bladder is completely empty. However, a very full bladder can also make interpretation difficult, as patient discomfort has the potential to increase patient movement during scan acquisition.

The patient should be aware that a patient safety questionnaire will need to be completed before entering the MR scan room. In addition, patient clothing should not contain any metal components because this would need to be removed.

An intravenous cannula should be positioned in the antecubital fossa before the patient enters the MR scan room. The cannula is used to administer an antiperistaltic agent, as well as intravenous contrast. The antiperistaltic agent should be given once the patient is settled on the scan table before the scan commencing. Intravenous administration of an antiperistaltic agent (eg, Buscopan) acts very rapidly but wears off relatively quickly and therefore some centers give a second intravenous dose before the dynamic contrast scan, if needed. Some centers administer an antiperistaltic agent intramuscularly, usually in the thigh given patient positioning on the scan table, and although the antiperistaltic effect starts more slowly, it lasts longer throughout the duration of the scan.[5]

Ideally, the patient should be positioned in the supine position, with the coil centered over the pelvis and where possible, to cover the upper abdomen. The patient should be made as comfortable as possible with cushioning and blankets used safely.

Some patients may prefer lying prone, particularly for those that are claustrophobic, and this can assist with the reduction of movement artifact.

The patient should be aware that most sequences will be acquired with the patient breathing quietly. The patient should be advised to avoid taking deep breaths but preferably should use gentle quiet breathing throughout the procedure. The patient should also be advised that there will be some sequences where breath holds are necessary and clear instructions for this should be given during the scan.

The pelvic phased array coil (or in some centers, a cardiac coil) is recommended. The coil should be centered on the pelvis. However, if a large coil is available, then coverage from the kidneys down to the pubic symphysis is ideal. The coil should be firmly strapped across the pelvis, if the patient can tolerate this, in order to reduce breathing and movement artifact.

A summary of patient preparation steps are included in **Table 1**.

Essential MR Imaging Sequences and Rationale

System field strength

Imaging may be acquired on either 1.5 or 3 T systems. There are advantages and disadvantages to both. A 3 T system may allow for faster acquisition times and thus thinner slices may be acquired in a reasonable time frame, even in larger masses. Improved signal-to-noise ratio may also be possible. However, this is balanced against the greater likelihood of artifacts related to bowel gas, movement, or metal from previous surgery (eg, hip arthroplasty or pelvic surgical clips), and reduced homogeneity of the field.

Table 1
Patient preparation

	Action	Purpose
Patient leaflet	Let the patient know what to expect; give a contact number and email Advise removal of any metallic items such as piercings	Clear instructions before attending the scan allows the patient to be fully prepared and gives an opportunity to ask questions, reducing anxiety
Guidance on menstrual cycle	Imaging may be performed at any stage in cycle Check risk of pregnancy	If pregnant, avoid contrast administration where possible
Fasting instructions	Fast for 3–4 h; some water allowed	To reduce bowel peristalsis
Bladder filling advice	Void bladder 30 min before scan	To ensure bladder is partially full but not overly distended
Safety questionnaire	Standard MR safety questions, including pacemaker and other implants, intrauterine contraceptive device, pregnancy, and contrast allergy	To allow planning for adjustments to made with regards to correct imaging investigation and any changes needed to MR protocol
IV cannula	Antecubital fossa	For administration of antiperistaltic agent and contrast infusion
Patient positioning/coil positioning	Ensure pelvic mass is center of coil when planning scan	To consider differences in size and position of mass
Pelvic strapping	Pads/cushioning to ensure limited respiratory excursion of abdominal wall	To ensure patient comfort and reduce movement
Breathing instructions	Ask patient to favor chest wall respiration and avoid significant abdominal wall movement during respiration	To reduce ghosting artifacts from movement of the anterior abdominal wall
Smooth muscle relaxant	IV or IM administration (usually determined by department standard of care) Intravenous administration is allowable but may need to be repeated before DCE to ensure continuing antiperistaltic effect	IV provides instant antiperistaltic effect but can be short-lived. IM effect takes longer to develop but lasts longer

The preference in many centers is to use a 1.5 T magnet as a robust workhorse to provide diagnostic quality images in most patients within a reasonable timeframe.

Imaging sequences

There is a standard set of sequences that are needed to ensure complete evaluation of an adnexal mass for the O-RADS MRI classification.[1,6] The exact parameters, including field of view (FOV) and slice thickness, may vary depending on the MR system being used and the size and position of the adnexal mass. The essential sequences with their suggested parameters are summarized in **Table 2**.

3-Plane localizer This preliminary sequence is very important because it gives the technician an idea of the location and size of the pelvic mass, to allow planning of the diagnostic sequences appropriately. For very large masses or those that lie high in the pelvis, adjustments may be needed to ensure adequate coverage (**Fig. 2**).

Table 2
MR imaging sequences for Ovarian-Adnexal Reporting and Data System MR imaging interpretation

		Center and Coverage	FOV (cm)	ST (mm)	Comment
1	3-plane localizer	Kidneys to pubic symphysis	35		For planning
2	Sagittal T2WI without fat saturation	Center on pelvic mass	26	3	High-resolution T2WI of the mass and uterus. Hip to hip in right left dimension. 3-mm slice thickness if possible, 4-mm slice thickness if needed.
3	Axial T2WI without fat saturation	Kidneys to pubic symphysis[a]	30	5	Axial T2 includes pelvis at 5-mm slice thickness matching the axial T1 Dixon and diffusion sequences of the pelvis. This large FOV T2 covers up to renal hila to evaluate para-aortic nodes and hydonephrosis
4	Axial T2WI	Center on pelvic mass	24	3	High-resolution T2WI of the mass
5	Axial 3D T1 Dixon	Center on pelvic mass[a]	30	5	
6	Axial Diffusion WI	Center on pelvic mass[a]	30	5	Low b value between 0 and 50. High b value between 900 and 1200
7	Axial 3D DCE T1WI with fat saturation	Center on pelvic mass	32	2–3	15-s time resolution. Continuous 4-min acquisition. Commence injection at 30 or 45 s from the start of injection, without pausing the acquisition. Injection rate 2 ml/s followed by 20-ml saline flush. Include in-line subtraction. May be acquired in sagittal or coronal plane for large masses
8	Axial 3D T1 Dixon postcontrast	Center on pelvic mass[a]	30	5	Optional as T1WI with fat saturation is available postcontrast as part of the DCE. However, this T1W Dixon is useful as an additional postcontrast sequence in case the DCE fails

This table provides a guide to the key sequences at 1.5 T or 3T. Final parameters will need to be optimized based on the MR scanner, as well as the position and size of the mass. The axial sequences covering the pelvis at 5-mm slice thickness.
Abbreviations: 3D, 3-dimensional; FOV, field of view; ST, slice thickness; WI, weighted image.
[a] Should all have the same positioning and FOV to allow direct comparison of the mass across the different sequences. This does not include the upper abdominal coverage, apart from the T2 that is extended to reach the renal hilum.

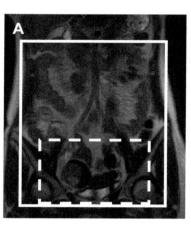
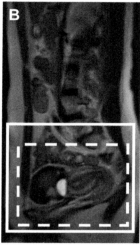
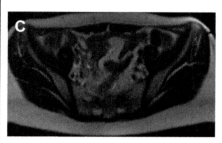

Fig. 2. Three-plane localizer on breath hold T2WI. (*A*) Coronal image with solid-bordered box demonstrating the large FOV used for the 5-mm axial T2-weighted image. (*B*) Sagittal image with solid-bordered box demonstrating the FOV for coverage of the 5-mm axial T1 Dixon precontrast and postcontrast and diffusion sequences. The white dashed box indicates the FOV for the high-resolution axial T2 and DCE sequences.

Sagittal T2-weighted sequence Sagittal T2-weighted imaging (T2WI) fast spin echo without fat suppression is acquired with 3 to 4-mm slice thickness and a maximum gap of 1 mm. The slice thickness is narrow to provide high spatial resolution (**Fig. 3**).

The FOV must cover the mass in the craniocaudal dimension and include the pelvis from one femoral head to the other in the right-left dimension.

The main aim of the high-resolution sagittal T2WI sequence is to evaluate the anatomy and morphology of the uterus and its relationship to the adnexal mass. It is used in conjunction with the other sequences to determine the site of origin of the mass.

Axial large field of view T2-weighted sequence A large FOV axial T2-weighted fast spin echo without fat saturation is acquired with 5-mm slice thickness and a maximum gap of 1 mm (**Fig. 4**). The craniocaudal coverage should extend from the renal veins down to pubic symphysis.

The pelvic component should directly align with the T1 and diffusion-weighted sequences (described in later discussion) to allow side-by-side comparison of the mass components (fluid and solid components) on the different sequences.

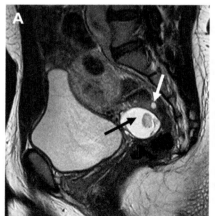
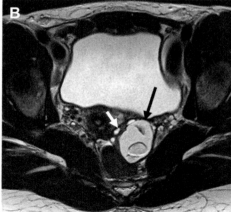

Fig. 3. High-resolution sagittal (*A*) and axial (*B*) T2WI with slice thickness of 3 mm with 1-mm gap. The left ovarian morphology is clearly seen with visualization of normal follicles (*white arrows*). The left adnexal mass, benign cystic teratoma, originates from the left ovary (*black arrows*).

The main aim is to assist with overall anatomic position of the mass and its site of origin. The large FOV allows for the identification of hydronephrosis, the ovarian pedicle, peritoneal deposits, and retroperitoneal lymph nodes.

Axial T2-weighted sequence high resolution
High-resolution axial T2-weighted fast spin echo without fat suppression is acquired using 3-mm slice thickness without slice gap, and the FOV is centered on the mass, ensuring complete coverage. In the setting of large adnexal mass(es), this sequence may sometimes require 2 acquisitions (see **Fig. 3**). This high-resolution T2WI may be acquired as a 3D T2-weighted sequence, if available on the MR system.

The main aim is to evaluate the fine morphology of the mass components, including the morphology of the wall, any septations, and any papillary formations.

Axial T1-weighted (Dixon) sequence Axial T1-weighted Dixon acquisition is acquired with 5-mm slice thickness in order to acquire T1 images that are in-phase, out-of-phase, water-only, and fat-only. Ideally, the sequence should be acquired as a 3D sequence to allow reformatting in any plane. If the Dixon sequence is not available, then axial T1WI should be done both as in-phase and with fat saturation (see **Fig. 4**).

The main aim of this sequence is to evaluate the various T1 signal intensities (SIs) of fluid and to identify the presence of fat components. These can be directly compared with the axial T2, diffusion, and the T1-weighted postcontrast sequences.

Axial diffusion-weighted sequence Axial diffusion-weighted sequence with 5-mm slice thickness and a maximum gap of 1 mm should have the same coverage and FOV as the T2-weighted and T1-weighted axial sequences above, to allow direct comparison of the different cystic and solid components on diffusion (see **Fig. 4**).

The low b value should be between b0 and b50. The high b value should be high enough to ensure that the urine in the bladder is suppressed sufficiently, such that any freely diffusing water is low in SI (**Fig. 5**). Depending on the MR system, the high b value should be between b1000 and b1400. The apparent diffusion coefficient (ADC) map should also be calculated and provided for review, mainly for the analysis of the cystic component.

How do you choose the optimal b value for your system? You can undertake several b values (eg, b900, b1000, b1200 to allow you to identify the level at which the urine in the bladder becomes dark. However, to be sure that there is enough signal, you can check the ovaries in a premenopausal woman to ensure that the normal moderate diffusion signal is still visible (see **Fig. 5**).

The main aim of the diffusion-weighted sequence is to identify the presence or absence of high SI of any solid tissue components of the adnexal mass on the high b value sequence. This information will allow classification of the "low T2, low diffusion," or so-called dark–dark masses. The high b value sequence also allows for the detection of peritoneal deposits and retroperitoneal lymph nodes with high sensitivity.

Dynamic contrast-enhanced T1-weighted sequence The dynamic contrast-enhanced (DCE) sequence is acquired as a 3D isotropic gradient echo. This should be done with high resolution, a slice thickness of 2 mm with 1-mm gap, and spatial resolution of 3 mm. The time resolution should allow for an acquisition every 15 seconds, at the most. The FOV should ensure complete coverage of the mass. Ideally, the sequence should be done in the axial plane to allow direct comparison with the other axial sequences. However, with large masses, it may not be possible to achieve this, and planning the DCE in either the coronal or sagittal plane should allow for the high resolution in both slice thickness and time (**Fig. 6**).

The acquisition should start and run continuously without breaks for 4 minutes from beginning to end. The contrast injection should start at 30 to 45 seconds, without break in sequence acquisition, in order to ensure that there are at least 2 precontrast sequences. The injection should be done using a pump-injector with a rate of 2 mL/s, followed by a 20-mL saline flush of the tubing. Imaging continues uninterrupted for 3 minutes following contrast administration, allowing for the evaluation of the curve shape and any washout-out that may occur. Routine subtraction sequences should be generated using the initial time-points before the injection.

If a fast DCE is not available on the scanner, then an axial 3D T1-weighted sequence with fat saturation and 3-mm slice thickness may be obtained at time 0, then postinjection at time 30, 60, 90, 120, and 150 seconds.

Axial T1-weighted (Dixon) postcontrast sequence This final sequence copies the T1-weighted Dixon acquisition that was done before contrast administration. This allows delayed review of contrast enhancement of the mass and other pelvic structures. This can be helpful in establishing the site of origin of a mass. In addition

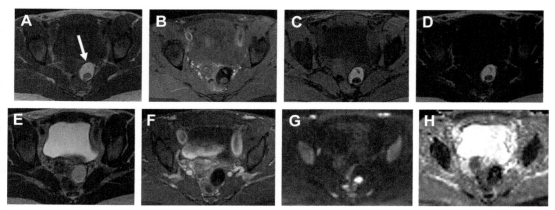

Fig. 4. Axial images of left adnexal mass, a benign cystic dermoid (*white arrow*), with 5-mm slice thickness. The FOV and slice thickness are similar for all sequences to allow colocalization on different sequences. A to D are the 4 parts of the T1 Dixon: (*A*) T1 in phase, (*B*) T1 water only (T1 fat saturated), (*C*) T1 out of phase, (*D*) T1 fat only, (*E*) Axial T2, (*F*) T1 water only postgadolinium, (*G*) diffusion-weighted b1000, (*H*) ADC map.

if there is a problem with the DCE acquisition, this provides another opportunity to review the presence of enhancement of any solid components. If the Dixon sequence is not available, then axial T1-weighted with fat saturation can be acquired. The postcontrast T1 with 5-mm slice thickness should line up exactly with the previous T2, diffusion and precontrast T1-weighted sequences (see **Fig. 4**).

The main aim of this sequence is to evaluate the presence of enhancement of solid components, allowing direct comparison to the axial T2, diffusion and the T1-weighted precontrast sequences.

Optional extension of the core protocol to include the upper abdomen In cases that are considered at higher risk of malignancy, or where time and capacity allow, the axial 5-mm sequences (T2, T1 Dixon precontrast, diffusion, T1 Dixon postcontrast) can be extended to include the upper abdomen, to identify more distant sites of peritoneal disease (**Fig. 7**). The additional "stations" can be stitched together with the pelvic sequence

to create a uniform block of slices from the diaphragm down to the pubic symphysis. The set of stitched sequences can be viewed together, aiding the detection of peritoneal disease, nodal disease, or other pathologic conditions.

In addition to the axial extension to the upper abdomen, it may help interpretation to include a short breath-hold T2-weighted sequence of the liver and diaphragmatic region in the coronal plane to assess the subdiaphragmatic peritoneal space (see **Fig. 7**). This is a quick sequence to acquire and gives an overview of the upper abdomen in another plane.

Technique for interpretation of the dynamic contrast-enhanced sequence: time-intensity curve and visual assessment

Time–intensity curves (TICs) allow accurate characterization of the enhancement pattern of solid tissue into low-risk, intermediate-risk, and high-risk enhancement, also previously known as type 1, 2, and 3 curves.[7] Visual assessment (VA) can be used when creation of a TIC graph is not possible but has some limitations (eg, only being

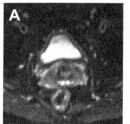
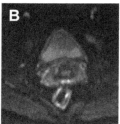
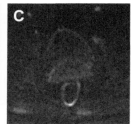
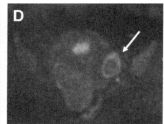

Fig. 5. Optimization of diffusion-weighted imaging sequence. (*A*) b0, the urine in the bladder is very-high signal intensity. (*B*) b800, the urine in the bladder is not fully suppressed. (*C*) b1000, the urine in the bladder is fully suppressed. (*D*) Moderate signal intensity is retained in this normal premenopausal ovary (*arrow*), indicating that there is sufficient residual signal.

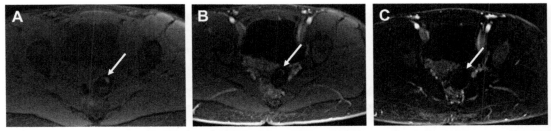

Fig. 6. Dynamic contrast-enhanced series T1FS with and without subtraction. (*A*) Before contrast injection, there is a focal area of high T1SI within the dermoid cyst (*arrow*). (*B*) The focus remains high in SI following contrast administration (*arrow*), rendering determination of postcontrast enhancement difficult. (*C*) Subtraction imaging effectively removes the precontrast area of high T1SI (*arrow*), demonstrating that there is no enhancing area within the cyst. This ability to subtract the precontrast high T1SI is critical for cases where there is a concern for enhancing solid tissue in a region of intrinsically high T1SI.

able to differentiate high-risk cases from all other enhancement types).[8]

Time–Intensity Curve Method

Region of interest placement: Using the nonsubtracted DCE, the TIC is measured by first placing a region of interest (ROI) within the outer myometrium (avoiding any adenomyosis, leiomyomata, or myometrial vessels). This initial ROI acts as an internal reference. A second ROI should then be placed on the earliest enhancing solid tissue within the adnexal mass. It can be helpful to review an early time-point when the contrast is just seen, to identify the earliest possible region of enhancement in the mass. This can be called the "hot spot." Identification of the "hot spot" can be helped in some cases by using a color map or heat map of enhancement, if available.

It is important to ensure that the vertical axis uses either relative enhancement or percentage enhancement, and not the absolute enhancement.

Subtraction: Automated subtraction DCE, whereby the precontrast series at time 0 or 15 seconds is subtracted from the later series, is very important, particularly in cases with high T1-weighted SI contents. Subtraction of the high T1 SI allows for an accurate identification of enhancement without the uncertainty of the precontrast high T1 SI.

Although it is important to review the subtracted images for areas of enhancement and to accurately identify the "hot spot," it is not correct to use the subtracted images for ROI placement for curve analysis, due to calculation difficulties and challenges related to the subtraction process.

Low-risk curve: This curve type demonstrates gradual increase in SI of the solid tissue and the curve has no well-defined shoulder (**Fig. 8**).

Intermediate-risk curve: This curve type demonstrates moderate initial increase in the SI of solid tissue but enhances more slowly compared with myometrium or enhances at the same time as the myometrium. In this curve, there is a definite shoulder followed by a plateau (**Fig. 9**).

High-risk curve: This curve type demonstrates a rapid initial increase in SI that is earlier than (faster than, or steeper than) the myometrium (**Fig. 10**).

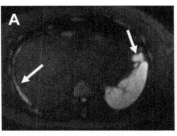
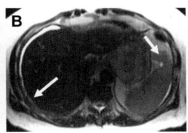
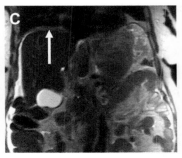

Fig. 7. Extension FOV to include the upper abdomen in patient with advanced disease. (*A*) b1000 diffusion-weighted image at level of the liver demonstrates high SI metastases adjacent to the liver and anterior to the spleen (*white arrows*). (*B*) Same level on T2WI. (*C*) Breath hold T2WI coronal image demonstrates disease beneath the right diaphragm (*white arrow*).

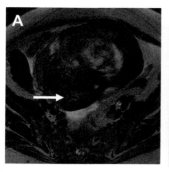
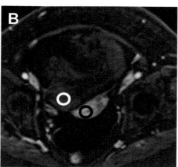
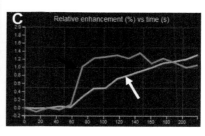

Fig. 8. Right ovarian fibroma. (*A*) T2WI demonstrates a lobulated overall low T2SI mass (*white arrow*) with a small region of mixed T2SI. (*B*) DCE image demonstrates relatively low-level enhancement in the mass (white region of interest) compared with the uterus (black region of interest). (*C*) Low-risk TIC (*white arrow*) is demonstrated. The myometrial enhancement curve is indicated by black arrow.

TIC interpretation post hysterectomy: In women who have previously had a hysterectomy, it is not possible to classify a curve as high-risk. However, it is possible to distinguish between an intermediate risk curve, which has a defined shoulder and plateau and a low-risk curve, which has no clear shoulder or plateau. This will allow the distinction between O-RADS MRI score 3 from those that must be classified as score 4.

Visual Assessment Method

Most modern scanners can perform the DCE as described in the technique section above, with a T1-weighted 3D gradient echo acquisition, 3-mm slice thickness, and 15-second time resolution. If a fast DCE is not available on the scanner, then an axial 3D T1-weighted sequence with fat saturation and 3 mm slice thickness may be obtained at time 0, then post injection at time 30, 60, 90, 120, and 150 seconds. In this case, or where there is no software available to do the TIC graph, it is possible to use VA of the enhancement.

To perform visual assessment, the radiologist needs to review the solid tissue in the adnexal mass, identify the earliest point of enhancement, and then assess whether this is earlier than the outer myometrium at 30 seconds and at 60 seconds.

High-risk enhancement on VA: The earliest part of the adnexal solid tissue is higher SI than that of the myometrium at 30 seconds (**Fig. 11**).

Intermediate-risk enhancement on VA: The earliest part of the adnexal solid tissue is lower SI than that of the myometrium at 30 seconds and higher at 60 seconds.

Low-risk enhancement on VA: The earliest part of the adnexal solid tissue is lower in SI than that of the myometrium at both 30 seconds and 60 seconds.

Comparison of Time–Intensity Curve and Visual Assessment

Using a TIC allows for higher accuracy in risk stratification of adnexal masses compared with VA overall, with 95.6% of malignant lesions having an intermediate or high-risk TIC, whereas only 75.8% malignant lesions have an intermediate or high-risk enhancement on VA.[8] However, the

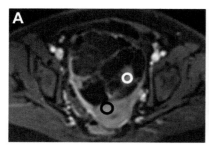
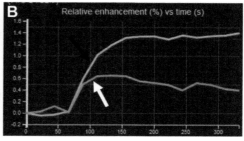

Fig. 9. Multiseptate adnexal cyst. (*A*) DCE demonstrates enhancement of solid tissue (white region of interest). A black region of interest is positioned over the myometrium. (*B*) The adnexal solid tissue enhances with an intermediate TIC (*white arrow*), with the up-stroke being the same as the myometrium (*black arrow*), with a clear shoulder.

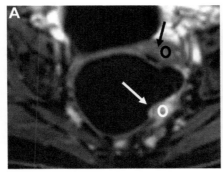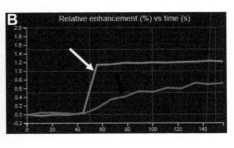

Fig. 10. Cystic solid adnexal mass. (*A*) DCE demonstrates an enhancing solid mural nodule (*white arrow*, region of interest white circle) and the adjacent myometrium (*black arrow*, region of interest black circle). (*B*) TIC demonstrates a high-risk enhancement curve of the mural nodule (*white arrow*), the nodule enhancing earlier than the myometrium (*black arrow*).

specificity of a high-risk enhancement on VA is very high for borderline or invasive malignancy (93%), is no different compared with a high-risk TIC (94%), and both can score as ORADS MRI score 5.

Using VA, 24% of all malignant cases have low-risk enhancement. Therefore, both low-risk and intermediate-risk enhancement must be classified as ORADS MRI score 4. It is not possible to assign low-risk enhancement on VA as ORADS MRI score 3 due to the substantial number of malignant cases that would fall into this category.[8]

The accuracy of TIC analysis is better than VA, and therefore, TIC analysis is always preferred when possible.[8]

Frequently Asked Questions

What do you do if a patient is uncomfortable lying on their back?
Patients can lie prone on their stomach if they are uncomfortable on their back. If the patient has a large mass, then lying on their side may be the most comfortable position. Adequate cushioning and strapping of the coil is advisable to ensure that the patient is in a comfortable position, in order to reduce the risk of movement artifacts.

How can abdominal wall movement artifact related to breathing be reduced?
Ideally, the patient should be instructed to breathe using their chest wall, minimizing the movement of the abdominal wall during respiration. This can be helped by ensuring that the coil that is positioned over the pelvis and lower abdomen is firmly strapped across the pelvis, though of course within the reasonable comfort of the patient. It is important to let the patient know that they should avoid excessive movement of the abdomen during the acquisition period.

How can bowel movement artifacts be reduced?
Ideally, an antiperistaltic agent should be given, as described above. Motion artifacts can result in ghosting, blurring, and reduced signal-to-noise

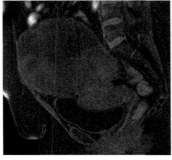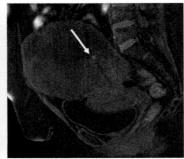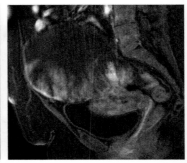

Fig. 11. Sagittal 3D T1W gradient echo sequence with fat saturation multiphase acquisition. (*A*) At baseline before contrast administration. (*B*) At 30 seconds following contrast administration. (*C*) At 60 seconds following contrast administration. A tiny blush of contrast is seen within the adnexal mass (*white arrow*) at 30 seconds (*B*) earlier than myometrial enhancement. In this case, an ORADS MR imaging score of 5 can be assigned.

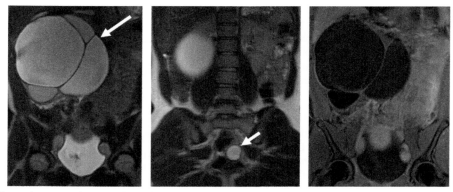

Fig. 12. Bilateral masses that could not be included in a single DCE series. (*A*) Coronal T2WI anteriorly demonstrates a large multiseptated cyst (long *white arrow*). (*B*) Coronal T2WI posteriorly demonstrates a left adnexal cystic mass (short *white arrow*, a benign dermoid cyst demonstrated in **Figs. 5** and **6**). (*C*) A large FOV coronal T1WI with fat saturation was obtained to cover the upper lesion. This was a right cystic dermoid cyst on a long pedicle.

ratio, and this is particularly problematic on images with longer acquisition, such as T2 or diffusion-weighted images (see **Fig. 1**).[9] However, if there is a contraindication, or if the patient declines, then asking the patient to lie prone may help reduce the effect of bowel movement on the images of the pelvis. In addition, it may help to ask the patient to fast for 4 to 6 hours before the scan, only allowing water for hydration and bladder filling.

What options are there to improve imaging if there are hip replacements or other metal artifacts?

Metal implants in the pelvis may be troublesome, particularly in relation to the diffusion-weighted sequences. Adjusting the FOV may allow avoidance of a metal implant. However, it is not always possible to avoid images being degraded by large metal implants such as hip replacements. It may be possible to adjust acquisition, depending on

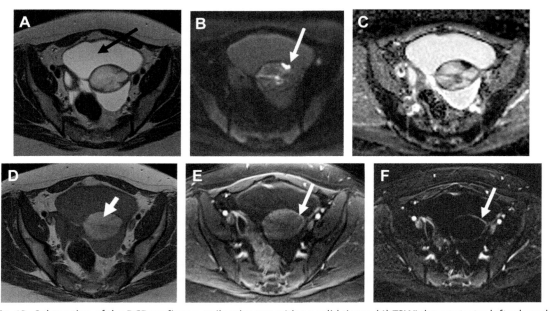

Fig. 13. Subtraction of the DCE confirms a unilocular cyst with no solid tissue. (*A*) T2WI demonstrates left adnexal lesion with internal low SI areas, surrounded by high T2SI fluid (*black arrow*). (*B*) b1000 demonstrates high SI anteriorly (*white arrow*), which is low on ADC map (*C*). (*D*) T1WI in phase demonstrates high T1SI within the lesion (short *white arrow*). (*E*) DCE postcontrast demonstrates possible enhancing irregularity of the inner wall of the lesion. (*F*) DCE subtraction image confirms smooth nature of the wall with no internal enhancement. The lesion was a benign organizing hemorrhagic cyst surrounded by a peritoneal inclusion cyst (*black arrow*).

the scanner type that is being used. Some techniques can be attempted including the use of long echo train lengths for the fast spin echo sequences, a high bandwidth, thin section selection, and increased matrix. The details of sequence adjustments are beyond the scope of this article but a review of this topic is available.[10]

What if the dynamic sequence fails?

The DCE may fail due to the contrast not being injected or because the DCE FOV has been incorrectly assigned, for example, if there are 2 masses and the scan focuses on one and the other is inadvertently excluded (**Fig. 12**). It may be that there is sufficient information to assign an O-RADS MRI score, for example, if there is peritoneal disease (score 5) or if the lesion is a classic dermoid or endometriotic cyst, or demonstrates "low T2 and low diffusion" in SI (all of which are score 2). Otherwise, the score may remain uncertain and a score 0 may need to be assigned.

If the dynamic injection fails for technical reasons and no contrast has been injected, then ideally it would be best to reinsert the intravenous line if needed and repeat the sequence following resetting of the pump injector.

How should enhancement be evaluated if there is high T1-weighted signal intensity in the mass before contrast administration?

In this case, it is important to ensure that subtracted DCE sequences are available. With subtractions sequences, the high T1-weighted SI precontrast is negated, allowing for adequate assessment of any enhancing solid tissue (**Fig. 13**).

SUMMARY

A standardized imaging protocol is essential for reproducible and accurate evaluation of adnexal masses using the O-RADS MRI classification. The use of the published lexicon ensures that radiologists are using the same terminology for each finding. In addition, using the ORADS MRI score allows for reproducible and evidence-based risk stratification. However, if the initial MR acquisition lacks a fundamental sequence, or if the scan is limited due to artifacts or poor planning of the scan, then diagnostic accuracy will be decreased. It is therefore of great value to pay attention to patient information, patient preparation, training MR technicians, and monitoring quality to ensure the highest possible accuracy in categorizing adnexal masses on MR imaging. This article should provide the recipe to achieve excellent MR imaging technique for adnexal mass evaluation.

CLINICS CARE POINTS

- Ovarian-Adnexal Reporting and Data System MR imaging (O-RADS MRI) has high diagnostic accuracy and reproducibility for characterizing adnexal masses and may be used to assist in treatment planning in cases of uncertainty.

- O-RADS MRI lexicon allows for reproducible language and scoring of adnexal masses and is recommended for reporting.

- Acquisition of the correct MR imaging sequences is essential for the interpretation of adnexal masses according to the O-RADS MRI risk score. Good patient information and preparation as well as technical expertise are needed to ensure the highest diagnostic accuracy.

- Enhancement should be assessed using a time intensity curve where possible because this is more accurate than visual assessment in adnexal lesions with solid tissue.

DISCLOSURE

The authors have nothing to disclose.

ACKNOWLEDGMENTS

Andrea Rockall acknowledges support from the Imperial National Institute of Health Research Biomedical Research Centre and the Imperial Cancer Research UK Centre.

REFERENCES

1. Thomassin-Naggara I, Poncelet E, Jalaguier-Coudray A, et al. Ovarian-Adnexal Reporting Data System Magnetic Resonance Imaging (O-RADS MRI) Score for Risk Stratification of Sonographically Indeterminate Adnexal Masses. JAMA Netw Open 2020;3(1):e1919896.
2. Sadowski EA, Rockall AG, Maturen KE, et al. Adnexal lesions: Imaging strategies for ultrasound and MR imaging. Diagn Interv Imaging 2019;100(10):635–46.
3. Reinhold C, Rockall A, Sadowski EA, et al. Ovarian-Adnexal Reporting Lexicon for MRI: A White Paper of the ACR Ovarian-Adnexal Reporting and Data Systems MRI Committee. J Am Coll Radiol 2021;18(5):713–29.
4. Thomassin-Naggara I, Belghitti M, Milon A, et al. O-RADS MRI score: analysis of misclassified cases in a prospective multicentric European cohort. Eur Radiol 2021;31(12):9588–99.

5. Gutzeit A, Binkert CA, Koh DM, et al. Evaluation of the anti-peristaltic effect of glucagon and hyoscine on the small bowel: comparison of intravenous and intramuscular drug administration. Eur Radiol 2012; 22(6):1186–94.

6. Sadowski EA, Thomassin-Naggara I, Rockall A, et al. O-RADS MRI Risk Stratification System: Guide for Assessing Adnexal Lesions from the ACR O-RADS Committee. Radiology 2022;303(1):35–47.

7. Thomassin-Naggara I, Aubert E, Rockall A, et al. Adnexal masses: development and preliminary validation of an MR imaging scoring system. Radiology 2013;267(2):432–43.

8. Wengert GJ, Dabi Y, Kermarrec E, et al. O-RADS MRI Classification of Indeterminate Adnexal Lesions: Time-Intensity Curve Analysis Is Better Than Visual Assessment. Radiology 2022;303(2):E28.

9. Johnson W, Taylor MB, Carrington BM, et al. The value of hyoscine butylbromide in pelvic MRI. Clin Radiol 2007;62(11):1087–93.

10. Talbot BS, Weinberg EP. MR Imaging with Metal-suppression Sequences for Evaluation of Total Joint Arthroplasty. Radiographics 2016;36(1):209–25.

Moving?

Make sure your subscription moves with you!

To notify us of your new address, find your **Clinics Account Number** (located on your mailing label above your name), and contact customer service at:

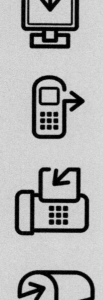

Email: journalscustomerservice-usa@elsevier.com

800-654-2452 (subscribers in the U.S. & Canada)
314-447-8871 (subscribers outside of the U.S. & Canada)

Fax number: 314-447-8029

Elsevier Health Sciences Division
Subscription Customer Service
3251 Riverport Lane
Maryland Heights, MO 63043

Printed and bound by CPI Group (UK) Ltd, Croydon, CR0 4YY

08/05/2025

01864724-0020